Modern Dispensing and Hospital Pharmacy

Modern Dispensing and Hospital Pharmacy

Dr. N. K. Jain
M. Pharm., Ph.D., LL.M., FIC
Professor
Department of Pharmaceutical Sciences
Dr. H. S. Gour Vishwavidyalaya,
Sagar – 470 003 (MP)

Dr. G. D. Gupta
M. Pharm., Ph.D.
Professor and Director
ASBASJSM College of Pharmacy
BELA (Ropar) - 140 111 (Punjab)

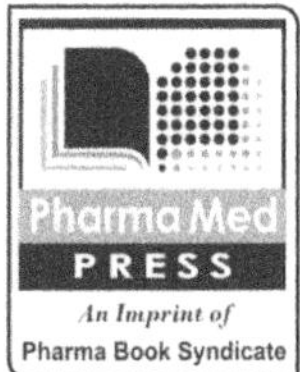

PharmaMed Press
An imprint of Pharma Book Syndicate

A unit of **BSP Books Pvt., Ltd.**

4-4-309/316, Giriraj Lane,
Sultan Bazar, Hyderabad - 500 095.

Published by

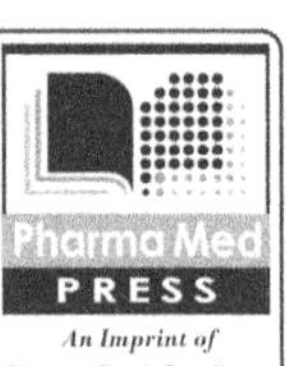

PharmaMed Press

An imprint of Pharma Book Syndicate

A unit of BSP Books Pvt., Ltd.

4-4-309/316, Giriraj Lane, Sultan Bazar, Hyderabad - 500 095.
Phone: 040-23445605, 23445688; Fax: 91+40-23445611
E-mail: info@pharmamedpress.com

ISBN : 978-93-52300-47-1 (HB)

Preface

Traditional practice as well as orientation of Dispensing and Hospital Pharmacy has undergone drastic changes. The spectrum of activities of the pharmacists involved in Dispensing and Hospital Pharmacy is widening with a greater focus and emphasis on health care delivery.

The book 'Modern Dispensing and Hospital Pharmacy' comprises of Section A and Section B. Section A consisting of Dispensing Pharmacy deals with four units and 15 chapters such as Genesis and Evaluation of Pharmacy, Principles of Dispensing, Prescription, Pharmaceutical Calculation, Posology, Mixtures, Solutions, Emulsions, Powders, Lotions and Liniments, Suspensions, Ointments and Miscellaneous Preparations, Extraction and Galenical Products, and Incompatibility. Section B is divided into four units and six chapters. This section deals with 'Hospital Pharmacy' including Organization of a Hospital Pharmacy, Drug Distribution, Drug Information Centre, Hospital Management and Records as applicable in modern hospital pharmacy.

The book has been prepared as per the syllabus of Jawaharlal Nehru Technology University, Hyderabad but caters to the syllabi of most of the universities in India. The main aim of writing this book is to present up to date knowledge to maintain a balance between the traditional and the modern techniques of dispensing and hospital pharmacy. An attempt has been made to include the newer concepts and latest knowledge relevant to a pharmacist as a member of health care delivery system.

Authors are open to suggestions for further improvement in the subject matter of this book and shall welcome criticism as well as feedback.

- Authors

Contents

UNIT - IV

SECTION - B

HOSPITAL PHARMACY

UNIT - V

UNIT - VI

UNIT - VII

UNIT - VIII

SECTION - A
DISPENSING PHARMACY

UNIT - I

CHAPTER 1

GENESIS AND EVALUATION OF PHARMACY

HISTORY OF PHARMACY

The Indian traditional systems of medicine have been *Ayurveda*, *Siddha* and *Unani*. *Ayurveda* and *Siddha* systems of medicine originated in India while *Unani* or Greco-Arabic medical system came form West Asia. Pharmacy profession has existed in an elementary form from time immemorial, probably from the dawn of civilization. Greeks were one of the first patrons of this profession. The word pharmacy originated from the Greek word *Pharmakon*.

It was in 9th century in the civilized world around Baghdad that the profession of pharmacy started acquiring shape. It slowly spread to Europe as alchemy and finally developed into chemistry. The first known chemical process was carried out by the artisans of Mesopotamia, Egypt, and China. However in the 19th century it completely sprouted out from medicine and started developing as a separate profession. This happened only when the role of pharmacist as a compounder of medicines was identified and differentiated from physician whose role was accepted as the therapist. The practice in those times was restricted to compounding, dispensing medication and manufacturing medicaments in bulk lots, not for general sale. The medicaments commonly produced included simple elixirs, spirits, and powders in contrast to the complex pharmaceutical remedies of the modern era. The 19th century witnessed various milestones being set in the field of pharmacy. In 1821, first school of pharmacy was established at Philadelphia in United States of America. The first U.S. pharmacopoeia was published in 1820. American Pharmaceutical Association was founded in 1852.The first National Formulary (U.S.) was published in 1888.

The inception of pharmacy profession in India was marked by the first class of the chemist and druggist conducted at the Madras Medical College in 1870s to train students to gain skills in pharmacy practice. Pharmacy education pattern was based on the instructions provided by the Pharmaceutical Society of Great Britain. A formal training of the compounders was started in 1881 in Bengal.

The pharmacy profession entered India almost simultaneously with U.S. but the growth in India remained very slow. For almost half a century not much progress was noticed, until B.Pharm course was started in 1932 at Banaras Hindu University, *Varanasi* and in 1944 at the Punjab University, Lahore (now in Pakistan). The B.Pharm course at BHU was industry oriented while that at Punjab University was oriented towards Pharmacy practice. Although the profession was oriented towards pharmacy practice at the introductory stage yet, as it grew, it became more industry oriented. This bent lead to the development of modern Indian pharmaceutical industry, which is now the 4th in terms of volume and 14th in terms of value. The future prediction for the Indian pharmaceutical industry is that it is expected to become the super power by the year 2020. As the pharmaceutical industry is becoming highly automatic the trend is again towards the pharmacy practice, like in rest of the world. The future of pharmacy is again in pharmacy practice. Thus history is repeating itself and pharmacy profession in India is going back to from where it started, the Pharmacy Practice.

Present Positions of Pharmacy Colleges/Institutes in India approved by AICTE

State	No. of Institutes	State	No. of Institutes
Madhya Pradesh	89	Chandigarh	01
Chhattisgarh	07	Haryana	21
Gujarat	73	New Delhi	04
Mizoram	01	Punjab	29
Sikkim	01	Rajasthan	46
Orissa	16	Andhra Pradesh	250
West Bengal	11	Pondicherry	01
Tripura	01	Tamil Nadu	39
Assam	01	Karnataka	73
Bihar	03	Kerala	16
Uttar Pradesh	105	Maharashtra	130
Uttranchal	14	Goa	02

Total Pharmacy Institutes in India: 934 (including both Diploma and Degree)

ORIGIN AND DEVELOPMENT OF PHARMACOPOEIAS

As the drug trade advanced, the necessity for legalized standards to define the character, establish the purity and regulate the strength of medicines was recognized by many civilized nations. The existing pharmacopoeias are the outcome of such recognition. A pharmacopoeia (Greek *Pharmacon,* 'a drug or medicine' and *poeio* 'to make') is accepted today as a book of standards. A national pharmacopoeia contains a list of drugs and formulae for medicinal substances/preparations with description, tests for these substances and the standards to which they must conform. A pharmacopoeia is issued under the authority of the government of a country. The countries, which have not developed their own pharmacopeias, allow the standards laid down by pharmacopoeias of some other countries. Likewise, if a substance or preparation is not included in a national pharmacopoeia, the standards laid down in some other national pharmacopoeia may be recognized in practice. Indian pharmacopoeia is the authorized book of standards in India but other pharmacopoeias have also been recognized under the Drugs & Cosmetics Act and Rules. By far the major role of pharmacopoeias is in the quality control, which facilitates the regulation of drugs trade by the Food and/or Drug Control Administration authority. Prior to the advent of pharmacopoeias the apothecary had to look for guidance and knowledge from books written by individuals who had achieved name and fame in medicine.

The Pharmacopoeia of India

The history of the Indian Pharmacopoeia goes back to 1833 when a Committee of the East India Company's Dispensary recommended the publication of a Pharmacopoeia, and Bengal Pharmacopoeia was published in 1844, which mainly listed most of the commonly used indigenous remedies. The Bengal Pharmacopoeia was published in 1844, nearly 20 years prior to the publication of the first BP. As on record, the first Pharmacopoeia of India was published in 1868 which was prepared under the authority of Her Majesty's Secretary of State for India in Council. It was divided into sections on vegetable, animal and inorganic materia medica and a separate section on products of fermentation and distillation. A supplement to the Pharmacopoeia of India was published in 1869. A catalogue of Indian synonyms of the medicinal plants, products, inorganic and organic substances was included in the pharmacopoeia, with explanatory and descriptive remarks, in fourteen Indian languages, in addition to English. Largely however, it was the BP which was considered as the book of standards during the pre-independence era. The first Indian and Colonial addendum to the BP 1868 was published in 1901. By turn of the nineteenth century the Pharmacopoeia of India ceased to attract attention and passed into oblivion. In 1902 Bose published the 'Official Indigenous Drugs of India', which was later published as enlarged edition in 1932 under the title 'Pharmacopoeia Indica'. The 'Indian Pharmacopoeial List' was published in 1946 by the Government of India, which served as a supplement to the British Pharmacopoeia and consisted mainly of crude drugs along with preparations and few synthetics like Urea Stibamine, which were of special interest to India. The Indian Pharmacopoeial Committee was appointed in 1948 to prepare a National Pharmacopoeia.

The first edition of the Indian Pharmacopoeia (Pharmacopoeia of India) was published in 1955. The reconstituted Pharmacopoeial Committee compiled a supplement to the First

Edition of the Indian Pharmacopoeia in 1960 in order to provide standards for some new drugs introduced into the market.

The Second Edition of the Indian Pharmacopoeia was published in 1966 i.e. after a gap of 11 years from the publication of the First Edition. A supplement to the Second Edition of IP was also published in 1975.

The Third Edition of IP appeared in 1985 followed by two addenda in 1989 and 1991. **The Fourth Edition** of IP became effective from 1 December 1996 and its Addenda were published in 2000, 2002, 2005 and the Veterinary Products Supplement in 2002. It contained 1149 monographs including 291 new monographs whereas 110 monographs were deleted and the titles of 142 monographs were changed.

The fifth edition of "Indian Pharmacopoeia 2007", effective from 1st April 2008 has been published recently by the Indian Pharmacopoeia Commission (IPC) on behalf of the Government of India, Ministry of Health & Family Welfare. The Government of India constituted the IPC on 22nd March 2005 as an autonomous body under the provisions of the Societies Registration Act, 1860. The functioning of the Commission is governed by the provisions of the approved Memorandum of Association, Rules and Regulations of the IPC. The Commission has its headquarters at the Central Indian Pharmacopoeia Laboratory (CIPL), Ghaziabad [UP].

The Indian Pharmacopoeia 2007 has been prepared in accordance with the principles and designed plan, decided by the Scientific Body of the Indian Pharmacopoeia Commission. In addition to the past practices of requesting for comments, the contents of revised appendices and monographs have been publicized on the website of the Indian Pharmacopoeia Commission, for collecting comments from various institutions and organizations. All the feedback and inputs have been reviewed by the relevant Expert Committee to ensure the feasibility and practicability of the standards and methods revised in this edition of the Pharmacopoeia, as well as the principle of "openness, justice and fairness" is kept in mind during compiling and editing.

The Indian Pharmacopoeia 2007 and Addendum 2008 have been considerably revised and improved in respect of General Notices, Requirements of Monographs, general Requirements for preparations of Appendices and New testing methods etc, by introducing advanced technology and experimental methods widely adopted in India and abroad. The contents of Appendices are by and large revised in consonance with those now adopted internationally for monitoring the quality of the drugs.

This is the fifth edition of the Indian Pharmacopoeia after independence. It supersedes the 1996 edition but any monograph of the earlier edition that does not figure in this edition continues to be official as stipulated in the second schedule of the drugs and Cosmetics Act, 1940.

The Indian Pharmacopoeia 2007 is published in three Volumes: Volume I deals with Notices, Preface, Indian Pharmacopoeia Commission, Acknowledgments, Introduction, General Notices, Test Methods, Reference Data, Reagents and Solutions, General Tests, Containers and Tables; Volume 2 mainly contains General Notices, General Monographs on Dosage Forms and Monographs on Drug substances, Dosage forms and Pharmaceutical aids Monographs (A to M); Volume 3 comprises of General Notices, Monographs on Drug substances, Dosage forms and Pharmaceutical aids Monographs (N to Z), Monographs on Vaccines and Immunosera for Human Use, Monographs on Herbs and Herbal Products, Monographs on Blood and Blood-related Products, Monographs on Biotechnology Products, Monographs on Veterinary Products and Index. It is hoped that the Indian Pharmacopoeia 2007 would be able to fulfill the Mission of the Indian Pharmacopoeia Commission to promote public health both in India and other countries using drugs manufactured in India. It is expected to play a vital role in initiating new perspectives for improving the quality of medicines and accelerate development of Pharma Sector in India. Defining the Mission, Vision and Objectives of the IP is a unique feature of the 2007 edition.

The Indian Pharmacopoeia Commission (IPC)

The Indian Pharmacopoeia Commission (IPC) has a three-tier structure comprising of the General Body of 19 members, Governing Body of 8-10 members and Scientific Body of 15-23 members from different related scientific fields; the number of members of the Scientific Body may vary from time to time. The Indian Pharmacopoeia is published in continuing pursuit of the Mission, Vision and Objectives of the IPC.

Mission: To promote public health in India by bringing out authoritative and officially accepted standard for quality of drugs including active pharmaceutical ingredients, excipients and dosage forms, used by health professionals, patients and consumers.

Vision: To promote the highest standards of drugs for use in humans and animals within practical limits of the technologies available for manufacture and analysis.

Objectives

1. To develop comprehensive monographs for drugs to be included in the Indian Pharmacopoeia; including active pharmaceutical ingredients, pharmaceutical aids and dosage forms as well as medical devices, and to keep them updated by revision on a regular basis.
2. To develop monographs for herbal drugs, both raw drugs and extracts and their formulations.
3. To accord priority to monographs of drugs included in the National Essential Medicines List and their dosage forms.
4. To take note of the different levels of sophistication in analytical testing/ instrumentation available while framing the monographs.

5. To accelerate the process of preparation, certification and distribution of IP Reference Substances, including the related substances, impurities and degradation products.
6. To collaborate with pharmacopoeias like the Eur Ph, BP, USP, JP, ChP and International Pharmacopoeia with a view to harmonizing with global standards.
7. To review existing monographs periodically with a view to deleting obsolete ones and amending those requiring up gradation/revision.
8. To organize educational programs and research activities for spreading and establishing awareness on the need and scope of quality standards for drugs and related articles/materials.

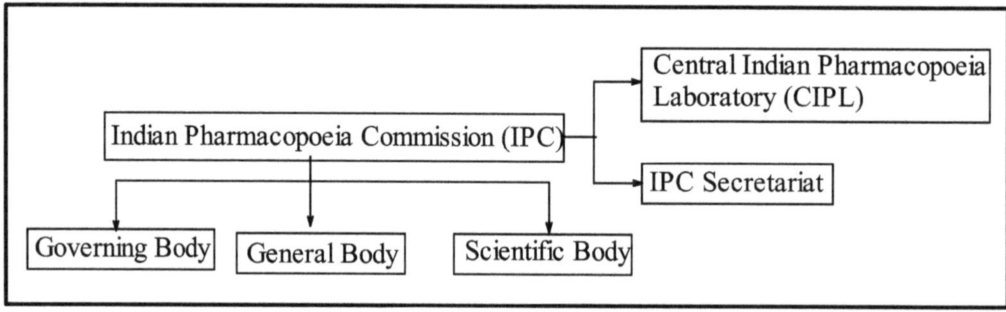

Chart 1.1 Organization chart of Indian Pharmacopoeia Commission (IPC)

A total of 12 items included in the 1996 edition of the Indian Pharmacopoeia have been deleted in the 2007 edition of IP while 186 new drug monographs, 4 biotechnological products, 15 blood and blood products, 23 herbs and herbal products, 36 vaccines for human use, and 7 veterinary monographs have been added.

To ensure that commercial formulations based on medicinal plants are safe, effective and of standard quality, the Regional Research Laboratory (RRL) Jammu, and the Indian Drugs Manufacturers' Association (IDMA), Mumbai have jointly published the Indian Herbal Pharmacopoeia in two volumes. The volume I published in 1998 contains 20 monographs and 1 Appendix. The volume II published in 1999 contains 20 monographs and 6 appendices.

To lay down the standards of quality for the drugs of A*yurvedic*, *Unani* and *Siddha* Systems of Medicine in the country, the Pharmacopoeial Laboratory for Indian Medicine was established in 1970 at Ghaziabad, UP.

The Ministry of Health and Family Welfare, Govt. of India published the first edition of the Ayurvedic Pharmacopoeia of India in three volumes. The Volume I published in 1990 contains 80 monographs and 7 Appendices, Volume II published in 1999 contains 78 monographs and 6 Appendices, and the volume III published in 2001 contains 100 monographs and 6 appendices.

An exhaustive list of legally recognized books pertaining to the various systems of medicine including the allopathic system has been given under the Drugs & Cosmetics Act and Rules.

Table 1.1 The Indian Pharmacopoeia

Edition	Year	Volumes
First	1955	One
Second	1966	One
Third	1985	Two
Fourth	1996	Two
Fifth	2008	Three

HISTORY OF AYURVEDA

Ayurveda, which literally translated means "the science or knowledge of life", is the traditional holistic medical system of India. The true history of Ayurveda starts from the time of the Holy books, the *Vedas*. Ancient mythology contends that the concept and essence of *Ayurveda* was revealed by the creator of the world himself – Lord *Brahma*. The *Vedas* were written approximately five thousand years earlier. There are four *Vedas*. They are –

1. Rig veda
2. Yajur veda
3. Sama veda
4. Adharva veda

They preach the philosophy of life. The *Atharvaveda* contains the principles of healing on which *Ayurveda* is based. '*Ayur*' means 'life' in *Sanskrit*. *Ayurveda* is the most ancient science of healing which enhances longevity. It has influenced many of the older traditional methods of healing including Tibetan, Chinese and Greek medicine. Hence, *Ayurveda* is considered by many as the 'mother of healing.' The hymns, the *mantras* and the medical information contained in the *Vedas* were contributions of *Rishis* and *Munis* or sages, over a period of time. Many of these sages were learned saints who devoted their life to understanding the world.

Before the advent of writing, the ancient wisdom of this healing system was a part of the spiritual tradition of the *Sanatana Dharma* (Universal Religion), or Vedic Religion. *VedaVyasa*, the famous sage, *shaktavesha* avatar of *Vishnu*, put into writing the complete knowledge of *Ayurveda,* along with the more directly spiritual insights of self realization into a body of scriptural literature called the *Vedas* and the *Vedic* literatures. There were originally four main books of spirituality, which included among other topics, health, astrology, spiritual business, government, army, poetry and spiritual living and behavior. These books are known as *Vedas*.

A diet and health plan is given to the individual according to the needs to correct the imbalance. The basis for all other concepts in *Ayurveda* is *Sankhya* (the analytical study of the elements that comprise the universe). Although the modern physicist would delineate well over one hundred elements, *Sankhya* states there are twenty-four elements, of which five are the foundation of the gross world: **Earth, Water, Fire, Air and Ether.**

Everything which is solid in the table of the elements is earth, water is everything liquid, and air is everything gaseous, ether is the field in quantum mechanics upon which everything rests, and fire is the transformer of one thing to another. These five elements, when joined in different combinations, make up the three *doshas* or 'biological modes' which are the *Prakruti* or nature of an individual and the nature of all things.

The combination of air and ether gives us *Vata* or the Kinetic Biological Mode. *Vata* is that which is electric in the body and causes all movement in and out of the system (breathing, urination, defecation, menstruation, etc.)

The combination of fire and water gives us *Pitta* or the Transformative Biological Mode. *Pitta* is that which mutates or transforms the outside elements of the macrocosm into the inside elements of the body (the microcosm). *Pitta* governs the digestion of physical, mental, and emotional elements.

Finally, the combination of earth and water gives us *Kapha* or the Structive Biological mode. *Kapha* is that which makes both lubrication (mucus, synovial fluid) and structure (bones, muscles, fat, joints, etc).

The *Rik Veda*, a compilation of verse on the nature of existence, is the oldest surviving book of any Indo-European language (3000 B.C.). The *Rik Veda* (also known as *Rig Veda*) refers to the cosmology known as *Sankhya*, which lies at the base of both *Ayurveda* and *Yoga*, contains verses on the nature of health and disease, pathogenesis and principles of treatment. Among the *Rik Veda* are found discussions of the three *dosas*; *Vayu, Pitta and Kapha*, and the use of herbs to heal the diseases of the mind and body and to foster longevity.

The *Atharva Veda* lists the eight divisions of Ayurveda :

The practical tenets of Ayurveda are divided into eight sections or branches. These eight sections are called *Astanga Ayurveda*.

1. Internal Medicine,
2. Surgery of Head and Neck,
3. Ophthalmology and Otorinolaryngology,
4. Toxicology,
5. Psychiatry,
6. Pediatrics,
7. Gerontology or Science of Rejuvenation, and
8. Science of Fertility.

The *Vedic* Sages took the passages from the *Vedic* Scriptures relating to *Ayurveda* and compiled separate books dealing only with *Ayurveda*. One of these books, called the *Atreya Samhita* is the oldest medical book in the world! The *Vedic Brahmanas* were not only priests performing religious rites and ceremonies; they also became *Vaidyas* (physicians of *Ayurveda*).

The sage-physician-surgeons of the time were the same sages or seers, deeply devoted holy people, who saw health as an integral part of spiritual life. It is said that they received their training of *Ayurveda* through direct cognition during meditation. In other words, the knowledge of the use of various methods of healing, prevention, longevity and surgery came through Divine revelation; there was no guessing or testing and harming animal. These revelations were transcribed from the oral tradition into book form, interspersed with the other aspects of life and spirituality. What is fascinating is *Ayurveda's* use of herbs, foods, aromas, gems, colors, yoga, mantras, lifestyle and surgery. Consequently *Ayurveda* grew into a respected and widely used system of healing in India.

Around 1500 BC, various authors took *ayurvedic* passages from the four scriptures and created *ayurvedic* texts for at least eight specific branches of medicine, divided into two main schools: *ATREYA*, or physicians, and *DHANVANTARI*, or surgeons. Through experimentation and research, these two schools transformed ayurveda from a primarily religious discipline to a scientific medical system. Scholars from China, Tibet, Egypt, Persia, Greece and Rome flocked to India's Ayurvedic schools to learn about this holistic medicine.

Over 1,200 years ago, masters of the two schools assembled their knowledge into essential texts. *Charak*, a doctor of the *Atreya* school, compiled information on diagnosis and prevention of disease, internal and external causes of illness, herbal prescriptions and anatomy. He stated that a disease - physical, mental and spiritual - is fundamentally caused by a separation from Divine Oneness. He also gave strikingly detailed descriptions of human fetal development month-by-month.

Sushrut, from the *Dhanvantari* school, classified functions of organs, nerves and joints, catalogued various kinds of wounds and described sophisticated surgical equipment used in technical procedures like amputation and plastic surgery. His text also includes the first mention of the science of massage using *MARMA* points, vital nerve intersections like those used in Chinese acupuncture.

After the flowering of ayurvedic knowledge came hard times. First, schools began splitting over technical interpretations. In the 1600s, the British East India Company took control over the subcontinent. By 1833, it had sufficient authority to ban all ayurvedic colleges and opened the first Western-style medical university. Ayurvedic medicine survived only in rural areas where local doctors treated those who could not afford Western medicine.

Only in 1920 did the discipline of ayurveda begin to regain its former respect. When India established independence in 1947, ayurvedic medical schools were once more officially accepted and allowed to open.

Today, well over 120 ayurvedic colleges in India grant degrees after a five-year program. More than 300,000 ayurvedic physicians belong to the All-India Ayurveda Congress, making it the largest medical organization in the world.

There are six tastes according to Ayurveda: Sweet, Sour, Salty, Pungent, Bitter and Astringent. Each is comprised of two elements

1. Sweet (earth and water) examples: wheat, sugar, milk, rice, dates
2. Sour (earth and fire) examples: yogurt, lemon, tamarind
3. Salty (water and fire) examples: sea salt, rock salt, kelp
4. Pungent (fire and air) examples: onion, radish, ginger, chilly
5. Bitter (air and ether) examples: dandelion root, rhubarb root, bitter melon
6. Astringent (air and earth) examples: plantain, pomegranate, apples

There are two other considerations in Ayurveda. First, whether a food's action is heating or cooling. The taste sweet, bitter, and astringent are cooling; sour, salty, and pungent are all heating. The second is the post-digestive effect or how the foods 'taste' to the tissues during and after assimilation. Sweet and salty are sweet in post-digestive effect. Sour is sour, and pungent, bitter, and astringent are pungent. Taste, action, and post-digestive effect are known is *Sanskrit* as *rasa, virya,* and *vipack*, respectively in Ayurveda. They are the keys to understanding food and herbs. With this knowledge, one can unlock the mysteries of the energetic dynamics of food and be able to make the right choices for oneself.

Recent History

Before Ayurveda began its recent renewal in the West, it went through a period of decline in India when Western medical education became dominant during the era of British rule. Ayurveda became a second-grade option used primarily by traditional spiritual practitioners and the poor. After India gained its independence in 1947, Ayurveda gained ground and new schools began to be established. More than five hundred Ayurvedic companies and hospitals have been opened in the last ten years, and several hundred schools have been established. Although Ayurveda remains a secondary system of health care in India, the trend toward complementary care is emerging, and Western and Ayurvedic physicians often work side by side.

Interest in Ayurveda in the West began in the mid 1970's as Ayurvedic teachers from India began visiting the United States and Europe. By sharing their knowledge they have inspired a vast movement toward body-mind-spirit medicine. Today Ayurvedic colleges are opening throughout Europe, Australia, and the United States.

SALIENT FEATURES OF IP, USP AND BP

International Pharmacopoeia

The International Pharmacopoeia (Pharmacopoeia Internationals) was published for the first time in 1951. It is published by the World Health Organization with the cooperation of the member countries of the United Nations. Although it recommends the international standards for drugs, it has no legal status. It is expected that different countries publishing their own pharmacopeias would use the information given in International Pharmacopoeia while revising their respective pharmacopeias. Since it is published with the team efforts of member countries of United Nations, it commands due recognition and respect.

In addition to the IP, BP, USP and International Pharmacopoeia, the pharmacopeias are also published by countries like France, Italy, Japan, East Germany, Norway and Russia. Those countries not publishing their own pharmacopeias recognize the pharmacopeias of other country(ies).

Besides the pharmacopeias, a number of countries including India also publish the National Formularies. These Formularies are significant in the sense that the pharmacopeias can include only a limited range of drugs and preparations. The formularies give details of substances in common use. The first National Formulary of India (NFl) was published in 1960. Many hospitals also publish their own formularies, which contain monographs/lists of drugs and preparations commonly prescribed in the respective hospital.

United States Pharmacopoeia (USP)

The first edition of the Pharmacopoeia of the United States (USP) was released on December 15, 1820. The title USP VIII was adopted for the ninth edition to indicate that it was the '8th Revision'. The USP of 1900, which was published in 1905 adopted average doses, the 'Purity Rubric', and 25°C as the standard temperature for specific gravity and solubility standards. USP IX added for the first time biological assays, biological products etc. and a chapter on the methods of analytical determination. The dipthhong was dropped in the word pharmacopoeia in USP XIV. USP XVIII (1970) included a new quality test (Dissolution test for tablets) so far not included in most of the other pharmacopoeias. Similarly a 'microbial limit test' was also incorporated for tablets to prevent the presence of *Salmonella* and *E. coli.* USP XIX (1975) was the last individual USP. In 1988, the American Pharmaceutical Association published the first national formulary under the title *The National Formulary of Unofficial Preparations.* The title was changed to *National Formulary* in response to the US Food and Drugs Act of 1906, when both the USP and NF standards were referenced. In 1975, USP acquired the NF and began publishing this compendium concurrently with USP in a single volume titled

USP-NF. *USP XX* (1980) first combined USP with NF. This approach helps to consolidate the standards for new drugs, eliminate duplicative text and permits a single index.

From 1820 to 1942 the USP was published at 10-year intervals, from 1942 to 2000 at 5-year intervals, and beginning in 2002, annually. USP 32 NF 27, 2009 is latest. Asian edition is also available for sale in prescribed Asian countries.

British Pharmacopoeia (BP)

The first British Pharmacopoeia (BP) was published in 1864. However the Pharmacopoeia Londinensis, which appeared for the first time in 1684, was the forerunner of BP. The first Edinburgh Pharmacopoeia in Scotland was published in 1699 and the first Dublin Pharmacopoeia appeared in 1807. The fusion of the above three pharmacopoeias resulted in the publication of the first BP in 1864. The earlier editions of the BP contained monographs mostly on the crude drugs but over the decades the BP, as like other pharmacopoeias, has undergone drastic changes in its contents. Presently BP is released annually latest being the BP 2010. The new edition comprises six volumes: Volumes I and II (Medicinal Substances), Volume III (Formulated Preparations. Immunological Products, Radiopharmaceutical Preparations and Surgical Materials, Volume IV (Appendices, Infrared Reference Spectra and Index), Volume V (BP - Veterinary) Volume VI [CD-ROM version of the BP 2010 and BP (vet) 2010] with three updates.

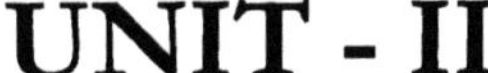

UNIT - II

CHAPTER 2

PRINCIPLES OF DISPENSING

In India only registered pharmacists are authorized to dispense, sell, or compound a drug or supervise the part of a Pharmacy where drugs are kept. Dispensing includes the selection, preparation, and transfer of one or more doses of a drug to a patient. The process of dispensing mainly comprises of the following components.

1. Technical Component

- receiving and reading the prescription,
- adjusting an order according to approved policy,
- entry of order,
- selecting the drug or determining the product to dispense,
- checking the expiry date,
- reconstituting a product as per the requirement,
- labeling a product,
- final physical check for accuracy of finished product,
- maintaining but not interpreting medication profiles, and
- maintaining, preparing and operating equipment.

2. Cognitive Component

- assessing the therapeutic appropriateness of a prescription,
- making a recommendation to a prescriber, and
- developing the formula for a drug that needs to be specifically prepared by a pharmacist;

Following activities do not constitute dispensing: a) administration of medications, b) repackaging of medications, c) supplying medications.

PRESCRIPTION PROCESSING

Following precautions are essential during the processing of a prescription

a. Collect the important information relating to the patient.
b. Carefully scrutinize the prescription for quantity and dose, therapeutic use and incompatibilities of ingredients.
c. Dispensed prescriptions should be compared with their originals for accuracy.
d. Check label of large quantity container.
e. Properly affix labels on container having necessary information.
f. Another pharmacist should finally check filled prescriptions.
g. Following information should be clearly recorded on all new prescriptions:
    - Name of patient
    - Age of patient
    - Weight of patient
    - Type of disease
    - Any allergic reaction
    - Identification of agent acting on behalf of patient.
    - Contact person on delivered prescriptions

Prescription records of Schedule X drugs and Narcotic Drugs and Psychotropic Substances must be maintained.

Important Instruction while working in the dispensing laboratory

a. Laboratory should be neat and clean.
b. All chemicals and other articles should be in proper place.
c. Electric points, washing and weighing area and working table should be arranged properly to reduce the risk of mistakes, errors and contamination.
d. Protect the clothes and reduce contamination of dispensed product using neat and clean white overcoat (apron), gloves, napkin etc.
e. Before dispensing, read the prescription carefully. In case of any doubt in understanding clarify the confusion with the prescriber.
f. For formula and quantity consult Pharmacopoeia or other reference book (do not apply any trial and error method or approximate quantity).
g. Following things are also checked –dose, number of doses prescribed, incompatibility.
h. Check the calculation of different ingredients used in prescription.
i. Selection of containers for dispensing.

j. Weighing, mixing, and other steps performed as per the process.
k. Label should have all information regarding product, instruction for use and storage.
l. Paste the label on the container properly.
m. Wrap the container according to suitability of transportation.
n. Check the finished product before delivery to the patient or consumer.
o. Ensure that the patient or his representative has followed the instructions regarding mode of administration and storage of the prescription.
p. Maintain the record of the prescription having all basic requirements.

SOURCES OF INFORMATION

The pharmacist should rely on following sources of information.

1. Official books

- Indian Pharmacopoeia [IP]
- United States Pharmacopoeia [USP]
- Extra Pharmacopoeia [Martindale]
- British Pharmacopoeia [BP]
- British Pharmaceutical Codex [BPC]
- European Pharmacopoeia [EP]
- International Pharmacopoeia

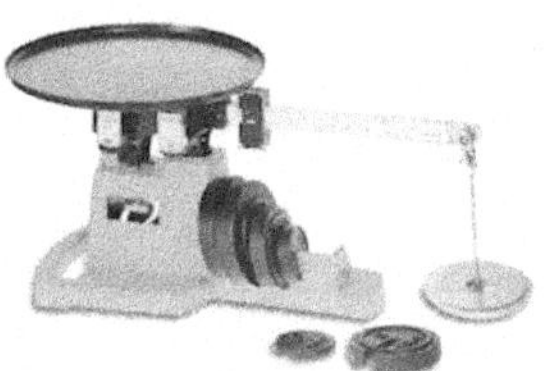

Mechanical Beam Balance

2. Reference books

- Remington's Pharmaceutical Sciences
- Pharmaceutical Handbooks
- National Formulary of India
- Drug Today
- Monthly Index of Medical Specialties [MIMS]
- Current Index of Medical Specialties [CIMS]
- Physician Desk Reference [PDR]
- Indian Drug Review [IDR]
- Indian Pharmaceutical Guide [IGP]

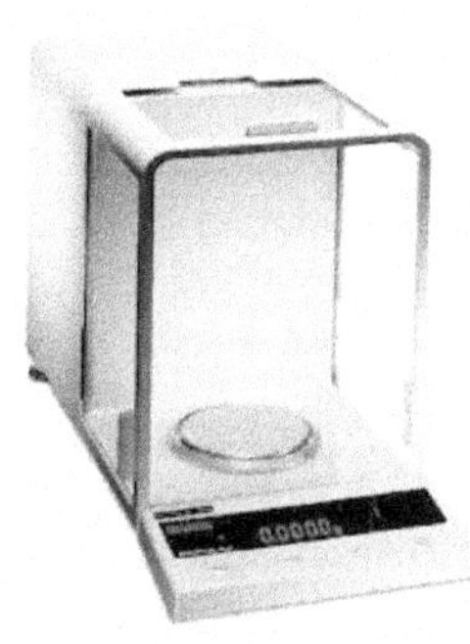

Analytical Balance

3. Journals

Name of Journal	Frequency of publication	Address
Bhartiya Vegyanic Avam Audhyogik Anusandhan Patrika	Half Yearly	The Sales and Distribution officer, NISCAIR, CSIR, Dr. K. S. Krishna Marg, New Delhi – 12
CSIR News	Bimonthly	The Sales and Distribution officer, NISCAIR, CSIR, Dr. K. S. Krishna Marg, New Delhi – 12
Current Literature of Science	Bimonthly	The Sales and Distribution officer, NISCAIR, CSIR, Dr. K. S. Krishna Marg, New Delhi – 12
Drugs and Pharmaceutical Industry Highlight	Weekly	Scientist-in-Incharge, Central Drug Research Institute, Chattar Manzil Palace, Lucknow-226 001
IDMA, Bulletin	Weekly	Indian Drug Manufacturer's Association 102-B, A-Wing, Poonam Chambers Dr. A.B.Road, Worli, Mumbai-400 018
Indian Drugs	Monthly	The Editor, Indian Drugs Indian Drug Manufacturers Association, 102-B, Poonam Chambers, Dr. A.B.Road, Worli, Mumbai – 400 018 [publications@idmaindia.com
Indian Journal of Chemical Technology	Bimonthly	The Sales and Distribution officer, NISCAIR, CSIR, Dr. K. S. Krishna Marg, New Delhi – 12
Indian Journal of Biotechnology	Quarterly	The Sales and Distribution officer, NISCAIR, CSIR, Dr. K. S. Krishna Marg, New Delhi – 12
Indian Journal of Chemistry Section B	Monthly	The Sales and Distribution officer, NISCAIR, CSIR, Dr. K. S. Krishna Marg, New Delhi – 12
Indian Journal of Pharmaceutical Education & Research	Quarterly	The Editor, Indian Journal of Pharmaceutical Education & Research,J.S.S. College of Phramcy, S.S.Nagar, Mysore – 570 015 (Karnataka) ijpeindia@lycos.com www.ijpe.org
Indian Journal of Pharmaceutical Sciences	Bimonthly	The Editor, Indian Journal of Pharmaceutical Sciences Kalina , Sanatacruz, (E), Mumbai – 400 098ijps 2002@rediffmail.com www.Indianpharma.org
Indian Journal of Pharmacology	Monthly	Publishers (Medknow Publications 12 Manisha Plaza, MN ROAD, Kurla (W) Mumbai- 400 070 [ijp@jipmer.edu, subscription@medknow.com]

Contd...

Indian Journal of Physiology and Pharmacology	Monthly	The Editor, Department of Physiology, All India Institute of Medical Sciences,Ansari Nagar, **New Delhi**-110 029
Indian Journal of Traditional Knowledge	Quarterly	The Sales and Distribution officer, NISCAIR, CSIR, Dr. K. S. Krishna Marg, New Delhi – 12
Journal of Scientific and Industrial Research	Monthly	The Sales and Distribution officer, NISCAIR, CSIR, Dr. K. S. Krishna Marg, New Delhi –12
Indian Journal of Natural Products	Quarterly	The Editor, Deptt. of Pharamcy, Dr. H. S. Gaur University, Sagar- 470 003 (MP)
Pharma Pulse	Weekly	The Editor,Indian Express Newspapers (Bombay) ,Ltd. First Floor , Express Towers , Nariman Point Mumbai – 021 Bpdsubscriptions@expressindia.com
Pharmabiz	Weekly	The Editor, iPharma India Pvt. Ltd. Rajmahal , 4th Floor, 84, Veer – Nariman Road, Church Gate, Mumbai – 400 020 (Mah.)
Pharma Times	Monthly	The Editor, Pharma Times Indian Pharmaceutical Association, Kalina, Santacruz (E) Mumbai – 400 089
Probe	Quarterly	The Editor, Dr. S.K.Mitra, Probe, The Himalaya Drug Company, Makali, Banglore – 562 123
The Indian Journal of Hospital Pharmacy	Bimonthly	The Editor, The Indian Journal of Hospital Pharamcy, R-566, New Rajinder Nagar, New Delhi – 110 060
The Indian Pharmacist	Monthly	The Circulation Manager The Indian Pharmacist, Bazaz Publications 507, Ashok Bhawan, 93, Nehru Place, New Delhi – 110 019 subscription@indianpharmacist.com
The Pharma Review	Bimonthly	The Editor, The Pharma Review, Kongposh Publications Pvt. Ltd. C-19 Commercial complex, SDA, New Delhi fpc@vsnl.com website: kbpub.com

4. Internet

In 21st centaury, Internet is one of the easiest and quickest method for collection of the literature and latest information news, discoveries and other scientific development in the field of pharmaceutical sciences. Some important Phrama-websites are listed below.

Website	Information
www.apti.org	Association of Pharmaceutical Teachers of India
www.aicte.ernet.in	All India council for Technical Education, New Delhi
www.pharmweb.net	Pharmacy Information
www.who.ch	World Health Organization
www.aaps.org	American association of Pharmaceutical Sciences
www.nih.gov	National Institute of Health, Bethesda
www.nlm.nih.gov	National Library of medicine
www.acs.org	American Chemical Society
www.pharminfo.com	Pharm. Infonet
www.chemport.org	Chemical Abstracts and Chemistry Journals
www.biomednet.com	Bio-medical Journals
www.ideallibrary.com	International digital electronic access library
www.pharmweb.net/pharmweb/ fip.html	International Pharmaceutical Federation (FIP)
www.isinet.com	Current contents
www.elsevier.com	Elsevier Publishing company
www.pharmweb.net/pharmweb/ pharmwebyp.html	List of Pharmaceutical Companies on the internet
www.pharmweb.net/pharmweb/ pharmpress.html	Pharmaceutical press
www.pci.ac.in	Pharmacy Council of India, New Delhi

OPERATIONAL ASPECTS

The following operations are commonly required in pharmaceutical dispensing:

1. Weighing
2. Measuring
3. Dissolution
4. Solubilization
5. Size reduction
6. Size separation
7. Mixing
8. Filtration

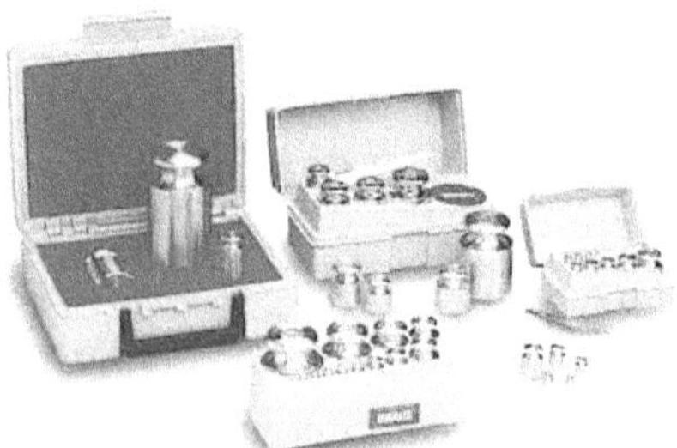

Weights

Weighing

Several varieties of dispensing scales and weight boxes are available. Three to four varieties of balances capable of weighing different quantities and of desired accuracies should be available in a pharmacy and a pharmacist exercises his choice for use while dispensing a prescription depending on the quantity to be weighed and accuracy desired. The balances should be installed on a heavy, stable platform in a corner free from drift of air or fumes. The balance meant for daily use may be installed at a suitable place on the working table. The balance should be adjusted in level with the help of a spirit level and checked for the null point and oscillations of the beam before use. While commissioning a new balance, the pharmacist should carefully read the literature supplied by the manufacturer and understand its operation and accuracy. Quantities lesser than 50 mg of ingredients and lesser than 100 mg of potent medicaments should be weighed on an analytical balance. After testing a balance, pieces of white paper should be placed under each pan. The weights should be handled and picked with the help of forceps and kept in the left pan of the balance. Solid is slowly added to the right pan or removed there from using a spatula of suitable size. Greasy and sticky substances are weighed by placing them on a greaseproof (butter or waxed) paper and then weighing using a counterpoise. After the weighing operation, the weights are rechecked while returning them to the weight box. The solid is then removed from the right pan, which is usually made of glass or stainless steel. Corrosive and oxidizing agents should not be put directly in a stainless steel pan but weighed in a watch glass providing a suitable counterpoise in the left pan. It may be borne in mind that weighing operation, if executed without care, may lead to serious errors.

Measuring

The devices used for this operation are measures and pipettes. The measures may be cylindrical or conical and between the two varieties the former are easier to read and more accurate and reliable. The latter are however, easier to clean, rinse and handle. Nature of meniscus and its reading influence the degree of measuring accuracy considerably. It is desirable that one acquires practice and experience in taking meniscus readings with different measures and liquids of different colours. A measure should rest on a flat surface perpendicular to the surface while taking readings and should be straight before the eyes to avoid parallax errors. Errors are also possible in removing the liquid from the measure. Viscous liquids may stick to the measure and deliver lesser volumes, the error sometimes being as high as 20%. In practice, one should use a clean, dry measure closest in volume to the quantity to be measured. The liquid from the bottle may be poured carefully in the measure upto the proper graduation from the side opposite to the label holding the bottle in the right hand The stopper of the liquid bottle should either be held in between two fingers of the right hand or placed on the table with the surface that touches the liquid pointing upwards so as to avoid the contamination by the wet surface coming in contact with the surface of the table top. After the requisite volume has been filled in the measure the container should be removed from the hand and stopper put back in position. The liquid may then be poured in the container or mortar as the case may be and rinsed if the liquid is viscous, adding the rinsing to the original lot. Small volumes can be accurately delivered with the help of graduated pipettes calibrated from 0.01 to 0.1 ml. Pipette should be of a proper size, clean and dry. A rubber teat should be attached to the upper end of the pipette. The air may be expelled by pressing the teat with right hand thumb and the lower end of the pipette immersed in the liquid to be sucked in. If excess liquid is sucked in, it can be removed by pressing the teat till the meniscus reads the required volume. The liquid inside the pipette can now be delivered to the container or mortar as the case may be. One can also remove the teat after sucking the pipette and can control delivery of the volume with the help of the thumb or the forefinger. Use of measuring pipettes based on vacuum (Vaccupet etc.) should be encouraged for reasons of accuracy and avoiding hazard while sucking the liquids through mouth.

Solubilization

It is the process of dissolving poorly soluble solute molecules in water in the presence of surfactants. Mc Bain introduced this term in 1937. The exact mechanism of solubilization is not clear yet. When surfactants with proper HLB values are added to a liquid in very low concentrations, the solution behaves as an ideal one. Surfactant molecules in the solution tend to orient themselves at the liquid-air interface. Addition of surfactant may be continued until all available space is saturated and beyond which the surfactant is forced back into the bulk of the liquid. At still higher concentrations, the surfactant molecules or ions tend to aggregate to form micelles. Thus micelles are the aggregates of 100 to 150 surfactant molecules. Solubilization concept has been profitably employed in pharmaceutical practice. Water insoluble substances are solubilized using various techniques of solubilization. Generally low toxicity soaps are used to provide micelles. Cholesterol can also be solubilized to an appreciable extent by soaps. Proprietary disinfectants such as Lysol, chloroxyxylenol solution and hexachlorophene liquid soaps are formulated on the basis of solubilization phenomenon. Lyophilic surfactants with HLB values higher than 15 are considered to be the best solubilizing agents.

Dissolution

It is presumed that a student is familiar with the theoretical aspects of solution. When a soluble solid is incorporated in a liquid, its physical form is changed. Essentially it is a phenomenon of mass transfer. After due scrutiny of the prescription, one should be able to envisage and assess whether the prescription would yield a clear product. Lack of comprehension may result into filtering out and rejecting the therapeutically active precipitate in an over enthusiastic attempt to supply a clear product. Such instances are not rare and it is vital that a pharmacist fully understands the likely reactions that may occur and act suitably. Once it is established that a solution will result he may take steps to affect it rapidly. Drugs in fine state of subdivision have a greater specific surface and dissolve faster than larger particles or crystals. Secondly, stirring the particles in the vehicle expedites dissolution as highly concentrated solution around the particle is replaced by dilute solution till the equilibrium is established. Raising the temperature usually accelerates the rate of solution. However, heating may not be advisable to if the drug is thermo-labile. Rise in temperature increases the diffusion coefficient and reduces the viscosity, two important factors that favor solution. As a rule, the pharmacist should not rely on his memory regarding the solubility of ingredients. It is advisable that he makes use of tables and texts for ascertaining solubility of the substances in given vehicle under the overall conditions of the prescription. When two substances are present to the optimum amount of their solubility, it is likely that the resultant product may not be clear. Further, the pharmacist should thoroughly examine the possibility of a chemical reaction resulting into precipitate formation. The drug is first powdered and the requisite quantity weighed. Stirring or shaking with a liquid may be done preferably in a conical flask large enough to prevent spilling during shaking. Another method for affecting solution of relatively less solute substances is to transfer the solid and a portion of the vehicle in a mortar and mixing with the help of pestle. Wherever volatile substances are prescribed, heating should be avoided as a precautionary measure and shaking done in a closed container with a suitable closure to prevent loss of volatile medicament. Whenever heating has been employed, the solution should be first cooled to room temperature, if need be, under running tap water. Filtration, dilution, making up the volume and transference to the container should be done thereafter.

Size reduction

In dispensing practice drugs and excipients are used in the preparation of dosage forms in specified size for effective result or action. Size reduction is necessary to some extent. 'Grinding', 'comminution' and 'milling' are the terms commonly used to signify size reduction of solids. Size reduction of a drug may include one or more of the operations e.g. cutting, slicing, chopping, rasping or grating, contusion, grinding, pulverizing, milling, micronizing etc. Selection of the processes and equipment depends on type of material, desired degree of size reduction, moisture content etc. in the material, mechanism of size reduction, stability of final product and economic and fast method of size reduction.

Some manual processes employed in the size reduction of substance used in the dispensing of prescription are explained below.

Trituration

The term trituration refers to the process of size reduction of substances to a fine powder but it is also applied for the process whereby a mixture of fine powders is intimately mixed in a mortar. The circular mixing motion causes blending and also breaks up soft aggregates of powders. Crushing or grinding can also be affected by means of application of the force on the pestle.

Pulverization by intervention

This is the process of powdering a substance with the help of another substance, which can be removed easily after the pulverization has been completed. Substances such as camphor, which are gummy and tend to re-agglomerate or which resist grinding, can be powdered by this method. Camphor cannot be pulverized by trituration because the particles tend to cohere as quickly as they are powdered. This difficulty is overcome by addition of a small amount of alcohol or other volatile solvent during trituration. The solvent can be removed after pulverization process is complete, by spraying the powdered camphor in a thin layer. Spermaceti wax may also be powdered in this manner. Iodine crystals may be pulverized with the help of a small quantity of ether. Picric acid is often mixed with 10 to 20% of water for safety in transportation. The water content serves a dual purpose. When picric acid is to be powdered for use in ointments, it prevents the dangerous explosion during comminution, and aids in the grinding process by intervention.

Levigation

A pharmacist often uses this process to incorporate solids into dermatological and ophthalmic ointments and suspensions. The term refers to the reduction of a substance to an extremely fine state of subdivision by rubbing it, in a glass mortar or on a slab with the aid of an insoluble liquid called the levigating agent. The process is one of wet grinding. Levigating agent should be selected on the basis of its ability to form a paste with the substance to be levigated, and its compatibility with other ingredients in the product. For instance, water cannot be used as levigating agent with zinc oxide, intended to be incorporated into an oleaginous ointment base. Liquid paraffin is the levigating agent of choice in this case.

PRINCIPLE OF SIZE REDUCTION

Size reduction involves four different mechanisms.

1. **Cutting:** This implies cutting of materials by means of sharp blade(s).
2. **Compression: This** is accomplished by application of force by a suitable device.
3. **Impact:** Impact implies hitting of a more or less stationary material by an object moving at high speed or striking the moving particles at a stationary surface. In either case, the material is shattered to small pieces.
4. **Attrition:** Attrition occurs when the material is subjected to pressure as in compression but the surfaces are mobile in relation to each other, resulting in shear forces, which break the particles. The mechanisms of impact and attrition may be combined as in ball mill and fluid energy mill.

Equipment in Small Scale : Mortars and pestles (China and Glass), Household mixer, Grinder, Hand mill and Laboratory mill

Large Scale Equipment

Following mill are commonly used in industry for size reduction. Selection of a mill is based on types of material, size required, cleaning, and mechanism of milling.

- Cutter mill
- Hammer mill
- Ball mill
- Rod mill
- Fluid-energy mill
- Roller mill
- Colloid mill
- Disc mill
- Edge runner mill
- ibration ball mill

SIZE SEPARATION

Control of particle size and size range is of great importance in dispensing pharmacy. Size reduction affected by the use of various types of equipments does not necessarily ensure the desired size distribution and therefore at times it is necessary to classify or grade the powdered materials. The process of fractionation of particles on the basis of size range is known as 'grading' or 'sifting'. Sieving has been used conventionally for the close control of particle size after size reduction. The wire sieves, used in sifting powdered drugs, are distinguished by numbers, which indicate the number of meshes (openings) included in a length of 2.54 cm, in each transverse direction parallel to the wires. It should be noted that it is the number of meshes that is specified and not 'the number of wires. Thus, a No. 20 sieve has 20 meshes per 2.54 cm in each transverse direction, but if there were 20 wires there would be 19 meshes only. According to I.P. 1996, "sieves for pharmacopoeial testing are of wire cloth woven from brass, bronze, stainless steel or other suitable material and not coated or plated. The wires are of uniform circular cross-section."

MIXING

Mixing is probably the most widely used operation in dispensing of medicine. Mixing may be defined as an operation, which tends to result in a state in which each particle of one material lies as nearly adjacent as possible to a particle of the other material. Mixing tends to minimize non- uniformity or gradients in composition, properties, or temperature of material in bulk. The desired degree of mixing depends on the purpose of the product and the objective of mixing depends on types of dosage form being dispensed.

Types of Mixtures

Mixtures are mainly three types -

1. **Positive mixtures:** This type of product results when there is an irreversible mixing of materials such as gases or miscible liquids.
2. **Negative mixtures:** These are more difficult to obtain and a higher degree of mixing efficiency is essential. Negative mixtures require work for their formation and the components of such mixtures separate out unless work is continually expended on them e.g. suspension.
3. **Neutral mixtures:** These mixtures are static in their behavior and the components neither have tendency to mix spontaneously, nor do they segregate after mixing. Examples are pharmaceutical mixtures e.g. pastes, ointments and mixed powders.

   Common Mixers used in Pharmaceutical Laboratories : Propeller mixers, Turbine mixers, Sigma-blade mixer, Triple-roller mill, Planetary mixer and Colloid mill

HOMOGENIZATION

Homogenization is the process, which renders a material to uniform quality, consistency or structure. The process is used in the preparation of fine suspensions, emulsions etc. Usually, in a homogenizer, the mixed phases of dispersion are passed through a finely ground valve and seat under high pressure, which causes atomization. This is further enhanced by the impact received by the atomized mixture as it strikes the valve seat.

a. **Hand homogenizer**: It is suitable for homogenizing small amounts of materials. This type of homogenizer is specially meant for laboratories and is moderately priced. It is probably the most efficient homogenizer apparently available to the prescription pharmacist.

b. **Silverson mixer-homogenizer**: Processes of mixing and homogenizing may be combined in some machines e.g. Silverson mixer-homogenizer. It consists essentially of an emulsifier head in which a set of rotor blades is surrounded by a fine-meshed stainless sieve. The materials are sucked through the mesh by the rotor blades and are reduced to a homogeneous dispersion before being expelled. The blades are adjusted so as to give a powerful shearing action. Two stage homogenizers are so constructed that the dispersion, after treatment in the first valve system, is passed on directly to a second one wherein it receives a second treatment.

FILTRATION

Filtration is a unit operation by which solid particles are removed from a fluid by passing the mixture through a porous, fibrous or glandular medium. The object of simple filtration is to obtain sparkling and optically transparent liquids, free from insoluble liquid drops whereas sterile filtration is aimed at the removal of microorganisms in addition to other foreign matter. When the solids are present in small proportions (not exceeding 0.15%), the process is usually spoken of as clarification. Filter media are the porous devices, which retain solids by mechanical separation and allow liquid to pass through. The accumulated layer of solids deposited on the filter medium during the filtration of a slurry or feed is known as filter cake. Slurry is a suspension of solids in a liquid to be filtered. It may also be referred to as feed. Filtrate is the clear liquid passing through the filter.

The mechanism of filtration basically involves a two-step operation -

(i) the flow of solid materials is resisted by the filter medium while the liquid is allowed to pass through; and

(ii) the solid material retained on the filter medium during the course of operation gradually builds up a filter cake which acts as a secondary, and sometimes as a more efficient filter medium.

Filtering Media

1. **Filter paper**: Filter papers are most commonly used for the retention of very fine solids and for the clarification of liquids containing only a small amount of solids. Rapid filtration rate is achieved because the pores on the paper are small and in a large number. As filtering medium may be a possible source of contamination in the finished product, a high quality of filter paper should always be used in pharmaceutical operations.

2. **Membrane filters:** These are employed for micro-filtration e.g. in the preparation of sterile solutions. These are made of pure cellulose or cellulose derivatives mainly cellulose esters or from nylon, teflon, polyvinyl chloride, or silver. Absence of fibers or particles in the integral structure is a particular advantage in the filtration of ophthalmic solutions. The thickness of the membrane filters ranges from 50 to 200µm with millions of pores per square meter of filtering surface. The pores are extremely uniform in size ranging from 0.05 to 14µm and may occupy up to 90 percent of filter volume. To avoid rapid clogging of membrane filler, because of surface screening characteristics, pre-filtration is often required. Thermo-labile materials can be economically and rapidly filtered/sterilized in one cycle by the membrane filtration process.

3. **Cotton filters**: Large particles of extraneous matter from a clear liquid may be removed by loosely inserting a small pledget of absorbent cotton wool in the neck of

the funnel. However, as fine cotton fibers may be frequently imparted to the filtrate, it is sometimes necessary to recycle the filtrate a number of times to attain transparency.

4. **Glass wool**: Filter paper, cotton-wool etc. are not suitable when solutions of highly reactive or corrosive substances as strong acids, alkalis and oxidizing agents are to be filtered. In such cases glass wool may be used as it is resistant to ordinary chemical action. Although it provides very effective filtration, glass wool may contaminate the filtrate with glass-fibers.
5. **Asbestos**: Asbestos pads are also used for the reasons stated above and placed under glass wool. They are prepared by compressing shredded asbestos lightly under pressure and are available in various size ranges. However, asbestos pads are of limited application because they impart an alkaline reaction to the filtrate. Calcium and magnesium ions released from the pads may cause incompatibility etc.
6. **Sintered glass filters**: These are made from borosilicate glass and the filtering medium is a flat or convex plate consisting of particles of Jena glass powdered and sifted to produce uniform solid granules, which are moulded or sintered together at a very high temperature. Depending upon the powder size used during sintering, these filters are available in different pore sizes.

Filtration Equipment

The selection of filtering equipment depends on the nature of the material, the volume to be filtered and the object of the operation. The one that satisfies all the requirements at the minimum overall cost is considered to be the most suitable process of filtration. Various types of filtering equipment may be conveniently discussed under the following three main headings:

A. Small Scale Filtration : Filter Funnels, Porcelain Funnel, Hot filtration and Sintered glass filter

B. Large Scale Filtration : Gravity filter, Pressure filter, Vacuum filter, Filter press, Leaf filter, Cartridge filter, Edge filter and Continuous rotary drum filter

C. Sterile Filtration : Candle filter, Seitz filter, Edge Filter, Sintered glass filter and Membrane filter

CLARIFICATION

Clarification is the process of removal of relatively small amount of suspended solid present, without the use of filters. The term applies when the solids do not exceed 0.15%. The filtrate clarity is seldom absolute even when brilliance is called for. The process is employed in the preparation of aromatic waters, fruit juices, syrups and honey. The selection of specific procedures and equipment for clarification depends on a number of factors.

i. the particle size of the suspended matter,
ii. the physical state of the suspended matter,
iii. the quantity of the suspended matter,
iv. the characteristics of the fluid medium, and
v. the speed of the operation.

Clarification methods

1. **Sedimentation and decantation**: Gravity sedimentation is the simplest method of clarification although it may not always be feasible. The method consists of allowing the suspension or slurry to stand in a suitable container until the suspended matter either settles down or rises to the top of the liquid, depending on the density of the suspended matter. Thus, if the suspended matter is colloidal or if its density is approximately equal to that of the liquid phase, the method cannot be used fruitfully. The insoluble matter can be separated from the clear liquid phase by siphoning, decantation or straining. Process of settling down can be accelerated by centrifugation. Simple batch sedimentation can be demonstrated in a laboratory by using graduated cylinders whereas for continuous sedimentation operations, thickeners and large sedimentation tanks are employed. Gravitational sedimentation is usually employed for clarification of fixed oils.

2. **Colation** (straining): In Latin colare means 'to strain'. Colation or straining is crude filtration. Like a filter, the strainer also acts by simple sieving action i.e. impeding the passage of suspended particles with diameters greater than that of the pores, while allowing the liquid to pass. The process consists of separating large, visible particles of a solid from liquid by pouring the mixture through a coarse cloth or a porous substance. Glass wool or asbestos is used for corrosive liquids such as potassium permanganate solutions, acids etc. The straining cloth may be freed from sizing materials e.g. starch glue, gelatin, albumin etc. by soaking it for a few hours in cold distilled water, rinsing thoroughly, and covering with distilled water or boiling for a few minutes. Final rinsing with distilled water will remove the last traces of sizing material.

3. **Siphoning**: It is an efficient method of removal of clarified supernatant liquid and students are expected to be familiar with basic principle underlying siphoning.

4. **Absorption and adsorption**: In addition to 'sieving' action of filter media, absorption and adsorption processes also help in efficient clarification. 'Soaking up' or trapping of the foreign particles within the media is called adsorption whereas adherence of foreign particles to the surface of the media is referred to as absorption. The absorption and adsorption properties may also be enhanced by addition of the filter

aids. Albumen, gelatin and some synthetic coagulants are used as clarifying agents. These agents convert the solids to be removed into a conveniently filterable size either by precipitation or coagulation followed by physical adsorption.

5. **Temperature**: If the suspended solids are free filtering, their characteristics may be improved by varying the temperature or pH of the medium. Increase in the temperature of a viscid liquid reduces its viscosity and specific gravity and hence the particles suspended into it separate readily. This process was formerly official for the clarification of honey.

CHAPTER 3

PRESCRIPTION

FORM OF PRESCRIPTION

A prescription is a written communication from a registered medical practitioner or other licensed practitioner to a pharmacist embodying salient instructions regarding the dispensing of prescribed medication. It designates a medication to be administered to a particular patient at a specified time. It is a means through which treatment is provided to a patient by combined skill and services of both the physician and the pharmacist.

The word "prescription" is derived from the Latin term *praescriptus* which is made up of two Latin words – *Prae* - a prefix meaning 'before' and *scribere*- meaning 'to write'.

Putting it all together (Prae + scribere), prescription means 'to write before' which reflects the historical fact that a prescription traditionally had to be written before a drug could be compounded and administered to a patient.

"A prescription is a written order for compounding, dispensing, and administering drugs to a specific client or patient and once it is signed by the physician it becomes a legal document"

Ancient prescriptions were generally noted for their multiple ingredients and complexity of preparation. The importance of the prescription and the need for complete understanding and accuracy made it imperative that a universal and standard language be used. Thus, Latin was adopted, and its use was continued until approximately 50 years ago.

Present day prescriptions are written in English, with doses given in the metric system, but often one still finds contracted Latin words (*Signatura*), Abbreviations (*tid, bid, Sig.*) etc. and Roman numerals intertwined.

Prescriptions are written in a blank of universally accepted format or may be made in pads. A typical prescription consists of the following parts.

1. **Physician (Prescriber) Information :** Information about physician is essential so that the doctor could be contacted in emergency to seek clarification and necessary instruction, missing words, confirmation etc. Following information is mentioned on the prescription:
   - Doctor's name, designation and Registration Number
   - Address with phone number and e-mail.
   - Date of issue of prescription.
   - Prescription number. (required when calling the pharmacy for a refill or for insurance purposes).
2. **Patient Information :** The name, address, age and sex of the patient help in identifying the prescription. Date of prescribing and date(s) of presentation for filling are necessary for keeping accurate records and ascertaining the needs of the patient. Age and sex of the patient, if mentioned, help the pharmacist to check the prescribed dose (s) of the medication.
   - Name of Patient : The prescribed medication is only for the patient whose name is on the label. Medications should not be given to another patient even if the other patient has similar symptoms.
   - Sex : Male / Female
   - Age and weight : For calculation of dose, dose frequency and route of administration.
3. **Superscription :** The *superscription* which consists of the heading where the symbol Rx (an abbreviation for recipe, the Latin for 'take thou' or 'you take', meaning you take) is found. Rx symbol comes before the inscription. The sign at the foot of the letter R is believed to represent the sign of Jupiter, the God of Healing. Some historians believe that the symbol Rx originated from the sign of Jupiter.
4. **Inscription :** The inscription (body of prescription) comprises an important part of prescription containing-
   - Name(s) of drug(s) and their quantities,
   - Other chief ingredients of the prescription with quantity,
   - Instruction regarding dosage form like tablet, capsule, suspension, mixture, etc., and
   - Dose and quantity of prescription
5. **Subscription :** The subscription gives specific directions for the pharmacist on how to compound the medication. Most of direction in usually expressed in contracted Latin or in the form of abbreviation. Instructions for preparation are also given such as: 'make a mixture', 'mix and make 10 tablets', or 'dispense 10 capsules'.

6. **Transcription or Signatura :** The signatura which gives instructions to the patient –
   - How, how much, When, and how long the drug is to be taken.

     These instructions are preceded by abbreviation 'Sig.' from the Latin, meaning 'mark.' The signatura should always be written in English; however, physicians continue to insert Latin abbreviations, e.g. '1 cap t.i.d. pc' which the pharmacist translates into

     English as 'take one capsule three times daily after meals'. It may also contain special instructions, warnings, followed by the signature of the prescriber.
7. **Renewal :** The number of times a prescription is to be repeated, is written by the physician under renewal instructions.
8. **Signature :** Finally the prescription must bear the signature of the prescriber to impart it the legal validity.
9. **Other Important Instructions**
   a. Refills — the label will show the number of refills permitted /no refills
   b. Qty : "quantity" or how much is in the package.
   c. Mfg. : "manufacturer" or who makes the medication.
   d. Expiry date : do not use the medication past this date. Do not save unused prescription. If same patient gets sick again, prescriber should be consulted.
   e. Take complete /full course : means that patient should finish taking the entire contents of the prescription even if feeling better especially patient taking antibiotics. This is to avoid recurrence of infection and development of resistance.
   f. Take with / without food : means whether the medication is to be taken after a meal or empty stomach. Some medications work better when the stomach is full while some medications work better when the stomach is empty.
   g. Take four times a day : means to take the medication four times in 24 hours with equal spacing of time. It is different than 'Take every four hours'. If any confusion, when to give the medications, one should consult doctor of pharmacist. Most medications do not have to be precisely timed to be effective, but some do.
   h. Take as needed as symptoms persist : means the medication can be taken when symptoms are present, without consulting the prescriber.
   i. The package may also have brightly colored warning labels with additional information. The following are examples:
      i. Safe storage instructions, such as 'keep refrigerated'.
      ii. Instructions for use, such as 'shake well before using'.
      iii. Possible side effects, such as 'may cause drowsiness'.

Prescription are known to be difficult to decipher and understood by a lay man. Initially, even a pharmacist requires effort and it is only after considerable experience that he can read the prescription. There are two reasons for it. Firstly, the busy physician always writes very swiftly and uses too many abbreviations, sometimes coined by himself, which a pharmacist alone can decipher. Somehow the physicians are known for a bad, illegible handwriting. The process of swiftness at times crosses all limits and physicians writing a letter or two only for the name of a drug are not too uncommon. Secondly, the use of Latin in prescription writing is traditional. Although teaching of Latin has slowly gone out of the curricula of medicine and pharmacy, some of the words and abbreviations have very deep roots and physicians still use them frequently. In earlier days, a prescription was a secret between the physician and the pharmacist and a mystery for the patient. With the increasing awareness about drugs no secrecy is now warranted. As such the patient has a right to know what medication has been prescribed and his interest is protected under the Consumer Protection Act. Some of the common Latin abbreviations are given below.

Note : (Latin Terms Commonly Used In Prescription Given In Chapter – 04)

A Model Prescription :

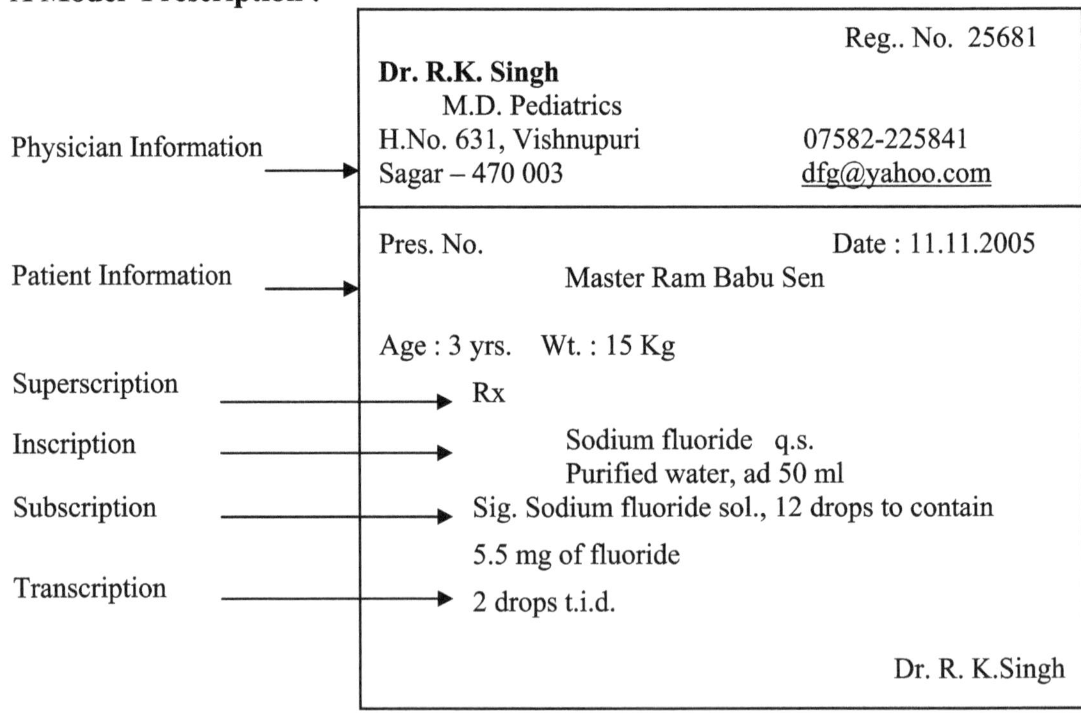

A practising pharmacist is expected to be thoroughly conversant with common systems of weight and measures, their inter-conversions and household equivalents; besides he ought to be well versed with such calculations as are applicable in his professional work.

The increasing use of manufactured dosage forms has gradually reduced the quantum of compounding to be handled by the pharmacist. However, he is ultimately responsible for dispensing the correct drug and accurate compounding. Whatever be the role of the pharmacist, he has to be constantly aware of the degree-of-accuracy due to absent mindedness, or negligence. A wrong drug may be dispensed on the one hand or mistakes in calculations or equivalents may occur. Such errors are inexcusable. To guard against them, it is desirable to check the labels of the ingredients at different stages of dispensing; while removing the container from the shelf, before weighing or measuring the drugs and at the time of replacing the container calculations must be thoroughly understood and doubly checked. If units are to be transferred from one system to the other, one should exercise great caution. Finally, care should be taken in writing and deciphering *decimal places*. Ultimate error in compounding is an outcome of the ± errors of weighing and measuring each ingredient and the final dilution. Dispensing balances are available for varying degrees of accuracy and varying quantities that can be weighed with their help. Usually, the selection of a balance depends on the degree of its accuracy desired. Also it is useful to ascertain the degree of sensitivity of the balance. Suppose the balance shows movement from the rest point only after a weight of 10 mg is placed on the pan, it is obvious that quantity less than 10 mg in weight can not be weighed by that balance. Secondly, one ought to fix the per cent error that can be tolerated. Suppose the sensitivity of a balance is 10 mg and the permissible error is ± 5%. The minimum quantity that can be weighed with such a balance will be 100 x 10/5 = 200 mg. In other words, the quantity by weight less than 200 mg should not be weighed with such a balance. If very small weights are to be taken, one may adopt solid : solid dilution by triturating the potent medicament with an inert diluent, both in suitable proportions; or a solid : liquid dilution by dissolving the drug in a solvent and making up to a volume. Appropriate quantity of such dilutions will represent the required quantity of the drug.

The following example may illustrate the point.

Rx

Atropine sulphate 0.5 mg

Send such 10 powders. To be used as directed.

The quantity of atropine sulphate required for 10 powders each of 0.5 mg shall be 5 mg. However the minimum quantity that can be weighed on the balance which is available is 10 mg. Therefore, a 10 mg : 10 mg dilution of atropine sulphate and lactose can be prepared. 10 mg of this triturate representing 5 mg of atropine sulphate should be weighed and thoroughly mixed with 90 mg of lactose, in geometric proportion, yielding a total weight of 100 mg (5mg of atropine sulphate and 95 mg of lactose). 10 powders each weighing 10 mg dispensed from the triturate will contain 0.5 mg of atropine sulphate and 9.5 mg of lactose each.

The equipment commonly used for measuring small volumes of liquids consists of either pipets or droppers. Larger volumes are measured with volumetric graduates. The measures may be graduated in milliliters, ounces, drachms or minims. The shapes differ from cylindrical to conical with a flat bottom. Volumetric apparatus may be meant either for delivering or containing desired volumes. The former class includes burettes, pipets and measuring glasses and the latter includes volumetric flasks and measures. Measuring glasses or graduated measures are used for both 'to contain' (TC) and 'to deliver', (TD) liquids. However, household measures for food etc. are not suitable for pharmaceutical compounding as these are likely to be inaccurate. Transference of highly viscous liquids leads to errors as some of the liquid is bound to remain sticking to the measure. Bottles bearing graduations should not be used to make up volumes as these graduations are not always reliable and may result into erroneous content. In general, one should use only such apparatus and appliances which are reliable for compounding accuracy.

The main purpose of correct weighing and measuring is to provide accurate dosage of the medication. The object stands defeated if the patient does not take quantities which represent accurate doses of the medicaments. It is desirable that proper guidance is provided to the patient and instructions given to withdraw proper volumes for administration. For solid dosage forms, the problems are limited as the medication is supplied in unit dosage form. For accurate delivery of liquid preparations, either dose marks should be affixed to the container or a plastic measure or dropper of appropriate size should be provided. Household measures are sometimes recommended e.g. tea, dessert and tablespoons; and tumblers of different sizes and nomenclature to deliver liquid medication. Unless these are available in standard sizes, it is not a good practice to use them. Use of droppers also needs care. Serious errors are possible due to difference in the construction of droppers, viscosity, density and surface tension of liquids in addition to personal factor. Polythene and glass droppers of the same aperture produce drops that are not uniform in size. A graduated dropper is the best answer in such cases.

HANDLING OF PRESCRIPTION

The scheme of dispensing may be considered from its beginning-receiving of the prescription-to the end delivery of the medication to the patient. Several steps are involved, some of them being procedural while others requiring compounding operations. The sum total of the scheme where compounding is not required can be briefly summarized as consisting of:

1. Receiving the prescription.
2. Reading and checking the prescription.

3. Packaging and labelling; if necessary.
4. Filing, pricing and delivery of the medication to the patient.

For compounded prescriptions the process is more elaborate and consists of:

1. Receiving the prescription.
2. Reading and checking the prescription.
3. Compounding, labelling and packaging.
    - (i) weighing and measuring
    - (ii) grinding and size reduction
    - (iii) solution
    - (iv) mixing
    - (v) filtering
    - (vi) finishing
    - (vii) checking and recording
4. Filing, pricing and delivery of the medication to the patient.

Receiving the prescription

A prescription should always be received by a pharmacist himself. The waiting area for the patients should be easily accessible, comfortable and clean, reflecting professional environment. Some magazines and other literature on health matters and current topics should be available to the patient during the waiting time. The patient should be informed about the likely waiting period. In large dispensaries, it is advisable to adopt some system of identification of the prescription like slip or token as practiced in banks. While receiving the prescription, a pharmacist should not make any comments or gesture either approving or disapproving it. A pharmacist should not even give a physiognomic expression to the patient that he is surprised or confused on seeing the prescription.

Reading and checking the prescription

A proper scrutiny of the prescription should not be attempted in the presence of the patient; it should be better examined behind the counter. Any difficulty in reading or ambiguity in the prescription may be solved by consulting senior pharmacists and if the solution is difficult to find, reference made to the prescriber. Problems of prescription reading and checking may be varied. With the increasing number of proprietary products and very little differences in the spelling of several drug names, a pharmacist's job has become very difficult. The illegible handwriting may make the situation worse. Prescription writing errors and omissions may range from missing quantities of the ingredients, units of weights and measures, strengths of solutions, vehicle, quantity to be supplied, directions for use etc., to errors in dosage of individual drugs and dosage regimen. Then, one frequently encounters incompatibilities in prescriptions. Although it falls under the domain of the pharmacist to detect and remedy the incompatibility yet there may be situations when reference to the physician may have to be made. In no circumstances should a pharmacist take liberties in situations of indecision or lend oneself in guesswork. This does not mean that the pharmacist should not take decisions at all but every issue must be judiciously looked into. In modern therapeutic practice, it is common to prescribe very high doses of medicaments in specific conditions. Calculation of doses of medicaments meant for children have to be done by the pharmacist and he should maintain standard tables and charts which may be referred to whenever necessary. At times a pharmacist has to receive prescriptions on telephone. It requires some experience and therefore it is desirable that a senior person receives the prescription as it may have to be taken down swiftly and in abbreviated form.

To guard against any error arising out of this practice, it is advisable that the prescription be repeated in parts or in full to the prescriber. A pharmacist sometimes comes across prescriptions written in foreign countries. In order to fill such prescriptions, he is expected to have knowledge of Latin and deciphering numerals in other scripts. Reference may be made to standard texts in foreign language maintained in the library.

Compounding, labelling and packaging

After reading and checking a prescription, the pharmacist proceeds to dispense it. Compounding, labelling and packaging should be carried out in a neat place. All the equipment etc. should be thoroughly cleaned and washed. In case a prepackaged medicine is to be dispensed under a manufacturer's label, the pharmacist may have to only wrap it and deliver to the patient. Sometimes, a smaller number or volume may have to be dispensed from a larger package. In such cases, he chooses a suitable container with a closure, or a package, and packs the requisite number or volume, affixes a label and delivers it duly wrapped. When compounding is to be done, a pharmacist has to perform a series of operations depending on the nature of the preparation he handles. This is the main area where his professional competence is required.

General aspects of compounding

Compounding should be done on a proper work table with suitable fittings. The pharmacist puts on his professional dress, a white overall, while engaged in his professional duties. Ingredients are arranged alphabetically on shelves to which he has an easy access. All equipment and apparatus necessary for compounding is within easy reach, properly arranged, duly cleaned and dried. More than one prescription should not be compounded at a time by a pharmacist. Since he has to work with concentration of mind, he should not be disturbed. But if it is inevitable, he should suspend compounding temporarily and restart only when he can pay undivided attention to his work. Labeling should be done immediately and under no circumstances two unlabeled containers of medication kept side by side to one another. Bottles of all the ingredients to be compounded should be assembled on the left hand side of the table with the dispensing balance in the centre. Labels should be read while removing the bottles from the shelf. Ingredients should be accurately weighed/measured and checked preferably by another pharmacist. The labels are read a second time while removing the quantity for weighing/measuring. After all the ingredients have been taken from the bottles, they should be kept on the right hand side of the balance in the order of their disposal after use. All the ingredients should then be compounded according to the directions of the prescriber or according to the pharmaceutical art. After compounding is over, the bottles should be replaced back on the shelf, again the label is read a third time. While removing and handling the containers and the ingredients, due care should be exercised not to soil the labels of the containers or spill the ingredients on the table or the floor.

The preparation, during processing, is expected to remain untouched by hand. The product is then filled in a suitable container and securely closed. Label of a suitable size is written or typed giving all the desired information in a clear-cut manner. Dropper or measure, when necessary, should be enclosed in the final package. Checking, recording and pricing should be done before delivery of the prescription. While delivering the prescription to the patient, the pharmacist should explain the mode of administration, storage etc. and repeat directions for use.

Labelling

Labelling is an important operation in dispensing practice. Information stated on the label is the only link between the patient and the pharmacist after the prescription has been delivered. It has to be interpreted by the patient who is not an expert and hence the direction should be stated in writing in simple and unambiguous words. Further, the label gives a face-lift to the prescription container and contributes to its elegance. Therefore the label design should be in artistic taste with regard to shape and size of the container, in quality and colour of the paper and printing thereupon. The label should be affixed with a strong adhesive so that it holds firmly in handing. Besides the information to the patient, the label bears other essential details so that on production of the container the prescription could be identified and its filling traced wherever necessary. A specimen label is written below, special labels if required for a product are affixed separately and prominently so that they do not miss attention of the patient.

Specimen label

Serial number	Date
Name of the patient	....
Name of the prescriber	....
Directions for use	....
Name and full address of the Pharmacy with its telephone number	

A label should be typed preferably with a machine having clear, narrow letters using computer so that the patient has no difficulty in reading it. A pharmacist is expected to type it himself. In case the label has to be written by hand it should be in clear print letters. While affixing it, the moistening should be done with a moistener and in no case with saliva. Use of saliva is both unhygienic and a non-professional practice. After affixing the label wrinkles, if any should be removed by smoothening with a soft paper. Affixing adhesive labels/stickers on glass surface is an easy operation but plastic and metallic surfaces are problematic in this respect. Special adhesives or lacquers may be needed for such surfaces. If the container is small to hold a label bearing all the directions, one may affix a small number on the container and enclose the container in a larger container with the same number and bearing all the information. Labels are sometimes intended to give a warning to the patient and taking special care while handling and using the medication. Such labels may be affixed separately to give prominence. Common examples of such labels are: 'Shake well before use', 'Do not use after.........days', 'Store in a cool place', 'Keep tightly closed', 'Not to be used internally', 'For external use only' etc. It is a good practice to avoid the use of word 'Poison' on the main or auxiliary label. The product should be finally checked at this stage from all angles - scientific such as colour, gas formation etc., safety and legal requirements etc. It should be on record that it has been checked and must bear the initials of the pharmacist who did the checking. During and after compounding a pharmacist makes a note of some important information which may be useful later for refilling the prescription or other reasons. These may include full words for illegible words, calculation if any, colour of the product, size of the capsule and its colour, procedure etc. The price charged should also find a place on the prescription so that the same price may be charged on a subsequent occasion. Some pharmacists maintain a record of their clients including the ailment and the medication supplied. This is a very desirable practice as it enables him to render a better service to his clients. The drug profile is readily available by a suitable filing system which should be consulted whenever necessary. Commonly the indexing is done on cards and preserved in cabinets for ready consultation.

Packaging

Final packaging of the container is done in a neat carton or bag which tightly hugs the container in proper shape. Sometimes corrugated paper is used to provide padding between the container and the carton. Loose paper bags are not suitable for packaging. Gaudy paper with dark colors should be avoided for external wrapping. Good quality paper in light colors or a paper bearing advertisement of the Pharmacy may encase the packet. A sticking tape is employed for affixing the wrapper in proper position.

SOURCE OF ERRORS IN PRESCRIPTION

Mistakes in the use of a medication are sometimes serious problem. Problems can include adverse reactions and interactions with other medications, and also basic administrative errors such as patients being given the wrong medication or wrong dosage. A less studied aspect of mistakes involving medications is the misdiagnosis of a disease when the real cause is a side effect of a medication. Children and infants are particularly at risk of medication errors mainly due to incorrect dosage, because of the need to modify dosages based on age and weight. The dosage modification may be either overlooked or miscalculated. Various studies have shown high error rates in doctors and nurses in calculating weight-dependent dosages in infants and especially neonates. Errors with medication can occur in hospitals, at the pharmacy, in the doctor's office, and even due to the patient.

The dispensing of prescription medications at the pharmacy can have various errors. The wrong medication can be given particularly when medications are named or packaged similarly. There are particular drugs that are known to have problems because their names are very similar. The pharmacy can also give out the wrong dosage of the drug in some cases.

Most studies of medication errors only analyzed hospital medication usage, and there is a large volume of medications prescribed in doctor's offices and dispensed by pharmacies.

The medications causing most problems were cytotoxics, cardiovascular drugs, antihypertensives, anticoagulants, and NSAIDs.

An **adverse drug reaction** (ADR) occurs when a patient suffers a reaction, side effect, or other injury from a medication. This can occur without an error, such as when a patient has an allergy to a medicine, but has never shown any signs or risk factors for this allergy previously. On the other hand, an error would occur if a previous allergy was known but the medication was still given to the patient.

The list of medications most frequently causing adverse reactions in order of incidence is given below.

- antibiotics,
- chemotherapeutic agents,
- anticoagulants,
- cardiovascular agents,
- anticonvulsants,
- antidiabetic agents,
- antihypertensives,
- analgesics,
- antiasthma agents,
- sedative-hypnotic agents,
- antidepressants,
- antipsychotic agents, and
- antiulcer agents.

Following types of errors are generally found in the dispensing of prescription.

- misdiagnosis (40%),
- medication error (28%),
- medical procedure error (22%),
- administrative error (4%),
- communication error (2%),
- incorrect laboratory results (2%),
- equipment malfunction (1%), and
- other error (7%).

Medication errors generally occur in following locations.

- hospital (48%),
- doctor's office (22%),
- operating room (7%),
- clinic (5%),
- emergency room (5%),
- pharmacy (4%),
- home (3%),
- medical laboratory (1%),
- nursing home (1%), and
- other (5%).

About 70% of all errors were believed to be preventable. The remainder were presumably non-preventable errors such as a patient reacting to a drug who had no previous history of an allergy to the drug.

Mistakes Occur

There are numerous ways that an error can occur in medical treatment.

- Self-treatment mistakes: Mistakes are very commonly when a patient tries to treat him/her self. Always professional medical advice should be sought.
- Wrong condition treated: i.e. from a misdiagnosis of the condition
- Wrong choice of treatment plan: the overall strategy used to treat condition might not be the best one.
- Wrong type of treatment given
- Delayed treatment: there must not be an undesirable delay in treatment, by choice or through non-diagnosis.
- Wrongly performed procedures: all medical events such as surgeries and tests performed wrongly can make things worse.
- Wrong medications

Prevention mistakes: The failure to prevent a condition is another type of medical failing. In certain cases, it is clear that preventive actions should be taken and failure to do so is a medical mistake.

- Failure to prevent known complications of a diagnosed disease.
- Failure to treat family members or others exposed to an infectious disease.
- Failure to address clear risk factors for various conditions

Surgery mistakes: Surgical procedures are often complex and subject to various errors. Administration of surgery can also lead to errors. In some cases, there are known complications or risks of surgery that are often unavoidable.

- Surgery administration mistakes: wrong-patient, wrong-site, wrong-organ, equipment left inside.
- Surgical mistakes: the surgeon might make a wrong cut or other mistake.
- Anaesthesia mistakes: too much, too little (waking up).
- Complications from surgery
- Infections from surgery: called **iatrogenic infections**
- Wrong blood type transfusion

Hospital mistakes: A hospital can make errors in any of its varied activities. There are many staff who can make human mistakes and overall system problems can also lead to errors.

- Hospital-caused infections: called **nosocomial infections**.
- Medication errors in hospitals: ordered medication not given, wrong medication, wrong dosage, wrong combinations, wrong patient given medication, and so on.
- Wrong procedures: failure to do ordered tests, wrong procedures or tests.

Medication mistakes: Errors in medication are a major source of medical mistakes. Medical error occur in hospitals or pharmacies, and the error may be made by any of the staff involved with choosing or dispensing medication.

- Inappropriate medication: the wrong medication given for a disease
- Wrong medication: the patient gets the wrong medication despite the doctor prescribing the correct one.
- Drug name mix-ups: several medications have similar-sounding names and can be mixed up by doctors or pharmacists.
- Wrong medication combinations: there are numerous types of medications that should not be mixed, because of side effects and cross-reactions when combined.
- Adverse reactions to medication: Some people have allergic or other adverse reactions to certain medications. These are risks and not necessarily avoidable mistakes if the person has no previous history of a particular adverse reaction.
- Side effects of medication: Almost all medications have some types of side effects. Some are mild, some nasty. It is almost impossible to know up front whether a person will have side effects from a medication.
- Non-compliance: the failure to follow prescribed medication regimen can be a mistake made usually by the patient.

Pharmacist errors: The dispensing of drugs by the pharmacy is a complex and busy activity. Various errors can occur at the pharmacist.

- Wrongly filled prescriptions
- Wrong drug supplied
- Wrong dosage supplied
- Drug name mix-ups: various drugs have similar names.

Pathology lab errors: Diagnostic testing done by a pathology laboratory can be subject to various errors. Some are administrative or human mistakes; other mistakes are inherent to the limitations of the type of test.

- Wrong biopsy results: visual inspection of cellular slides
- Administrative errors: mixing samples, etc.
- Known test errors and risks: almost all tests have a small percentage of unavoidable errors (false positives, false negatives).
- Known limitations of tests

Equipment failure errors: Physical failures with medical equipment can occur.

- IV drips dislodged
- Dead batteries in equipment

Unnecessary medical treatment: Excessive medical care can be a form of mistake for medical professionals and institutions. This can occur with good intentions (to ensure correctness) or for cynical reasons (to increase income).

- Unnecessary procedures
- Unnecessary tests

CARE REQUIRED IN PRICING, FILING AND DELIVERY OF THE PRESCRIPTION

Pricing a prescription is a very difficult task. Public in general feels that the price charged is high. When the pharmacist is alleged or interrogated in this regard, he finds himself in an embarrassing situation. He should be extremely polite and truthful when confronted with allegations of excessive profit making. The reasons for the price charged should be convincing. One of the reasons for a differing price structure is due to constant change in the prices of the ingredients and drugs as well as services. The society ignores such facts and looks at the pharmacist at times with extreme feelings of disfavour and unfriendliness. Remarks at times amount to accusing him as a profiteer and exploiter. The main reason for this unsympathetic attitude is great variation in the prices charged by different Pharmacies for the same prescription particularly if it happens to be a compounded one. It is not true that the price charged is always high but may be lower at times when dispensing has been done by the same Pharmacy. A pharmacist while pricing should have a clear policy and work within a framework of rules and rationalize the prescription price. By so doing, he is in a strong position to justify the price and convince the patient. There are several inputs that govern the price of prescriptions. These include cost of ingredients, labour cost, cost of containers, cost of professional services and other overhead expenses and lastly the profit. Cost of ingredients should be calculated without profit and tables stating the price of small quantities of each substance should be maintained and consulted to save time of the pharmacist. Container cost should be calculated taking into consideration the damage or breakage in storage and handling as well as rejections. Usually the cost of labour involved in compounding is dependent on the time required for the purpose. In western countries where the profession of pharmacy is highly developed, norms have been computed for compounding or dispensing prescriptions of different classes. According to an estimate the average time required for dispensing of a non-compounded prescription is 8 minutes and the dispensing of a compounded prescription requires 14 minutes. In India, such norms do not exist and it would be well worth if the profession works out the time-cost schedule of different types of prescriptions. Public is also likely to disregard the professional fee which is included in the prescription price. There has to be a charge for professional service rendered apart from the dispensing time. In addition to the price of knowledge and skill, the advantage derived from the advice by the pharmacist has to be compensated for and not expected to be free. Overhead expenses differ from Pharmacy to Pharmacy and establishment to establishment. These charges embody all such payments that are unavoidable to run an establishment e.g. rent of the premises, electricity bills, insurance, advertising, interest on the capital invested, furniture and fittings etc. In the aforesaid charges profit is not included and has to be charged extra. Profit calculation is dependent on the profit philosophy of the Pharmacy. Net profit expected for each prescription is added to arrive at the price chargeable for a prescription. Following example may illustrate the calculation of Price chargeable from the patient:

Cost of ingredients	Rs. 15/-
Cost of container	Rs. 1/-
Labour	Rs. 3/-
Overhead charges	Rs, 1/-
Professional service charges	Rs. 1/-
Profit	Rs. 3/-
Total price	Rs. 24/-

Filing of prescription in some way or the other is an essential requirement for a variety of reasons e.g., future service to the patient, calculating statistics and for situations legal in nature should complications arise as a result of dispensing the prescription. It has been pointed out earlier that all pharmacists should fully understand the implications of legal requirements prevailing in the country. Filing systems are adopted or evolved by the Pharmacy taking into consideration the nature of the establishment. Filing and maintaining the record depends upon how frequently and expediently one has to refer to it. At present three systems prevail in India. In some Pharmacies and Government hospitals, the original prescriptions are not retained by the pharmacist. The patient is allowed to take it with him. On authorization by the physician the patient presents it for refilling, with modifications if need be. A register is maintained in which all prescriptions dispensed are date wise and serially recorded in the order these prescriptions are presented to the pharmacist. The register has the requisite number of columns for recording the salient features. These columns are usually for serial number, date, name of the patient and the inscription. Tracing back a prescription after the lapse of a long time is difficult unless the original prescription or a reference regarding the date or serial number is available. It is possible to trace the same if the container bearing the date or serial number is presented. Another method is to retain the original prescription. This practice is prevalent in private dispensaries which are attached to a consulting physician. Larger establishments maintain a record of the prescription by photocopying or microfilming, the original prescription being returned to the patient. Whichever be the system, the object is to preserve bonafide information as a record in the hospital or retail pharmacies.

Even for proprietary preparations dispensed in the manufacturer's package, it is necessary that a record is maintained by the pharmacist. Pharmacies and pharmacists would be immensely benefited by the use of computers in keeping records of prescriptions and data retrieval.

For delivering the medication to the patient, two systems prevail-the direct and the indirect. In the direct system of delivery the pharmacist is able to establish a direct contact with the patient or his agent and thus while delivering the medication he can answer questions or at his own initiative explain the salient directions etc. and make certain -that the patient has understood "the manner in which the drug is to be administered and the precautions if any, that he has to take". This minimizes the possibilities of error in drug administration. The indirect system does not provide for a dialogue between the pharmacist and the patient. It can be classified in three categories. The delivery can be affected at a window where the patient collects the medication. Secondly, the medication is delivered at the residence of the patient i.e. home delivery. Thirdly, the medication can be sent to the patient by post. In all the three forms of indirect delivery the patient gets the directions and guidance through written information only and is not in a position to make enquiries from the pharmacist. Finally, in the process of compounding, dispensing and sale of medication, a pharmacist is to be guided by ethics of his profession and a sense of service to the sufferer and his approach is expected to be in the best interest of his clients.

Legal Provisions

Supply of drugs to a patient on prescription is the exclusive domain of a pharmacist which also has a legal sanction. Provisions of the Drugs and Cosmetics Rules, 1945 relating to dispensing and supply of medication are briefly summarized below.

In context with the supply of drugs the Rules provide as follows.

(i) The description 'Drug Store' shall be displayed by such licensees who do not require the services of a 'qualified person.'

(ii) The description 'Chemists and Druggists' shall be displayed by such licensees who employ the services of a **qualified person** but who do not maintain a 'Pharmacy' for compounding against prescription.

(iii) The description 'Pharmacy', 'Pharmacist', 'Dispensing Chemist' or 'Pharmaceutical Chemist' shall be displayed by such licensees who employ the services of a 'qualified person' and maintain a 'Pharmacy' for compounding against prescription.

['Qualified person' means a person who i) holds a diploma or degree in pharmacy or pharmaceutical chemistry of an approved institution, or it) is a registered pharmacist under the Pharmacy Act, 1948]

Following licenses are provided to sell, stock or exhibit for sale or distribution of drugs by **retail :**

a. drugs specified in Schedule C, C(1), and X;
b. drugs specified in Schedule C and C(1) excluding those specified in Schedule X; and
c. drugs specified in Schedule X.

Those holding the licenses for retail sale of drugs must satisfy the following conditions :

1. If any drug is compounded or made on the licensee's premises such operation should be conducted by or under the direct and personal supervision of a 'qualified person'.
2. The supply of any drug on the prescription of any Registered Medical Practitioner (RMP) shall be affected only by or under the personal supervision of a 'qualified person'.
3. The supply of any drug (other than those specified in Schedule X) on a prescription of a RMP shall be recorded at the time of supply in a prescription register specially maintained for the purpose and the serial number of entry in the register be entered on the prescription. The following particulars shall be entered in the register :
   a) serial number of the entry;
   b) the date of supply;
   c) the name and address of the prescriber;
   d) the name and address of the patient (or the owner of the animal);
   e) the name of the drug or preparation and the quantity or in the case of a medicine made up by the licensee the ingredients and their quantities;
   f) in the case of a drug specified in Schedule C or Schedule H the name of the manufacturer of the drug; its batch number and the date of expiry of potency, if any;
   g) the signature of the qualified person.

   In the case of drugs which are not compounded in the premises and which are supplied from or in the original containers the particulars specified in items (a) to (g) above may be entered in a cash or credit memo book maintained for this purpose.

   In the case of **refill prescriptions**, it shall be sufficient if the new entry in the prescription register includes a serial number, the date of supply, the quantity supplied and a reference to the earlier entry in the register. It shall not be necessary to record the above details in the register or cash or credit memo, particulars in respect of-

   i. drugs supplied against prescription under the Employee's State Insurance Scheme if all the above particulars are given in that prescription, and

ii. any drugs other than those specified in Schedule C or Schedule H if it is supplied in the original unopened container of the manufacturer and if the prescription is duly stamped at the time of supply with the name of the supplier and the date on which the supply was made.

The option to maintain a prescription register or a cash or credit memo book in respect of drugs and medicines supplied from or in original container, should be made in writing to the Licensing Authority. However, the Licensing Authority may require records to be maintained only in prescription register.

4. The supply by retail, otherwise than on a prescription of a drug specified in Schedule C shall be recorded at the time of supply either;

   (i) in a register specially maintained for the purpose in which the following particulars shall be entered :

      (a) serial number of the entry,

      (b) the date of supply,

      (c) the name arrd address of the purchaser,

      (d) the name and quantity of the drug,

      (e) in the case of a drug specified in Schedule C, the name of the manufacturer, the batch number and the expiry date; or

   (ii) in a cash or credit memo book, serially numbered and containing all the particulars specified in items (b) to (f) under (i) above,

The supply by retail of any drug shall be made against a cash or credit memo which shall contain the following particulars :

a. name and address and sale number of the order;
b. serial number of the cash/credit memo;
c. the name and quantity of the drug supplied,

The licensee should also maintain carbon copies of cash/credit memos as record.

Records of purchase of a drug intended for sale or sold by retail shall be maintained by the licensee and such records shall show the following particulars :

a. the date of purchases,
b. the name and address of the person from whom purchased and the number of relevant license held by him,
c. the name of the drug, the quantity and the batch number, and
d. the name of the manufacturer of the drug.

Purchase bills including cash or credit memos should be serially numbered by licensee and maintained in a chronological order.

5. All registers and records are open to inspection by Inspector and should be preserved for a period of not less than two years from the date of the last entry therein.

6. It shall not be necessary to record any particulars in a register specially maintained for the purpose if the particulars are recorded in any other register specially maintained for the purpose under any other Act for the time being in force.

7. Substances specified in Schedule H or Schedule X **shall not be sold by retail except** on the prescription of a RMP and in the case of substances specified in Schedule X, prescriptions shall be in duplicate, one copy of which shall be retained by the licensee for a period of two years.

   The supply of drugs specified in Schedule M or Schedule X to RMPs, hospitals, dispensaries and nursing homes shall be made only against the signed order in writing, which shall be preserved by the licensee for a period of two years.

   A prescription for Schedule H or Schedule X drugs shall

   i. be in writing and be signed by the person giving it with his usual signature and be dated by him;
   ii. specify the name and address of the person for whose treatment it is given, or the name and address of the owner of the animal if the drug is meant for veterinary use;
   iii. indicate the total amount of the medicine to be supplied and the dose to be taken.

8. The person dispensing a prescription containing a drug specified in Schedule H and Schedule X shall comply with the following requirements in addition to other requirements of the Rules-

   (a) the prescription must not be dispensed more than once unless the prescriber has specified otherwise.

   (b) at the time of dispensing there must be noted on the prescription above the signature of the prescriber the name and address of the seller and the date on which the prescription is dispensed.

9. No person dispensing a prescription containing substances specified in Schedule H or X may supply any other preparation whether containing the same substance or not in lieu thereof.

10. Substances specified in Schedule X kept in retail shop or premises used in connection therewith shall be stored –

(a) under lock and key in cupboard or drawer reserved solely for the storage of these substances; or

(b) in a part of the premises separated from the remainder of the premises and to which only responsible persons have access.

11. A substance specified in Schedule E sold by retail shall be labelled with word "Poison" in such language or languages as the State Government may prescribe by notification in the Official Gazette.

12. The licensee shall maintain an Inspection Book in Form 35 to enable an Inspector to record his impressions and the defects noticed.

13. No drug shall be sold or stocked by the licensee after the date of expiration recorded on its container, label or wrapper, or in violation of any statement or direction recorded on such container, label or wrapper.

14. The supply by retail of any drug in a container other than the one in which the manufacturer has marketed the drug, shall be made only by dealers who employ the services of a 'qualified person' under the direct supervision of the 'qualified person' in an envelope or other suitable container showing the following particulars on the label :

(a) *name* of the drug,

(b) quantity supplied and

(c) name and address of the dealer,

15. The supply of drugs specified in Schedule X shall be recorded at the time of supply in a register specially maintained for the purpose and separate pages shall be allotted for each drug. The following particulars shall be entered in the said register:

- date of transaction;
- quantity received; if any, the name and address of the supplier and the number of the relevant license held by the supplier;
- name of the drug;
- quantity supplied;
- manufacturer's name;
- Batch No. or Lot No.;
- name and address of the patient/purchaser;
- reference number of the prescription against which supplies were made;
- Bill No. and date in respect of purchases and supplies made by him;
- signature of the person under whose supervision the drugs have been supplied.

CHAPTER 4

PHARMACEUICAL CALCULATION

WEIGHTS & MEASURES

In our day-to-day life as well as in the practice of pharmaceutical profession, it is always necessary to have some unit to measure a quantity. The science, which deals with weights and measures, is called **Metrology**. As each and every pharmaceutical operation implies the fundamental knowledge of metrology, it appears appropriate to acquaint us with various aspects of metrology.

The need for a system of weights and measures might have been felt as a basis for comparison in day-to-day dealings and therefore mechanical devices like balances or scales were devised. Historically, the ancient standards referred to various parts of human body e.g. fathom, cubit, span, foot and nail etc. Later, the objects around human beings like grains or wheat were preferred for comparison. As the facilities for trade and transport widened and the geographical barriers crossed, a need was realized to bring about uniformity in the system of weights and measures which might have started initially on a regional basis and developed through provincial to a national and international basis. Such an attempt to adopt an uniform, scientific and methodical system naturally culminated in most of the civilized countries of the world having adopted the metric system of weights and measures which is certainly the simplest and the best. However most of the elder physicians still don't follow the metric system in prescription writing and hence it is desirable that a pharmacist should be acquainted with other systems of weights and measures normally encountered in prescription writing. The Indian system of weights and measures having the units *tola, masha* and *ratti* etc. is no more official since April 1,1956 when the Government of lndia recognized the metric system as the only official one. In India the Standards of Weights and Measures Act controls the weights and measures and the Pharmacopoeia of India has also recognized the metric system.

Mass is a constant based on inertia while weight changes with altitude, latitude, temperature and pressure. The measure of the gravitational force acting on a body is directly proportional to its mass and is known as *weight*. The unit of weight is Gram, which is equal to 1/1000 of the mass of the International Prototype Kilogram. The extent of volume of a body is called *measure*. The units commonly employed are litre and metre for capacity and length, respectively.

The Standards of Weights and Measures Act, 1976 provides for the reference standard, secondary standard and working standard for calibration of weights and measures. The Act also provides for the preparation of national prototypes of the kilogram and metre by the Central Government. The Standards of Weights and Measures Act, 1976 provides the calibration standard of weights and measures. Under the Act, 'International Bureau of Weights and Measures'means the Bureau International des Poids at Sevres in France. 'International prototype of the kilogram' is defined as the prototype sanctioned by the First General Conference on weights and measures held in Paris in 1889, and deposited at the International Bureau of Weights and Measures. Kilogram is recognized as the base unit of mass and is equal to the mass of the International prototype of kilogram. **Metre** is recognized as the base unit of length and is equal to 1650763.73 wavelengths in vacuum of the radiation corresponding to the transition between the levels $2p_{10}$ and $5d_5$ of the krypton-86 atom.

The Act also provides for the preparation of national prototypes of the kilogram and metre by the Central Government.

English System: The earlier units were based on the weight of 32 grains of wheat, which equaled a silver penny (Sterling), 20 penny weights (Pence) made an ounce, twelve ounces a pound and eight pounds made a gallon of wine, etc. The word 'haberdupois' was used first in English laws in 1303. The 'troy' weight has still earlier origin. Troyes is a French city in which great fairs were held during 8th and 9th centuries. However these systems caused great inconvenience to buyers and sellers of medicines. In 1790 Washington recommended the establishment of uniformity in currency, weights and measures; and in 1836 the troy pound (5760 grains), the avoirdupois pound (7000 grains) along with yard were introduced.

Metric System: In 1783, James Watt first proposed the use of decimal system and the commensurability of weight, length and volume. Metric weights were officially recognized in Great Britain in 1864, in United States in 1866 and in India in 1956. The principal attributes of this system are its simplicity, brevity and adaptability to everyday needs. It is the system of decimal progression meaning thereby that every unit is multiplied or divided by the same number (i.e. 10) to obtain various denominations. Latin prefixes like *milli, centi, deci,* etc. are used to indicate subdivisions while Greek prefixes like *deca, hecto, myria,* are used to denote multiples of the principal units.

A brief account of different systems of weights and measures and relationships relevant to a pharmacist are given below.

a. Measures of Mass

The difference between weight and mass is that the weight changes with the altitude, as it is dependent on the gravitational force, whereas mass remains unchanged.

The unit of weight is the Gram, which is defined as 1/1000 of the mass of the International Prototype Kilogram. e.g.

1 Tonne (T)	1,000 kilograms (Kg or kg or kilo)
1 Quintal	1000 kilograms
1 kilogram	1000 grams (g, G or Gm or gm)
1 Hectagram (Hg)	100 grams
1 Dekagram (Dg)	10 grams
1 Desigram 9dg)	1/10 gram.
1 Centigram (cg)	1/100 gram
1 Milligram (mg)	1/1000 gram
1 Microgram (mcg), μg	1/1000 mg or 10^{-6} g
1 Nanogram	1/1000 μg = 10^{-9} g
1 Picogram	1/1000 of a nanogram = 10^{-12} g

b. Measures of Length

The unit of length is the Meter (M), which is defined as the length of the International Prototype Meter bar

1 Kilometer (Km)	1000 meters (m.)
1 Centimeter (cm)	1/100 meter [0.01]
1 Millimeter (mm)	1/1000 meter
1 Micron (μ)	1/1000 mm
1 Millimicron (mμ)	10^{-6} mm
1 Micromicron (μμ)	10^{-9} mm

c. Measures of Capacity

The unit of capacity is the litre or liter (l. or L.) that is defined as the volume of 1 kg of water at 4°C. There is difference between millilitre and cc. 1 ml is the volume occupied by 1 g of water at 4°C whereas 1 cc is the volume of a cube each side of which is 1 cm length. 1 cc = 0.99984 ml or 1 litre = 1000.028 cc.

However, for all practical purposes ml and cc are taken as the same

1 Hectolitre	100 litres
1 Millilitre	1/1000 litre
1 litre	1000.028 cc = 1000 ml
1 Microlitre (μl)	0.001 ml = 10^{-6} litre
1000 litres	1 cubic meter

Imperial System

Imperial system of weights and measures, commonly known as Avoirdupois system was recognized in the British Pharmacopoeia, though at present UK also has switched over to the metric system.

i. Avoirdupois Weights and measures

Measures of mass

437.5 grains (gr.)	1 ounce (oz)
16 ounces	1 pound (lb.)
14 pounds	1 stone
112 pounds	1 hundredweights (cwt)
20 hundredweights	1 ton.

Measures of Capacity (Volume)

60 minims (min)	1 fluid drachm (dram) (fl.dr.)
8 fluid drachms	1 fluid ounce (fl.oz)
20 fluid ounces	1 pint (pt.)
2 pints	1 quart
4 quarts or 8 pints	1 gallon

Relationship of capacity to mass

- 1 Gallon = the volume of 10 pounds or 70,000 grains of distilled water at 62°F
- 1 Fluid ounce or 480 minims = the volume at 62°F of 1 oz. or 437.5 grains of distilled water
- 109.71 minims (taken as 110 minims) = the volume at 62°F of 100 grains of distilled water.

ii. Apothecaries' Weights and Measures

Measures of Mass

Grain is the same in both Avoidupois and Apothecaries systems.

20 grains	1 Scruple	
3 Scruples	1 drachm (dram)	
8 Drachms	1 ounce	
12 Ounces	1 pound	lb

The measures of volume are the same in both the systems. In Avoirdupois system the abbreviations are fl.dr and fl.oz while in Avoirdupois system they are and for dram and ounce, respectively.

United States of America : Weights and Measures

1 Fluid ounce (480 minims) = 454.6 grains at 25°C (USA standard) = 437.5 grains at 16.7°C (Imperial Standard)

1 pint =16 fl.oz. (USA) = 20 fl oz. (Imperial)

1 Gallon = 128 fl. Oz. (USA) = 3.7853 liters

1 Gallon = 160 fl.oz. (Imperial) = 4.5436 litres

1 hundredweight = 100 pounds (USA) = 112 pounds (Imperial)

1 ton = 2000 pounds (USA) = 240 pounds (Imperial)

Household Measures

The accepted approximate dose equivalents for the household measures are given below-

Household measure	Apothecaries measure	Metric measure
1 Drop	1 minim	0.04 ml
1 Teaspoonful	1 fl.dr	5 ml
1 Dessertspoonful	2 fl.dr.	8 ml
1 Tablespoonful	4 fl.dr.	15 ml
1 Wineglassful	2 fl.oz.	60 ml
1 Teacupful	4 fl.oz.	120 ml.
1 Tumblerful	8 fl.oz.	240 ml.

The drops of various liquids vary in size and it is therefore necessary to calibrate the dropper to get the correct dose of a potent liquid preparation.

Use of Equivalents

A pharmacist is sometimes required to convert a formula from one system to the other or to dispense prepared dosage forms like mixtures, lotions, ointments etc. in a suitable equivalent dose.

Imperial system	Approximate metric system	Exact metric equivalent
15 minims	1 ml	0.924 ml
16.23 minims	1 ml.	1.0 ml.
60 minims (1 fl.dram.)	4 ml.	3.697 ml
480 minims(1 fl.oz.)	30 ml.	29.573 ml.
33.8148 or 33.815 fl.oz.	1 litre	1 litre
1 gallon (177.27 cubic inches)	4.5 L.	4.5436 L.
1/60 grains	1 mg.	1.1 mg.
1 pound (lb)	454 g	453.59 g
1 grain	60 mg	64.7989 mg or 64.8 mg
7.5 grains	0.5 gram	0.4864 g.
10 grains	0.6 g.	0.6480 g.
15 grains	1 g.	0.972 g
15.432 grains	1 g.	1.0 g.
60 grains = 1 dram	4 g.	3.888 g
437.5 grains = 1 oz.	28 g.	28.3495 or 28.35 g
480 grains = 1 ounce	30 g.	31.1035 g.
32.151 Apoth. ounces	1kg.	1 kg.
35.274 Av. Ounces (2.2046 lbs)	1 kg.	1 kg.
16 Av. Ounces (1 lbs.)	450 g.	453.5924 g.
1 Inch	2.5 cm.	2.54 cm.
1 Cubic Inches	16 cc	16.3872 cc
39.37 inches	1 meter	1 meter
1.196 sq. yards	1 sq. meter	1 sq. meter
1 mile	1.6 km.	1.6093 km.
0.6214 mile	1 km.	1 km.

Uncalibrated teaspoons may vary from 2.4 to 7 ml and tablespoons may vary from 13.4 to 27.2 ml. In pharmaceutical practice the teaspoonful and tablespoonful should be taken to be 4 ml and 15 ml, respectively. It is the duty of the pharmacist to educate the general public regarding the use of calibrated spoons for the measurement of medicinal preparations. As such the manufacturers usually supply calibrated spoons along with the packages and therefore the use of household spoons must be discouraged.

Following points must be borne in mind to avoid confusion and to facilitate memorizing:

1. The pharmacist uses avoirdupois system of weights (1 oz = 437.5grains) to buy and sell merchandise other than on prescription.
2. The pharmacist uses apothecary system of weights (1 oz = 480 grains) to dispense prescriptions and compound formulae.
3. The term 'ounce' or its abbreviation 'oz' means an Avoirdupois ounce. The avoirdupois ounce (abbreviated as oz) is 42.5 grains lighter than apothecary ounce.
4. The Apothecary or Troy pound is not used in pharmacy.
5. One pound avoirdupois (lb) (7000 grain) is heavier than one pound apothecary (lb apoth) (5760 grain) by 1240 grain.
6. The avoirdupois and apothecary grain are exactly equal (both abbreviated as gr).
7. The abbreviations for apothecary system are represented by the signs as mentioned in table.
8. Measures of volume in apothecary and avoirdupois systems are same and hence differ from US measures of volume.
9. The US fluid ounce or minim equals 1.04 imperial fluid ounce or minim, respectively.
10. The US gallon contains 128 fl oz whereas the imperial gallon contains 160 fl oz.
11. The US pint weighs 1.04 avoirdupois pound.
12. The apothecary fluid ounce weighs 453.6 grains while imperial fluid ounce weighs 437.5 grains at 25°C and 15.6°C, respectively.
13. The standard of capacity is the litre which is the volume of 1 kg of distilled water at its maximum density (approximately 4°C). A millilitre is the volume occupied by 1 g of water at 4°C whereas a cc is the volume occupied by a cubic each side of which is 1 cm in length. Actually 1 cc = 0.99984 ml.
14. The denomination scruple exists only in the Apothecaries system and there is no counterpart in the Avoirdupois system.
15. Drachm and dram should not be confused. Dram is 1/16 of the Avoirdupois ounce and is equivalent to 27.34375 grains whereas a drachm contains 60 grains.
16. The unit 'one' is often expresed by the letter. When two or more units are to be used, the first one is expressed as j, e.g. 3ij, 3iij, 3vj.

Practice Exercise

1. Convert the following

   a. 205 mg to grain   b. 180 mg to grain   c. 2.5 gram to grain

   d. 25 pounds to gram   e. 5 pounds to kg

2. Convert the following

   a. 2.5 scruple to grain   b. 5 dram to scruple   c. 32 dram to ounce

   d. 2.5 pound to ounce   e. 60 grains to scruple

3. Fill in the blank –

   a. gr i = ______ mg   b. 1 gal = ______ ml   c. 1 oz = ______ g

   d. 1 kg = ______ lbs   e. 1 pint (pt) = ______ ml   f. fl oz i = ______ ml

   g. 1 lb = _____ g   h. 1 qt = _____ ml   i. 1 oz = _____ gr

   j. 1 g = _____ gr   k. 1 (teaspoonful) tsp = ______ml

4. Convert the following

   a. 1750 grains to ounce   b. 2.5 kg to pound   c. 26 gram to grain

   d. 155.5 gram to ounce   e. 66 ounce to pound

5. Convert the following

   a. 24 ml to fluid drachm   b. 50 ml to minim   c. 352 fluid ounce to liter

   d. 2841 millilitre to fluid ounce   e. 185.9 millilitre to minim

6. Convert 1 gallon, 1 pint and 2 fluid ounce to ml.
7. A specific gravity bottle filled with water weighed 121.0 g, when 12.0 g of an insoluble powder was introduced and then filled with water the sp. gr. bottle weighed 123.0 g. The weight of empty bottle is 21.0 g. Calculate the sp. gr. of the powder
8. What is the capacity in litres of a cylindrical percolator that is 3 feet high and 0.5 feet in diameter?(Capacity of a cylindrical percolator = $\pi r^2 h$).
9. The dose of a liquid is 10 minims. How many doses are contained in 4 f3 of the liquid?
10. 308 tablets each containing 1/2gr of a drug are to be prepared. How many gram of the drug will be required?
11. If a 3 feet deep, 6 feet long and 4 feet wide tank is filled with a liquid preparation, how many 2 oz. bottles can be filled out of it?

12. How many grains of a chemical are left in a bottle after ʒii are dispensed from it?
13. A pharmacist prepared 5000 tablets each containing 1/200 grain of a drug. How many grains of the chemical are left if the pharmacist started with 1/4 oz. of the drug?
14. A solution has been prepared by dissolving 32 grains of a drug in 1 fl oz. How many grains of the drug are contained in 200 mL of the solution?
15. A tank is 6 ft long, 4 ft wide and 2 ft deep and is filled with a cough syrup. How many 4 oz. bottles can be filled out of it?
16. Tetracycline suspension contains 250 mg of tetracycline per five cc's. How much of the suspension would be required to give a patient 125 mg of tetracycline? Give the answer in household equivalents.
17. Pyrantel pamoate is given as treatment for roundworms in a single dose of 1 ml for 10 pounds of body weight. What would be the dose in milliliters for a 44-lb child?
18. Meperidine hydrochloride injection contains 50 milligrams of meperidine HCl per milliliter of injection. How many milliliters must be administered to give a patient 75 milligrams of the drug?
19. Calculate the number of 1/2-grain phenobarbital capsules that can be made from 4 ounces of phenobarbital.
20. To lower a patient's elevated blood pressure, a physician has prescribed 500mg of methyldopa to be taken each day. Tablets are supplied in 250-mg. How many tablets must be dispensed to give the patient a 30-day regimen?
21. How many 30-mg doses can be made from one ounce of a drug?

Answers

1. a. 3.416 gr. b. 3.0 g c. 37.5 gr. d. 11339.75 g e. 2.26795 kg

2. a. 50 g b. 15 scruple c. 4 ounce d. 30 ounce e. 3 scruple

3. a. 65 b. 3785 c. 28.4 d. 2.2 e. 473
f. 30 g. 454 h. 946 i. 437.5 j. 15.432 k. 4 or 5

4. a. 4 b. 5.5 c. 401.23 d. 5.485 e. 5.5

5. a. 6.76 b. 845 c. 10 d. 100 e. 11

6. 5176.62 ml (1 one fl oz = 28.41 ml) **7.** 1.2 **8.** 16.72 litres

9. 24 doses **10.** 10.0 g **11.** 8976 bottles **12.** 317.5 grains

13. 84.4 grains **14.** 14.2 grains **15.** 11965 bottles **16.** 1/2 teaspoonful

17. 4.4 ml **18.** 1.5 ml **19.** 3484 **20.** 60 tablets **21.** 945 doses

INTRODUCTION TO LATIN TERMS

Table 4.1 Terms Related to Dosage Forms

Latin terms	Abbreviation	English meaning
Aurinarium	aurin.	An ear cone
Auristillae	auristill.	Ear drops
Buginarium	buginar.	Nasal drops
Capsula	caps.	A capsule
Casula amylacea	caps. amylac.	A cachet
Capsula gelatina	caps. gelat.	A gelatin capsule
Cataplasma	cataplasm.	A poultice
Cereolus	cereol.	An urethral bougie
Collunarium	collun.	A nose wash
Collutorium	collut.	A mouth wash
Collyrium	collyr.	An eye lotion
Cremor	crem.	A cream
Emulsio	emul.	An emulsion
Gargarisma	garg.	A gargle
Gelatina	gelat.	A jelly
Guttae	gtt.	Drops
Haustus	ht.	A draught
Inhalatio	inhal.	An inhalation
Injectio	inj.	An injection
Insufflatio	insuff.	An insufflation
Linctus	linct.	A lictus
Linimentum	lin.	A liniment
Lotio	lot.	A lotion
Mistura	m., mist.	A mixture
Nebula	neb.	A spray solution
Oblatum	oblat.	A cachet
Pasta	past.	A paste
pastillus	pastill.	A pastille

Table 4.1 ***Contd…***

Pessus	pess.	A pessary
Pigmentum	pigm.	A paint
Pilula	pil.	A pill
Pulvis	pulv.	A powder
Conspersus	consper.	A dusting powder
Sternutamentum	sternut.	A snuff
suppositorium	suppos.	A suppository
Tabletta	tab.	A tablet
Trochiscus	troch.	A lozenge
Unguentum	ung.	An ointment
Nomen Proprium	n.p.	Proper name

Table 4.2 Terms used in preparation of dosage Forms

Latin terms	Abbreviation	English meaning
Fiat	ft.	Let (it) be made
Fiant	ft.	Let (them) be made
Misce/misceatur	m.	Mix
Misce fiat mistura	m.ft.m.	Mix to make a mixture
Misce secundum artem	m.s.a.	Mix pharmaceutically, Mix according to the art
Divide/dividatur	div.	Divided
Dividatur in partes aequales	div. in pt. aeq.	Divide into equal parts
Fiat pulvis subtilis	ft.pulv subtil.	Make a fine powder
Tere / teratur	ter.	Rubbed
Tere bene simul	ter. bene simul	Rubb well together
Duplum	duplum	Twice the quantity
Mitte	mitt.	Send
In phiala		In a bottle
Phiala prius agitata	p.p.a.	The bottle being first shaken
Quantitas duplex	qt. dx.	Twice the quantity
Talis/Tales/Talia	tal.	Such
Capiendus	capiend.	To be taken

Table 4.2 ***Contd...***

Dandus	dand.	To be given
Deglutiendus	degult.	To be swallowed
Infricandus	infricand.	To be rubbed in
Inhaletur	inhal.	Let be inhaled
Instillandus	instilland.	To be dropped in
Miscendus	miscend.	To be mixed
Sugendus	sugend.	To be sucked
Sumendus	sum.	To be taken
Ut antea	u.a.	As before
Utendus	utend.	To be used

Table 4.3 Common Terms Used in Dose, Administration and Parts

Latin terms	**Abbreviation**	**English meaning**
Bis in die / bis die	b.i.d./b.d.	Twice a day
Ter in die / Ter die	t.i.d. / t.d.	Three times a day
Qauter in die /Quarter die	q.i.d. / q.d.	Four times a day
Bis terve in die	b.t.i.d.	Two or three times a day
Ter quaterve die	t.q.d.	Three or four times a day
Quotidie / indies	quot./indies	Daily
Prima luce / primo mane	prim. luc. / prim. m.	Early in the morning
Mane	m.	In the morning
Omni mane	o.m.	Every morning
Jentaculum	jentac.	Breakfast
Omni nocte	o.n.	Every night
Hora decubitus	h.d.	At bedtime
Nocte maneque	n.m.	Night and morning
Hac nocte	hac noct.	To-night
Omni hora / omni singula	o.h. /o.s.	Every hour
Omni altena hora / Quaque alterna hora	o. alt.h. / qq. alt. h.	Every alternate hour
Omni quarta hora	o.q.h.	Every fourth hour
Anti cibos	a.c.	Before meals

Table 4.3 ***Contd…***

Ante cibum	a.c.	Before food
Post cibos	p.c.	After meals
Post cibum	p.c.	After food
Inter cibos	i.c.	Between meals
Lente		Slowly
More dicto / modo dicto	m.d.	As directed
Pro re nata	p.r.n.	Occasionally
Si opis sit	s.o.s.	When required; when necessary
Tussi urgente	tuss.urg.	When the cough is troublesome
Parti affectae / Partibus affectis	p.a.	To the affected part
Parti affectae applicandus	p.a.a.	To be applied to the affected part
Sinister / Laevus	sinist. / laev.	Left
Oculis	ocul.	For the eyes

PERCENTAGE SOLUTION

Percentage rate per hundred is a convenient means of expression of the concentration of a solute in solution or amount of a potent drug in a dosage form or the quantity of an ingredient in a mixture. The common types of percent solutions or mixtures in Pharmacy are classified as follows-

1. Percentage of solid in liquid usually expressed as % *w/v*
2. Percentage of solid in solid usually expressed as % *w/v*
3. Percentage of liquid in solid usually expressed as % *v/w*
4. Percentage of liquid in liquid usually expressed as % *v/w*
5. Miscellaneous mixtures

Percentage of solid in liquid

The true percentage of solid in liquid is expressed as weight in weight e.g. 10% Solution of sugar in water means 10 g of sugar dissolved in sufficient water to make up 100 g of solution or 10 grains of solution dissolved in sufficient water to make up 100 grains of solution.

In this type where the percentage strength is expressed as weight by weight (W/W) the solutions are to be done by weighing solids and liquids. It is not easy to weigh the liquids. It is also necessary to take into consideration the specific gravity of the solvent and the final solution when finding the amount of a substance in equal volume of two solutions of the same substance.

Useful Tips

1 fl oz of 1% *w/v* solution requires 4.375 grains of solute
1 pint of 1% *w/v* solution requires 87.5 grains of solute
1quart of 1% *w/v* solution requires 175 grains of solute
1 gallon of 1% *w/v* solution requires 700 grains of solute.

1 pound = 16 ounce
1 fl oz = 8 fl drachm
1 pint (568 ml)=20 fl oz
1 quart = 40 fl oz or 2 pint
1 gallon =160 fl oz or 8 pint or 4 quart
1 pound = 453.59 grams

Practice Exercise

1. How many grams of glucose will be required to prepare 10 litre of 2.5% *w/v* solution?
2. How many 5 grains tablet would be required to prepare 5 gallons of 2.5% *w/v* solution?
3. Calculate the amount of potassium permanganate to prepare 5 litres of 1 in 4000 solution.
4. How many grams of a drug are required to make 3 L of a 1 in 500 solution?
5. How many grains of glucose are required to make 6 fl oz of 0.4% w/v solution?
6. A mixture contains 2% boric acid and 1 in 2000 mercuric chloride. How many grains of each are contained in 4 fl oz?
7. How many grains of a substance should be dissolved to make 6 fl oz of a solution so that one fl dr. of it when diluted to a pint gives 1 in 4000 solution?
8. Calculate the weight of nux vomica seeds containing 1 % strychnine required to prepare 10 gallons liquid extract containing 1.5% strychnine.
9. How many g of a drug are required to make 8 L of a 1 in 500 solution?
10. How many grains of Pot. Permanganate are required to make 8 fl oz of a solution so that 2 fl dr when diluted to a quart makes a 1 in 500 solution?
11. How many ml of a 0.1% *w/v* solution of mercury bichloride can be prepared from 50 tablets each containing 0.47 g. of the drug
12. Fifty fl oz solutions have been prepared by dissolving 75 grains of scopolamine hydrochloride. What is the % *w/v* strength of this solution?

13. How many 5 grains tablets would be required to prepare 10 gallons of 5% *w/v* solution?
14. Calculate the % *w/v* strength of a solution prepared by dissolving 0.5 lb. of a salt in sufficient water to make one pint.
15. A sunsceen lotion contains 5% *v/v* of methyl salicylate. How many ml of methyl salicylate should be used to prepare 3 pints of the solution.
16. A pharmacist has in stock 200 grains of bichloride of mercury. How many ml of a 0.25% *w/v* solution of bichloride of mecury can the pharmacist prepare from his stock?
17. An inhalation aerosol contains 0.25% *w/v* of isoproterenol hydrochloride. If each actuation of the aerosol valve delivery 0.12 mg of the drug. How many doses are contained in a 28 ml aerosol package?
18. How many grains of a substance should be dissolved to make 8 fl oz. of a solution so that 1 fl dr. of it when diluted to a pint gives 1 in 2000 solution?
19. 850 g of sucrose are dissolved in sufficient water to make 1000 ml of syrup having sp. gr. of 1.313. Calculate the % *w/v* strength of the syrup.
20. An ophthalmic ointment contains 2 mg/10 g of mercury bichloride. Calculate the % w/v strength of mercury bichloride in the ointment.
21. Syrup is 85% *w/v* solution of sucrose in water and has specific gravity of 1.3131 g/ml. How many ml of water should be used to prepare 500 ml of syrup?
22. Ten pound of a cosmetic cream is to be preserved using a 0.04% mixture of methyl paraben (70 parts) and propyl paraben (30 parts). Calculate the quantities in grams of methyl and propyl parabens required.
23. How much 95 % alcohol is required to prepare 10 L of 70% alcohol?
24. How many grams of crystal violet should be used in preparing 5 gallons of a 0.025% *w/v* solution?
25. How many grains of gentian violet should be used in preparing of 8 fl oz of a 0.25% *w/v* solution
26. A pharmacist has to dispense 450 g of a 15 % *w/w* solution of zinc sulphate. How many grams of zinc sulphate should be used?
27. How many lit. of 2% solution can be made from 4 oz of a solid?
28. How many Lt. of 0.9% solution can be prepared from 500 g of sodium chloride?
29. How many grams of drug are needed to make 5 L of a 1 in 500 solution?
30. How much of a drug is required to make 2 quart of a 1 in 1200 solution?

31. How much solute is required to prepare 12 oz of a solution so that 3 teaspoonfuls to a quart will make 1/8% solution?
32. How much solute is required to prepare 8 oz. of a solution so that 1 tablespoon to half a gallon will make a 1 in 500 solution?
33. How much solute is required to make 4 oz. of solution so that 2 teaspoonfuls diluted to a pint will make a 1 in 1000 solution.
34. Rx

    Pot. permanganate : 3.0 g

    Distilled water 120.0 ml

    Sig. Dilute 2 teaspoonful to one quart calculate the % strength of the dilution

    How many grains of $KMnO_4$are required?

Answers

(1) 250 grams	**(2)** 1750 tablets	**(3)** 1.25 g	**(4)** 6.0 g	**(5)** 10.5 gr
(6) 35 grains and 0.88 grains	**(7)** 105 grains	**(8)** 150 lbs.	**(9)** 16.0 g.	**(10)** 1120 gr
(11) 23500 ml	**(12)** 33.33%	**(13)** 7000	**(14)** 48% w/v	**(15)** 85.2 ml
(16) 5184 ml	**(17)** 583 doses	**(18)** 280 gr.	**(19)** 64.7%	**(20)** 0.02%
(21) 231.5 ml	**(22)** Methyl para 12.5 g, Propyl Para 5.475 g.			
(23) 8.4211	**(24)** 5.67g.	**(25)** 8.7 grains		**(26)** 67.5 g.
(27) 5.67 L.	**(28)** 5.5 Lt.	**(29)** 10 g.	**(30)** 1.59 g.	**(31)** 700 gr.
(32) 1120 gr.	**(33)** 140 gr.	**(34)** 700 gr.		

PROOF SPIRIT

Alcohol is an excellent solvent. It is used for many purposes in pharmaceutical practice and in formulation of cosmetic etc. In the United States Pharmacopoeia, all alcohol concentrations are expressed as volume-in-volume, based on the quantity of absolute alcohol present, as determined at 15.56°C. Proof spirit was official in B.P. 1885. London Proof spirit mean that mixture of ethyl alcohol and water which weighs exactly $12/13^{th}$ part of an equal volume of distilled water at 51°F. Proof spirit has a sp. gr. of 091976 at 15.5°C and contains 57.1% *V/V* of ethyl alcohol to 100 volume of proof spirit.

Proof spirit is therefore an aqueous solution containing 57.1% *v/v* of absolute alcohol. Any alcohol solution, which contains 57.1% v/v alcohol, is a proof spirit and it is said to be 100^0 Proof.

Over proof (°O/P) means strength of alcohol above the proof strength.

Under proof (°U/P) means strength of alcohol below proof strength.

Thus 25 (°U/P) mean that 100 volume of such alcohol are equivalent to 100-25 = 75 volume of proof sprit. 35 (°O/P) mean that 100 volume of such alcohol are equivalent to 100 + 35 = 135 volume of proof spirit.

In India the rates of excise duty are prescribed in terms of rupees per litre of proof alcohol.

Example: Convert 90% V/V alcohol into proof spirit.

As 57.1 volume of ethyl alcohol = 100 volume of proof spirit

1 volume of ethyl alcohol = 100/57.1 = 1.7513 volume of proof spirit

90 volume of ethyl alcohol = 90 X 1.7513 volume of proof spirit

Hence Proof strength of 90% *v/v* alcohol = (90 X 1.7513) – 100 = 57.6°O/P

Similarly Proof strength of 30% v/v alcohol can be calculated as follows.

Proof strength of 30% V/V alcohol = (30 X 1.7513) – 100 = -47.5 or 47.5°U/P

Thus 70 °O/P = 100 + 70 / 1.7513 = 97% *v/v* of ethyl alcohol, and

70 °U/P = 100 - 70 / 1.7513 = 17.13% *v/v* of ethyl alcohol.

Practice Exercises

1. Convert the following degrees of Proof into percentage strength of ethyl alcohol by volume? a. 12.1(°U/P), b. 17.1 (°U/P) c. 21.5 (°U/P) d. 54.8 (°U/P) e. 75.0 (°U/P)
2. Convert the following degrees of Proof into percentage strength of ethyl alcohol by volume? a. 44.6 (°O/P) b. 44.0 (°O/P) c. 35.3 (°O/P) d. 24.0 (°O/P) e. 18.4 (°O/P)
3. How many proof gallons are contained in 5 gallons of 70% of ethyl alcohol?
4. How many gallons of 20 % *v/v* of ethyl alcohol would be equivalent to 20 proof gallons?
5. On the first of Dec. 1997 a hospital pharmacist had on hand a drum containing 54 gallons of 95 % alcohol. During the month he used the following amount

   a. 10 gallons in the manufacture of bathing solution

   b. 15 gallons in the manufacture of soap solution

   c. 8 gallons in the manufacture of medicated alcohol and at the end of month.

   How many proof gallons of alcohol did he have on hand?
6. On the first day of the month a hospital pharmacist had two drums (108 gallons) of 95 % alcohol and 10 pints of absolute alcohol (100%) on hand. During the month he prepared 25 gallons of 70% *v/v* of ethyl alcohol and .25 gallons of 50% *v/v* alcohol. He also dispensed two pints of absolute alcohol. How many proof gallons of alcohol did he have on hand at the end of the month?
7. How many proof gallons are represented by 50 wine gallons of 90% *v/v* alcohol?

8. 20 gallons of 70% *v/v* alcohol and 30 gallons of 50 % *v/v* alcohols were mixed. Calculate the proof strength in the mixture.
9. Five gallon proof spirit was diluted with two gallons of water. Calculate the alcoholic strength of the mixture
10. An alcoholic inventory shows 30 gallons of 95% and 7.5 pints of absolute (100%) alcohol. How many proof gallons of alcohol are represented in the inventory?
11. In what proportion should 95% and 25% alcohol be mixed to prepare 70 litre of 40 (°U/P) alcohol?
12. If the excise duty payable on spirit is Rs. 3.85 per LP gallon, calculate the duty to be paid on 25 gallons of rectified spirit containing 90% *v/v* alcohols
13. On a purchase of 10 gallons of rectified spirit containing 94% alcohol, hjgh a manufacturer paid Rs. 288 as excise duty. Calculate the rate of excise duty per Proof Litre

Answers

(1) a. 50.14% b. 47.29% c. 44.78% d. 25.78% e. 14.26%

(2) a. 82.49% b. 82.14 % c. 77.18% d. 70.73 % e. 67.54%

(3) 6.13 gallons (4) 57.1 gallons (5) 34.39 (6) 128.9 proof gallons

(7) 28.8 Pg (8) 50.78 % (9) 40.78 % (10) 51.5 proof gallons

(11) 95% -9.22 lt., 25% alcohol-60.78 lt (12) Rs.727.65 (13) Rs. 3.85

REDUCING AND ENLARGING RECIPES

It is common practice to reduce a recipe for dispensing or enlarge the recipe as required for the purpose of patient. This is required when a manufacturing formula is to be taken from the laboratory scale to a manufacturing floor and a formula for the large scale manufacturing is to be adopted for prescribing to a patient. Such calculations may also involve conversions from one system of weights and measures to another.

The following rules are generally useful in such system

Rule 1. To convert a recipe in imperial system to metric system

"Write grams in place of grains, divide the minims by 1.1 and write the result as milliliters. For large batch, read avoirdupois ounce as grams and fluid ounces as milliliters"

Rule 2. To convert a recipe in metric system to imperial system

"For a small batch write grains in place of grams and multiply the milliliters by 1.1 and write the result as minims. For large batch, write ounce in place of grams and fluid ounce in place of minims"

Example 1

Rx

Sodium hypophosphite gr. xx

Sulphuric acid fl dr. I

Cinnamon water q.s. ad fl.oz. ii

Dispense 50 ml

Calculation : Convert to metric system

Sodium hypophosphite 20 g. = 20 X 50/872.7 = 1.15 g

Sulphuric acid 60/1.1 = 55.5 ml = 55.45 X 50 / 872.7 = 3.2 ml

Cinnamon water q.s. ad 2 X 480/1.1 = 872.5 ml = 50 ml

Dispense 50 ml

However, the simpler solution of the problem would be to retain the original recipe and prepare 2 fl. oz. of the mixture, which corresponds to about 60 ml. Out of 2fl.oz, 60 ml, could be dispensed and the rest rejected.

Example 2

Rx

Pt. Nitrate

Sod. Chloride

Camphor of each 3 g

Tincture opium 15 ml

Alcohol to make 200 ml.

Dispense 4 fl.oz.

Solution:

4 fl oz of the prescription is to be dispensed hence quantities can be converted to Imperial system.

R

Pt. Nitrate

Sod. Chloride

Camphor each 3 grains

Tincture opium = 15 X 1.1 = 16.5 minims

Alcohol = 200 X1.1 = 220 minims

4 X 480 = 1920 minims

Quantity of Pt. Nitrate, Sod. Chloride and Camphor = 3X 1920/220 =26.2 grains

So to avoid this we can prepare 9 times the formula1980 minims and dispense 4 fl.oz and reject 60 minims

Example 3

Calculate the amounts of ingredients required to make 50 ml of calamine lotion.

Rx

Calamine 150 g

Zinc oxide 50 g

Bentonite 30 g

Sodium Citrate 5 g

Liquefied Phenol 5 ml

Purified water, q.s. 1000 ml

Dispense 50 ml.

Solution :

Formula is to be reduced by 50/1000 = 1/20, hence each quantity is to be multiplied by 1/20

Thus the calculated quantities of the ingredients will be –

Ingredient	Quantity for 50 ml
Calamine	150 g X 1/20 = 12.5 g
Zinc oxide	50 g X 1/20 = 2.5 g
Bentonite	30 g X 1/20 = 1.5 g
Sodium Citrate	5 g X 1/20 = 0.25 g
Liquefied Phenol	5 ml X 1/20 = 0.25 ml
Purified water, q.s. 1000 ml	1000 ml 1/20 = 20 ml

Practice Exercises

1. Calculate the quantity for making 50 ml of the given formula.

Rx

Opium tincture 50 ml

Benzoic acid 5 g

Camphor	3 g
Anise Oil	3 ml
Alcohol (60%) q.s.	100 ml

2. How many grams of each ingredient are required to make 100 ml of lotion?

Rx

Calamine	150 g
Zinc oxide	50 g
Bentonite	30 g
Sodium citrate	5 g
Liquefied phenol	5 ml
Purified water q.s.	1000 ml

3. Calculate the quantity of each ingredient required to prepare 1 ounce of the ointment.

Rx

Benzoic acid	6 parts
Salicylic acid	3 parts
PEG ointment	91 parts

4. An antihistamine tablet contains the following ingredients. How many grains of each ingredient are required to prepare a batch of 2.5 million tablets?

Rx

Reserpine	100 mcg
Hydralazine hydrochloride	25 mcg
Hydrochlorthiazide	15 mg

A mixture contains 7.5 g of a drug per 100 ml. How many pounds of the drug will be required to make 5 gallons of the mixture?

5. From the following formula, calculate the quantity of each ingredient required to make 8 litres of the lotion

Rx

Witch Hazel	4 parts
Glycerine	1 parts
Boric acid solution	15 parts

6. Calculate the quantities of each ingredient needed to make 2 lb of the mixture from the following formula:

   Rx

Potassium citrate	30.0 g
Hyoscyamine tincture	30.0 ml
Tween 20	0.4 ml

   Distilled water q.s.

7. A formula for 1000 capsules contains 5.0 g of amphetamine, 325 g of thyroid, 1 g of thiamine hydrochloride, 40 g of Phenobarbital, and enough lactose to make 500g.

   How much of each ingredient should be used in preparing 76 capsules?

8. Prepare 2 pints of the mixture

   Rx

Zinc oxide	2 g
Talc	2 g
Milk of Magnesia	3 ml
Bentonite magma	5 ml
Lime water qs ad	16 ml

9. What quantities will be required for 8 fl oz of the following recipe?

   Rx

Glycerine	25%
Zinc oxide	25%
Lanolin	50%

10. From the following formula, calculate the quantity of each ingredient that should be used in preparing 10 lb of the ointment base.

    Rx

Stearic acid	14 g
Triethanolamine	1 g
Cetyl alcohol	4 g
Glycerine	8 g
Water	63 g

11. From the following quantities to make 6 fl oz. Of an infusion of digitalis form the following preparation.

Rx

Powdered digitalis	15 g
Alcohol	100 ml
Cinnamon water	150 ml
Boiling water	7000 ml
Cold water, to make	1000 ml

12. From the following formula, calculate the quantity of each ingredient required to make 10 lb of the powder.

Rx

Bismuth subcarbonate	8 parts
Kaolin	15 parts
Magnesium oxide	2 parts

13. Calculate the quantity of each ingredient to make 500 ml.

Rx

Boric acid	3.5
Sodium chloride	5.0
Glycerin	3.0
Camphor water	13.0
Purified water	75.5

14. Calculate the quantity of each ingredient required to make 25 ml of the following recipe.

Rx

Ammonium bicarbonate	25.0 g
Strong ammonia solution	67.5 ml
Lemon oil	0.5 ml
Nutmeg oil	0.3 ml
Alcohol (90%)	37.5 ml
Purified water q.s.	1000.0 ml

Answers

1. Opium tincture – 25 ml, Benzoic acid – 2.5 g, Camphor- 1.5 g Anise Oil –1.5 ml Alcohol (60%) q.s. 50 ml.
2. Calamine -15 g, Zinc oxide- 5 g, Bentonite-3.0 g, Sodium citrate- 2.5 g. Liquefied phenol-2.5 ml, Purified water q.s. 100 ml.
3. Benzoic acid-300 g, Salicylic acid-150 g, PEG ointment –4550 g.
4. Reserpine-225 g, Hydralazine hydrochloride –62.5 g, Hydrochlorthiazide –37.5 kg. 0.75 lbs.
5. Witch Hazel-1.6 pint, Glycerine – 1 parts, Boric acid solution- 6 pint.
6. Potassium citrate- 9.6 oz, Hyoscyamine tincture-9.6 oz, Tween –1 fl oz, Distilled water to make 2 lb.
7. amphetamine-0.38 g, thyroid-24.5 g, thiamine hydrochloride-0.76 g, Phenobarbital-3.04 g, lactose-38 g.
8. Zinc oxide – 118.28 g, Talc – 118.2 g, Milk of Magnesia-177.42 ml, Bentonite magma-295.70 ml, Lime water – 2 pint.
9. Glycerine- 2 fl oz, Zinc oxide- 2 oz, Lanolin-4 oz.
10. Stearic acid-706 g, Triethanolamine-50 g, Cetyl alcohol-202 g, Glycerine-404 g Water-3178 g.
11. Powdered digitalis-39.5 gr, Alcohol- 4fl dr 48minims, Cinnamon water-7 fl dr 12 minims, Boiling water-4 fl oz 1 fl dr 36 minims, Cold water-6 fl oz.
12. Bismuth subcarbonate-1.4528 kg, Kaolin-2.724 kg, Magnesium oxide-363.2 g.
13. Boric acid-17.5, Sodium chloride-25.0, Glycerin-15.0, Camphor water-65.0 Purified water –377.5.
14. Ammonium bicarbonate-0.625 g, Strong ammonia solution-1.6875 ml, Lemon oil-0.0125 ml, Nutmeg oil-0.0075 ml, Alcohol (90%)-0.9375 ml, Purified water q.s.25 ml

ALLIGATION

Alligation is a rapid arithmetic method used to solve problems that involve mixing two products of different strengths to form a product having a desired intermediate strength. The term alligation has its origin in Latin, *alligatio* which means the art of attaching and therefore refers to lines drawn during calculation to bind quantities together.

Alligation medial is used in calculating the strength of the mixture of two or more components of different strengths. It gives the weighed average percentage strength of a mixture resulting from components of known quantities and concentration.

Alligation method is used to calculate:

a. The amount of diluent that must be added to a given amount of higher strength preparation to make a desired lower strength.
b. The amounts of active ingredient that must be added to a given amount of lower strength preparation to make a higher strength.
c. The amount of higher and lower strength preparations that must be combined to make a desired amount of an intermediate strength.

It is often more practical to dilute a known strength preparation than it would be to compound an entire preparation. Sometimes, a simple calculation using alligation allows us to calculate the amount of diluent to be added to an already prepared higher strength preparation to form the strength desired.

Sometimes, it is necessary to increase the strength of a preparation by adding an active ingredient for example if 1% coal tar ointment is available and required strength is 2 %, it can be accomplished by adding an unknown amount of coal tar (100 percent).The unknown amount may be found by using alligation method.

Procedure of Calculation

a. Draw a problem matrix
b. Insert quantities as shown
c. Subtract along the diagonals
d. Read along the horizontals

The desired strength always goes in the center square of the matrix. The desired strength is the strength of the preparation that one wishes to make.

Example: In what proportions should a preparation containing 15% of drug be mixed with one containing 30% of drug to prepare a mixture of 20% strength.

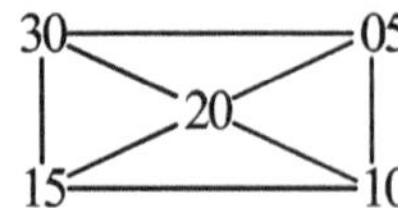

Thus 5 parts of 30% and 10 parts of 15% drug mixed together will give a mixture of 20% drug strength.

Proof of alligation Method

Suppose a product of X percentage strength is to be prepared by mixing constituents of percentage Y (Higher) and Z (lower).

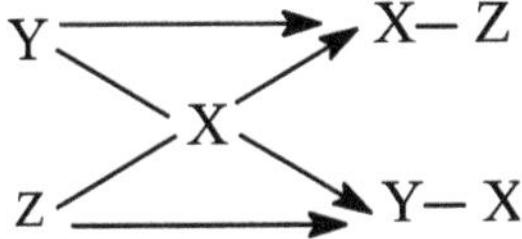

Hence desired percentage strength of X. can be obtained by mixing together (X- Z) parts of Y and (Y-X) parts of Z

$$(X-Z) \times Y + (Y-X) \times Z = [(X-Z) + (Y-X)] \times X$$

Solving the equation-

$$XY - ZY + YZ - XZ = [X - Z + Y - X] \times X$$

$$XY - XZ = [Y - Z] \times X = XY - XZ$$

This equation proves the line diagram method of alligation is correct and most suitable in such calculation

Example 1

What is the % of alcohol in a mixture obtained by mixing 5 L of 25%, 1L of 50% and 2 L of 95% alcohol?

Solution

(1 Litre = 1000 ml)

5000 ml × 25% = 1250

1000 ml × 50% = 500

2000 ml × 95% = 1900

8000 ml 3650

3650 : 8000 : : X × 100

$$X = \frac{3650}{8000} \times 100 = 45.6\%$$

Final mixture concentration = 45.6%

Example 2

What is the strength of zinc oxide in an ointment prepared by mixing 400 g of 10%, 100 g of 20% and 50 g of 5% ointment?

400 g	× 10%	= 40
100 g	× 20%	= 20
50 g	× 5%	= 2.5
550 ml		62.50

62.50 : 550 : : X × 100

$$X = \frac{62.50}{550} \times 100 = 11.36\%$$

Final mixture concentration = 11.36%

Example 3 :

How many parts of 70%, 60% 40% and 30% alcohol should be mixed to get 50% alcohol.

Calculation

Strength	Required	Parts
70		20
60		10
	50	
40		10
30		20

or

Strength	Required	Parts
70		10
60		20
	50	
40		20
30		10

Answer : 20:10:10:20 or 10:20:20:10

Example 4 :

In what proportion should 12%, 8% and 3% alcohol be mixed to get 5% alcohol?

Solution

Strength	Required	Parts
12		2
8		2
	5	
3		7 + 3 = 10

Answer : 2 : 2 : 10 (1:1:5)

Practice Exercises

1. What is the percentage of borax in an ointment prepared by mixing 50 grams of 5% ointment 100 grams of 15% ointment and 300 grams of 8% ointment?
2. 500 ml each of 20% dextrose and 50% dextrose solutions are mixed. Calculate the strength of the mixture.
3. In what proportion of alcohol 70% and 40% should be mixed to get 50% alcohol?
4. In what proportion 10%, 6% and 3% alcohol be mixed to make 5% alcohol?
5. 400 g of 20%, 240 g of 43% and 350 g of 66% sulfuric acid are mixed. How much water should be added to make a 10% solution of sulfuric acid?
6. How many parts of 80%, 60%, 40% and 30% alcohol be mixed together to get 50% alcohol?
7. How many ml of water should be mixed with 30 gm. of 40% w/w Sulphuric acid and 50 gm. of 60% w/w sulfuric acid to make 10% w/w acid?
8. How many g. of strong ammonia sp. gr. 0.880 be added to 40 g. of ammonia water sp. gr. 0.97 and 35 g. of ammonia water sp. gr. 0.98 so that the mixture may have sp. gr. 0.95?
9. One pound of a concentrated acid of sp. Gr. is overdiluted with twice its volume of water. What volume of additional acid must be added to yield an acid with sp. Gr. 1.3?
10. How much water has to be added to 700 ml of 92%, 850 ml of 86% and 600 ml of 26% alcohol to bring the strength of the mixture down to 20%?
11. Find out the quantity of pure silver nitrate to be added to a mixture of 125 g. of 8% and 75 g. of 6 % silver nitrate solution so as to make 10% solution.
12. One pound of concentrated acid with sp. gr. 1.62 in over diluted with twice its volume of water. What volume of additional acid must be added to yield an acid with sp. gr. 1.3?

Answers

1. 9.21%
2. 35%
3. 10 parts of 70% and 20 parts of 40% (1:2)
4. Proportion 2:2:6 or 1:1:3
5. 3152 g
6. 10:20:30:10 or 20:10:10:30

7. 340 ml
8. 25.7 grams
9. 0.9375 lb
10. 5504 ml
11. 6.11 g
12. 0.9375 lb.

ISOTON1C SOLUTIONS

Solutions of drugs administered by parenteral and ophthalmic routes enter into the respective body fluids i.e. blood and tears or lachrymal fluid. Hence these solutions must be physiologically acceptable. The greatest determinant of this physiological acceptability is osmotic pressure. Thus a drug solution having osmotic pressure equal to that of blood will be physiologically acceptable. Similarly, a drug solution having the osmotic pressure matching with the lachrymal secretion will also be physiologically acceptable. If the properties of drug solution are not matched with the body fluid in solution, the irritation and cell destruction may occur.

Osmotic pressure and freezing point depression are the colligative properties i.e. they depend on the number of solute particles in the solution irrespective of whether these are large or small or ions or molecules.

Two solutions having the same osmotic pressure are called *iso-osmotic* or *isotonic*. Solutions which do not have the same osmotic pressure are called paratonic. Paratonic solutions can be either hypertonic or hypotonic. *Hypertonic* solutions contain more quantity whereas *hypotonic* solutions contain less quantity of solute(s) than required for making them isotonic. Generally a pharmacist receives prescriptions for isotonic solutions but rarely he may also have to deal with a paratonic prescription. Intravenous solutions should be isotonic with blood while ophthalmic solutions should be isotonic with tears, Blood serum and tears have the same osmotic pressure.

The osmotic pressure of a 1.8% solution of urea and 0.9% sodium chloride solution are same as that of body fluids including blood and lachrymal fluid. Thus 0.9% sodium chloride solution is isotonic with physiological fluids. Isotonic and iso-osmotic are not necessarily equivalent. It is possible that an iso-osmotic solution may cause hydrolysis of RBCs upon injection. This happens because the solutes diffuse through the membranes of the cells.

Adjustment of tonicity calls for the addition of some inert material compatible with drug substance. In practice the following methods are used for calculation of isotonicity.

Methods for Calculating Isotonicity

1. **Freezing Point Method:** The lachrymal secretion contains several solutes in it and has a freezing point of -0.52°C. All solutions, which freeze at -0.52°C, will be isotonic with the lachrymal fluid. Human blood plasma also freezes at this temperature and hence solutions having freezing point at -0.52^0C will be isotonic with blood plasma as well. Adjustment of tonicity is simplified if the freeing points of the medicament and the inert salt (adjusting substance) are known for various strengths of their solutions. Freezing points are usually expressed in terms of 1% solutions and one can calculate the quantity by multiplying the freezing point with the factor.

   The following, equation is useful :

Freezing point of tear secretion or human Blood plasma	=	Freeing point of drug + freezing point of the adjusting substance

   Therefore the amount of adjusting substance required may be calculated from the equation

   $$W = \frac{0.52 - a}{b}$$

   where

   W = the weight, in g, of the added substance in 100 mL of the final solution;

   a = the depression of the freezing point produced by the medicament already present in solution, calculated by multiplying the value for the medicament by the strength of the solution expressed as a percent age w/v; and

   b = the depression of the freezing point of water produced by 1% of the adjusting substance.

   Example 1

   Two hundred ml of an eyewash containing 1% boric acid are to be dispensed.

   (F.P. of 1% boric acid at - 0.29°C and F.P. of 1% solution of sodium chloride =-0.58°C).

   Applying the above equation-

   $$W = \frac{0.52 - 0.29}{0.58} = 0.39 \text{ g/100 ml or } 0.39\%$$

   Thus the working formula for for 200 mL of the eyewash will be:

   Boric acid (1%, for 200 mL) = 1 g x 2 = 2 g.

   Sodium chloride (0.39%, for 200 mL) = 0.39 x 2 = 0.78 g.

   Purified water q.s. 200 mL.

Answer

However if the pharmacist has been asked to supply 200 ml of eyewash of boric acid', the calculation will be as follows:

Lowering of 0.29°C in F.P. is caused by 1 g of boric acid

Lowering of 0.52°C in F.P. will be caused by

$$\frac{1.0 \times 0.52}{0.29} = 1.8 \text{ g}$$

Therefore 1.8 g of boric acid is required to make 100 ml of eyewash and the working formula will be :

Boric acid (1.8%, for 200 ml) = 1.8 x 2 = 3.6 g. Purified water, q.s. 200 mL. Ans.

The freeing points of common substances used for adjusting the isotonicity are given in the following table.

Table 4.4 Freezing Points (°C) of 1 % solution of common substances

Substance	Freezing Point °C
Amethocaine hydrochloride	-0.109
Atropine sulfate	-0.074
Boric acid, Borax	-0.288, 0.241
Calcium chloride ($2H_2O$)	-0.298
Calcium chloride ($6H_2O$)	-0.200
Calcium gluconate	-0.091
Cinchocaine hydrochloride	-0.074
Cocaine hydrochloride	-0.090
Codeine phosphate	-0.080
Copper sulfate	-0.098
Dexamethasone sodium phosphate	-0.095
Emetine hydrochloride	-0.062
Homatropine hydrobromide	-0.096
Pethidine hydrochloride	-0.124
Pilocarpine hydrochloride	-0.134
Pilocarpine nitrate	-0.131
Potassium chloride	-0.439
Potassium nitrate	-0.323

Table 4.4 ***Contd...***

Procaine hydrochloride	-0.122
Quinine hydrochloride	-0.077
Silver nitrate	-0.190
Silver protein	-0.047
Sodium benzoate	-0.232
Sodium bicarbonate	-0.381
Sodium chloride	-0.576
Sodium nitrite	-0.481
Sodium sulfate	-0.148
Sulfacetamide sodium	-0.133
Sulfadiazine sodium	-0.137
Thiamine hydrochloride	-0.139
Zinc chloride	-0.354
Zmc sulfate	-0.085

2. **Molecular Weight Method :** Freezing point of a solute depends on the concentration of the solute dissolved therein. Greater the concentration of the solute, lower is the freezing point. In other words it depends on the number of ions (more correctly, the number of effective ions), the weight of the substance and its molecular weight. The concentration for 0.9% solution of sodium chloride can be expressed in the following manner:

$$\frac{g \times n}{m} = \text{Isotonic factor or Isotinicty}$$

Where

g = No. of gram of sodium chloride (g)

n = No. of effective ions (n)

m = molecular weight of sodium chloride (m)

i.e. isotonicity factor for sodium chloride is 0.03.

Since 0.9% solution of sodium chloride (normal saline) is isotonic with body fluids, 0.03 will be the isotonicity or tonicity factor for tear secretion and blood plasma as well. Thus quantities for making eye solutions can be calculated by equating the value of 0.03 with the tonicity contributed by the drug and the additive(s).

The following equation is employed for calculating the quantity of the additive(s):

$$0.03 = \frac{g \times n}{m} + \frac{g_1 \times n_1}{m_1} + \frac{g_2 \times n_2}{m_2}$$

where g, n and m denote the weight in gram, effective ion concentration and molecular weight of the medicament, respectively. Values followed by subscript 1 or 2 in the equation above refer to the first additive or the second additive (if present). Effective ionic concentration can be ascertained form the following generalizations;

$n = 1$ for non-ionisable substances, e.g. dextrose

$n = 1.5$ for partially ionisable solutes in two ions, e.g. silver nitrate

$n = 2$ for highly ionisable solutes in two ions e.g. sodium chloride

$n = 2$ for partially ionisable solutes in three ions, e.g. sodium sulfate

Example 2

Send 100 mL of eye drops of silver nitrate.

Solution

$$0.03 = \frac{0.03 \times m}{n} = \frac{0.03 \times 169.8}{1.5} = 3.4 \text{ g/100 ml} \quad \text{Answer}$$

Suppose the above exercise were to be read differently, 'supply 100 ml of 1% eye drops of silver nitrate' then the calculation will be as follows:

$$0.03 = \frac{g \times n}{m} + \frac{g_1 \times n_1}{m_1}$$

$$0.03 = \frac{1.0 \times 1.5}{169.8} + \frac{g_1 \times 1.5}{85}$$

$g_1 = 1.26$ g/100 mL

It may be noted that the substance to be used for rendering the solution isotonic is sodium nitrate because it is compatible with silver nitrate and not sodium chloride which, if added, will result into the precipitation of silver nitrate. Thus for making 100 ml of the eye drop solution containing 1% silver nitrate, the working formula will be:

Silver nitrate	1.00 g
Sodium nitrate	1.26 g
Purified water, q.s. ad	100.0 ml

Whereas it is desirable to make solutions isotonic with lachrymal secretion, it may be remembered that paratonic solutions within the range of 0.7 to 15% of sodium chloride or its equivalent in relation to other substances are easily tolerated by the eye.

3. **Sodium Chloride Equivalent Method :** This is the simplest method and is based on the sodium chloride equivalents of various drugs. Sodium chloride equivalent of a drug represents the amount of sodium chloride equivalent to 1 g of the drug. The method avoids tedious calculation. Sodium chloride equivalents of some common drugs are given in the following table.

Table 4.5 Sodium Chloride Equivalents

1 g (or grain) of drug	Equivalent g (or grain) of sodium chloride
Adrenaline acid tartrate	0.18
Adrenaline hydrochloride	0.29
Aminophylline	0.17
Ampiciilin sodium	0.16
Atropine sulfate	0.13
Bacitracin	0.05
Borax	0.42
Boric acid	0.50
Calcium chloride ($2H_20$)	0.51
Calcium chloride ($6H_20$)	0.35
Cephaloridine	0.07
Cephazoline sodium	0.13
Chloramphenicol	0.10
Chlortetracycline hydrochloride	0.10
Cocaine hydrochloride	0.16
Copper sulfate	0.18
Dexamethasone sodium phosphate	0.17
Emetine hydrochloride	0.10
Ephedrine hydrochloride	0.30
Ephedrine sulfate	0.23
Fluorescein sodium	0.31
Fructose	0.18
Gentamycin sulfate	0.05
Homatropine hydrobromide	0.17
Imipramine hydrochloride	0.20

Table 4.5 ***Contd...***

Kanamycin sulfate	0.07
Lignocaine hydrochloride	0.22
Morphine hydrochloride	0.15
Morphine sulfate	0.14
Neomycin sulfate	0.12
Oxvtetracvcline hydrochloride	0.14
Physostigmine salicylate	0.16
Physostigmine sulfate	0.13
Pilocarpine hydrochlonde	0.24
Pilocarpine nitrate	0.23
Povidone	0.01
Procaine hydrochlride	0.21
Resorcinol	0.28
Silver nitrate	0.33
Sodium borate	0.42
Sodium chloride	1.00
Streptomycin sulfate	0.07
Sulphacetamide sodium	0.23
Terbutaline sulfate	0.14
Tetracycline hydrochloride	0.14
Timolol maleate	0.13
Urea	0.59
Warfarin sodium	0.17
Zinc chloride	0.61
Zinc sulfate	0.15

It can be memorized that 0.27 g of sodium chloride makes 30 mL of a 0.9% solution and that 4.1 grain of sodium chloride makes 1 fl oz. of a 0.9% solution.

Example 3

Calculate the number of g of sodium chloride, which should be added to 20 mL of 0.5% solution of pilocarpine hydrochloride to make it isotonic.

Solution:

Wt. of pilocarpine hydrochloride contained in the prescription = 120 x 0.5% = 0.6 g

Sodium chloride eq. of pilocarpine hydrochloride = 0.22

Hence the amount of sodium chloride represented by pilocarpine hydrochloride contained in the prescription = 0.6 x 0.2 = 0.132 g.

120 mL of 0.9% sodium chloride would contain 120 x 0.9 = 1.08 g of sodium chloride

This is the amount of sodium chloride required to make 120 mL of isotonic solution in absence of pilocarpine hydrochloride.

Hence the no. of g of sodium chloride required = 1.08 g - 0.132 g = 0.948 g Answer

Example 4

Calculate the no. of g of sodium chloride needed to render 30 mL of physostigmine salicylate solution isotonic.

Solution :

Wt. of physostigmine salicylate contained in the prescription = 30 x 0.5 = 0.15 g

Sodium chloride eq. of Physostigmine salicylate =0.14

Hence Physostigmine salicylate present in the prescription is equivalent to – 0.15 x 0.14 = 0.0210 of sodium chloride.

30 mL of a solution containing 0.9% sodium chloride will contain 30 x 0.9% = 0.27 g of sodium chloride if sodium chloride alone were present in the prescription.

No. of g of additional sodium chloride needed =0.27 g - 0.0210 g = 0.2490 g Answer

4. **Isotonic solution V-Values :** Another method for adjusting tonicity is based on V-values. The isotonic solution V-values for some of the commonly used drugs are given in the following Table. The V-value of a drug is defined as the volume of water in mL to be added to 0.3 g of the drug to make an isotonic solution. The addition of an isotonic vehicle (diluting vehicle) to make 30 ml yields a 1% solution (0.3 g drug in 30 ml). Solutions prepared by this method are iso-osmotic with 0.9% sodium chloride.

Table 4.6 Isotonic Solution V-values

Drug (0.3 g)	Water (mL) needed for isotonicity
Ammonium chloride	37.3
Ascorbic acid	6.0
Atropine sulfate	4.3
Bacitracin	1.7
Boric acid	16.7

Table 4.6 *Contd...*

Cocaine hydrochloride	5.3
Ephedrine hydrochloride	10.0
Ephedrine sulfate	7.7
Ephedrine bitartrate	6.0
Epinephrine hydrochloride	9.7
Homatropine hydrobromide	5.7
Neomycin sulfate	3.7
Oxytetracycline hydrochloride	4.3
Pilocarpine hydrochloride	7.0
Pilocarpine nitrate	7.7
Potassium chloride	25.3
Scopolamine hydrobromide	4.0
Silver nitrate	11.0
Sodium acetate	15.3
Sodium bisulfite	20.3
Sodium borate	14.0
Sodium thiosulfate	10.3
Streptomycin sulfate	2.3
Sulphacetamide sodium	7.7
Tetracaine hydrochloride	6.0
Tetracycline hydrochloride	4.7
Viomycin sulfate	2.7
Zinc chloride	20.3
Zinc sulfate	5.0

Example 5

Calculate the v-value for streptomycin sulfate. Given that sodium chloride equivalent of streptomycin sulfate is 0.07.

Solution

$$\frac{100\text{ mL}}{0.9\text{ g NaCl}} \times \frac{0.07\text{g NaCl}}{1\text{ g drug}} \times 0.3\text{g of drug} = 2.33$$

v = 2.33 mL water/0.3 g drug Answer

Practice Exercises

1. Give a formula for 1 oz. of 1% solution of silver nitrate made isotonic with lachrymal secretion, using potassium nitrate.
2. Give a formula for 4 fl oz of a 0.25% solution of cocaine hydrochloride containing 0.25% zinc sulfate and 2% boric acid made isotonic with lachrymal secretion
3. Find out the weight of sodium chloride required for 100 mL of solution isotonic with blood serum (Mol, wt. of sodium sulfate = 322, Mol. wt. of sodium chloride = 58.5).
4. Calculate the amount of sodium chloride required for dispensing this prescription

   Rx

Cocaine hydrochloride	0.15
Sodium chloride	q.s.
Purified water ad	15.0

   Make Isotonic solution

   Sig. : one drop in left eye.
5. Send 1 oz. of a solution containing 1/2 gr. of morphine hydrochloride in 20 minims, rendered isotonic with blood serum, using sodium chloride.
6. Calculate the amount of sodium chloride needed to render 4 fl 02 of 1/2 % solution of Procaine hydrochloridc, isotonic with blood serum.
7. Give the formula for 40 mL of a 2% solution of Procaine hydrochloride containing 0.5% phenol. (Molar concentration .of blood serum= 0.030%; Mol. wt. of Procaine HC1 = 272.6; Mol. wt.of phenol = 94; Mol. wt. of sodium chloride = 58.5).
8. How many grams of sodium chloride are needed to make 1 pint of 5% w/v dextrose solution isotonic?
9. Calculate the number of grains of sodium chloride to make 2 fl. oz. of 1% w/v solution of Pilocarpine HC1 isotonic.
10. A solution of anhydrous dextrose contains 20 g in 400 mL of water. Calculate the freezing point of the solution, (Mol. wt. of anhydrous dextrose = 180)
11. If the v value of silver nitrate is 1.0 calculate its sodium chloride equivalent.
12. Rx

Pilocarpine nitrate	1.75%
Dist-water q.s.	20 ml

    Mix and make isotonic buffered solution.

    Sig.2 drops in each eye q 4 h.

    V-value ofpilocarpine nitrate = 7.7 = 7.7 ml water/0.3 g drug

Answers

1. Silver nitrate- 4.375 gr; Pot nitrate- 4.46 gr; Water q.s.40mL,
2. Cocaine HC1- 4.5 gr.. Zinc sulfate- 45 gr;Boric acid- 3.5 gr.J
3. 2.31g
4. 0,105 g
5. Morphine HC1- 12 gr.. Sodium chloride- 2 gr, Water q.s 1 oz j
6. 14 gr.
7. Procaine HC1- 0.8 g; Phenol- 0.2 g, Sodium Chloride-0,116 g. Water to 40 mLJ
8. 0.473 gf
9. 6.22 grj
10. -0.52°C
11. 0.33
12. 8.99 mL

Note: For calculation of doses for children please refer next chapter.

DISPLACEMENT VALUE CALCULATION

Suppositories are prepared by incorporating medicaments in a molten base and the density of the two being unequal, it becomes necessary to calculate the displacement value of the medicament to ensure its correct amount in the suppositories. The displacement value of a medicament is defined as that proportion which displaces one part of the standard calibrating substance (oil of theobroma or cocoa butter). The displacement values as reported in literature are with reference to the oil of theobroma an hence when other bases are used such as gelato-glycerin, polyethylene glycols et. The displacement value are to be calculated accordingly.

Displacement value of medicaments

The quantity of medicament that displaces one part of cocoa butter is called displacement value. The volume of particular suppository mould is uniform but fill weight will vary according to the density of medicaments as compared with cocoa butter with which the mould was calibrated.

Determination of Displacement value

Weight of six suppositories of theobroma oil or any other base = a g

Weight of six suppositories containing, say 40 percent of drug(s) = b g

Calculate weight of theobroma oil = 60 / 100 × b = c g

Calculate drug(s) = 40/100 × b = d g

(a – c) g = the weight of theobroma oil displaced by d g of drug substances

Displacement value of the medicament = d / (a – c)

Table 4.7 Displacement Values (DV) of Solid Medicaments

Medicament	DV	Medicament	DV	Medicament	DV
Alum	2.0	Hydrocortisone	1.5	Phenol	1.0
Aminophyllin	1.5	Ichthamol	1.0	Quinine HCl	1.0
Bismuth oxynitrate	5.0	Iodoform	4.0	Resorcinol	1.5
Bismuth subgallate	2.5	Lead acetate	3.0	Salol	1.5
Boric acid	1.5	Lead Iodide	5.0	Silver Proteinate	1.5
Chloral hydrate	1.5	Mercury ointment	1.5	Tannic acid	1.0
Cinchocaine	1.5	Morphine HCl	1.5	Zinc oxide	5.0
Cocaine HCl	1.5	Opium	1.5	Zinc sulphate	2.0
Hydrocortisone	1.5	Peptone	1.5		

Example 1

Supply 12 suppositories of boric acid each weighing a 4g and containing 300 mg of boric acid.

Solution

Boric acid required for 12 suppositories = 300 x 12 = 3600 mg or 3.6 g

The displacement value of boric acid = 1.5 (given in table)

The total amount of cocoa butter displaced by boric acid = 3.6 / 1.5 = 2.4 g

Hence the quantity of the base required = (12 x 4) – 2.4 = 45.6 g

The formula for 12 suppositories would be :

Boric acid : 3.6 g

Cocoa butter : 45.6 g

Example 2

Send 12 suppositories each weighing 2 g and containing 200 mg of zinc oxide and 300 mg of bismuth oxychloride.

Solution

The displacement value of zinc oxide = 4.0

The displacement value of bismuth oxychloride is not known

The total weight of zinc oxide required = 12 x 0.2 = 2.4 g

This would displace = 2.4 / 4.0 = 0.6 g of cocoa butter

The total weight of bismuth oxychloride = 12 x 0.3 = 3.6 g

This may be taken to displace an equal weight of the base.

Thus the total weight of the base required = (12 x 2) – (0.6 + 3.6) = 19.8 g

The formula for 12 suppositories would be :

Zinc oxide	:	2.4 g
Bismuth oxychloride	:	3.6 g
Cocoa butter	:	19.9 g

Practice Exercises

1. How much of glycerin is required to produce 20 glycerin suppositories each weighing 1 g and containing 300 mg of peptone. (DV of peptone as compared with theobroma oil is 1.4 and sp. gr. of glycerin = 1.25).
2. Send 13 cocoa butter suppositories each weighing 15 g and containing 2 gr of bismuth subgallate, 1 gr of zinc oxide and balsam of peru each, and a sufficient quantity of base. (DV of bismuth subgallate – 2.7, zinc oxide – 4.0, peru balsam – 1.1).
3. Give a working formula for 12 suppositories (2 g sige) of tannic acid each containing 300 mg of tannic acid. (DV of tannic acid =1.6).

Answers

1. Peptone – 6.0 g, glycerin – 14.87 g
2. For 15 suppositories, Bismuth subgallate – 30 gr, Zinc oxide – 15 gr, Balsam of peru – 15.0 gr, theobroma oil – 196.5 gr.
3. Tannic acid – 3.6 g, Theobroma oil – 21.75 g

CHAPTER 5

POSOLOGY

The term posology (Greek *posos*, how much; and *logos*, science) is the science of doses. All Pharmacopoeias prescribe the doses of drugs for internal use. The dose is usually expressed as a range. The minimum dose or the lower limit of the dose is essential for eliciting an intended therapeutic response whereas the maximum dose or the higher limit of the dose is the amount of the drug substance that can be tolerated by an average individual. These doses are prescribed for the guidance of the prescriber. The pharmacist is much concerned with the maximum limit of the doses which, if exceeded, may cause untoward effects in the patient. The actual dose of a drug is to be decided by the prescriber depending on patient's, age, sex, symptoms, his medication history and the factors like tolerance, idiosyncrasy, route of administration etc.

Factors affecting the dose and action of drugs

These factors are discussed below.

1. **Age**

   In general, children require smaller doses than adults. Either Young's formula (based on age) or Clark's formula (based on weight) can be used for calculating the doses for children but the formula based on body surface area is more reliable.

2. **Sex**

   This is particularly important in the case of treatment with sex hormones. Female adults generally require smaller doses than males due to the presence of more body fat.

3. **Body weight**

   The usual doses for drugs are mentioned generally for 70 kg adult. The drug concentration at site of action is based on the ratio between the amount of drug administered and size of the body. The dose calculations for abnormally thin or obese patients are required to calculate on the basis of body weight.

4. **Severity of disease**

   It is a common experience that dull headache may be relieved by a single tablet of aspirin whereas severe headache may necessitate administration of 2-3 tablets of the same drug. But this is no true in all cases. For example, in case of iron deficiency anemia, the dose of iron salt administered orally remains the same irrespective of severity because there is a limit to which iron can be absorbed from the intestine daily and incorporated in haemoglobin.

5. **Health and nutrition**

   Debilitated and anaemic patients are, in general, more sensitive to the toxic effects of drugs and hence they are given in smaller doses. Persons with severe anaemia associated with hookworm infestation are more susceptible to the toxic effects of tetrachloroethylene. Myxoedematous patients are known to show less response to drugs like amphetamine because of low cellular metabolism.

6. **Pathological state**

   If the organs, through which biotransformation or excretion takes place, are diseased then smaller dose is indicated. For example, in case of renal insufficiency, phenobarbitone (mainly excreted by the kidneys) should be given in smaller dose and in case of patients suffering from liver diseases, morphine should be given in smaller dose (morphine is mainly inactivated in liver). Aspirin has no effect on normal body temperature but lowers the body temperature in fevered patients. Quinine precipitates black water fever more often with falciparum malaria than otherwise.

7. **Tolerance**

   Some children can tolerate relatively large doses of arsenic, belladonna and calomel. Tolerance can be acquired as a result of repeated administration of some drugs e.g. morphine, heroin and cocaine.

8. **Simultaneous administration of two or more drugs**

   a. **Addition :** When two or more drugs given together produce the same effect is the algebric sum of their individual effects e.g. carbachol and acetycholine.

   b. **Synergism :** In synergism, the effect produced is greater than the algebric sum of the effects due to individual drugs e.g. adrenaline and cocaine.

   c. **Antagonism :** When two drugs having opposite effect e.g. the use of amphetamine to correct partially the sedation caused by anticonvulsant does of phenobarbital and the administration of ephedrine to correct hypotension resulting from spinal anesthesia.

9. **Route of administration**

   In general, the rapidity of absorption of a drug decreases with route of administration in the following order:

   Intravenous > Intramuscular > Subcutaneous > Oral

   Thus, in general, intravenous (intravenous) dose of a drug is smaller than its intramuscular (intramuscular) or subcutaneous or oral dose.

   Example : Doses of ergotamine for various routes are as follows.

   Oral : 2 to 5 mg

   Intramuscular : 1 mg (about to 1/2 of oral dose)

   Intravenous : 0.25 mg (about to 1/8 of oral dose and ¼ of IM dose)

10. **Time and frequency of drug administration**

    Biological half-life of a drug i.e. the time required for the blood level to drop down to 50 % of the initial peak level, is the main factor governing frequency of drug administration. For example, if the biological half-life of sulphadiazine is 4 hours, 1 g of the drug has to be given every 4 hours after initial dose of 2 g. But in certain instances e.g. reserpine as a tranquiliser, biological half-life of a drug has no relation to frequency of administration.

11. **Idiosyncracy**

    Morphine normally it depresses central nervous system but may produce excitation in some individuals, specially women

12. **Allergy**

    Penicillin may produce anaphylactic shock (sudden fall of blood pressure) in allergic patients but not in normal patients.

    The doses of commonly used drugs are given in the Indian Pharmacopoeia.

CALCULATION OF DOSE

Dose represents the amount of a drug to be administered or taken by the patient for therapeutic effect. The dose may be expressed as –

Single dose : The amount of drug taken one time.

Divided dose : The amount of drug is taken two or more times in a day depending on the characteristics of the drug, types of diseases and severity of diseases.

Total dose : The amount of drug is taken during the complete therapy.

Dose calculation varies with age, weight, sex, surface area, disease condition etc. of the patient. Because of these variables the Pharmacopoeia prescribe the “average adult dose” or the "usual adult dose" for official drugs. Therefore the adult dose as mentioned in the Pharamcopoeia may also vary depending on the various factors to be considered by the prescriber, the physician.

For calculating the doses for children the following methods are used :

I. Methods based on age of child :

A. Young's Formula: The formula is most useful for the calculating the doses for children under 12 years of age.

Formula :

$$\frac{\text{Age in Years}}{\text{Age} + 12} \times \text{Adult dose} = \text{Dose for the child}$$

Example 1:

If the usual adult dose of drug is 60 mg, what is the dose for (a) a child of 6 years (b) a child of 8 years

According to Young's Formula

[a] Dose of child $= \frac{6}{6+12} \times 60 = 20$ mg

[b] Dose of child $= \frac{8}{8+12} \times 60 = 16$ mg

Answer (a) 20 mg (b) 16 mg

B. Dilling's Formula : The formula is most useful for the calculating the doses for children in between 4 to 20 years of age.

Formula : $\frac{\text{Age in Years}}{20} \times \text{Adult dose} = \text{Dose for the child}$

Example 2:

If the adult dose of Allopurinol is 200 mg, what is the dose for (a) a child of 12 years (b) a child of 16 years

According to Dilling's Formula

[a] Dose for child $= \frac{12}{20} \times 200 = 120$ mg

[b] Dose for child $= \frac{16}{20} \times 200 = 160$ mg

Answer (a) 120 mg (b) 160 mg

C. Cowling's Formula

Formula : $$\frac{\text{Age at next birthday in years}}{24} \times \text{Adult dose} = \text{Dose for the child}$$

or $$\frac{\text{Age in years} + 1}{24} \times \text{Adult dose} = \text{Dose for the child}$$

Example 3:

The maximum daily dose of a drug is 120mg . How much of it should be given to a child of (a) 11 years (b) 15 years

(a) Dose for the child $= \frac{11 + 1}{24} \times 120 = 60$ mg

(b) Dose for the child $= \frac{15 + 1}{24} \times 120 = 80$ mg

Answer (a) 60 mg (b) 80 mg

D. Fried's Formula: The formula is most useful for the calculating the doses for children under 2 years of age.

Formula : $$\frac{\text{Age in months}}{150} \times \text{Adult dose} = \text{Dose for the child}$$

Example 4:

The adult dose of a drug is 50 mg. How much of it can be to (a) a 6 month old infant (b) a 24 months old infants

(a) Dose for the child $= \frac{6}{150} \times 50 = 2.0$ mg

(b) Dose for the child $= \frac{24}{150} \times 50 = 8.0$ mg

Answer : (a) 2.0 mg (b) 8.0 mg

E Bastedo's Formula :

Formula : $$\frac{\text{Age in years} + 3}{30} \times \text{Adult dose} = \text{Dose for the child}$$

Example 5:

The adult dose of a drug is 100 mg. How much of it can be given to a patient of (a) 9 years (b) 12 years

According to Bastedo's Formula

(a) Dose for the child $= \frac{9 + 3}{30} \times 100 = 40$ mg

(b) Dose for the child $= \frac{12 + 3}{30} \times 100 = 50$ mg

Answer (a) 40 mg (b) 50 mg

II. Method Based on weight of the child

Clark's Formula

Formula : $\frac{\text{Weight in pounds}}{150} \times \text{Adult dose} = \text{Dose for the child}$

Example 6:

The adult dose of nimesulide is 100 mg. How much of it can be administered to a child weighing (a) 12 lbs (b) 15 lbs

According to Clark's Formula

(a) Dose for the child $= \frac{12}{150} \times 100 = 8$ mg

(b) Dose for the child $= \frac{15}{150} \times 100 = 10$ mg

III. Method based on body surface

The body surface area is widely used in two types of patient groups

i. Chemotherapy receiving cancer patient

ii. Pediatric patients of all childhood except premature and full-term newborns

Formula : $\frac{\text{Body surface area of a child}}{\text{Body surface area of adult}} \times \text{Adult dose} = \text{Dose for the child}$

In general the adult body surface area of an adult is considered as 1.73 m^2

$$\frac{\text{Body surface area of a child}}{1.73} \times \text{Adult dose} = \text{Dose for the child}$$

Table 5.1 Calculation of doses for children on the basis of Body Surface Area

Weight in kg	Surface area in Square meters	Percent of adult dose
2	0.15	9
3	0.20	11.5
4	0.25	14
5	0.29	16.5
6	0.33	19
7	0.37	21
8	0.40	23
9	0.43	25
10	0.46	27
15	0.63	36
20	0.83	48
25	0.95	55
30	1.08	62
35	1.20	69
40	1.30	75
45	1.40	81
50	1.51	87
55	1.58	91

Problems for Practice

1. If the dose of a drug is 100 mg, how many doses are contained in 2.0 g?
2. A cough syrup is 50 ml. The cough syrup is to be taken two teaspoonful two times a day. How many days are suitable for the given quantity?
3. A liquid medicine is prescribed three times daily by the physician, and if 120 ml are to be taken in 4 days, how many teaspoonfuls should be prescribed for each dose.
4. A liquid medicine is prescribed three times daily by the physician, and if 200 ml are to be taken in 4 days, how many teaspoonfuls should be prescribed for each dose while 5 ml of liquid medicine is loss in a day during handling of product.
5. If a cough syrup contains codeine 0.20 g in 100 ml of product. How many milligrams of codeine are contained in two teaspoonfuls?
6. One teaspoonful of elixir contains 5 mg of drug. How many milligrams drug are present in 120 ml?

7. If the usual adult dose of drug is 15 mg, what is the dose for (a) a child of 8 years (b) a child weighing 40 lbs.
8. Maximum daily dose of calomel is 250 mg. How much of it should be given to a child of (a) 12 years of age (b) weighing 35 lbs?
9. The dose of drug is 0.25 mg/kg weight/day. How many mg should be prescribed for an adult weighing 145 lbs for three days?
10. How many chloramphenicol capsule each containing 250 mg are needed to provide 25mg/kg/day for a week a patient weighing 175 lbs?
11. The dose of piperazine citrate is 50 mg/kg body weight once daily for seven consecutive days. How many ml of piperazine citrate syrup containing 500 mg/teaspoonful should be prescribed for a child weighing 33 lbs?
12. A drug is to be administrated at the rate of 0.09g /kg body weight as 2% solution. How much of the drug will be required and what quantity of solution of the given strength will be necessary for a single administration for a patient weighing 130 lbs?
13. A cough formula contains diphenhydramine HCl 14.08 mg; ammonium chloride 0.138g; sodium citrate 57.03 mg; menthol 1.14 mg and alcohol 0.0625 ml. Recommended dose for a child is 1 teaspoonful every 4 hours. Calculate the quantity of each ingredient for one-week supply.
14. A nasal solution contains xylometazoline HCl as 1% w/v solution. It is recommended to be used as 3 drops into each nostril 4 times daily. What volume of the solution should be supplied for 15 days and how much xylometazoline HCl will be required?
15. A cough formula contains 14.08 mg diphenhydramine HCl in each teaspoonful dose. How many grams of the drug will be required to prepare 5 litres of the preparation?
16. Each 15 ml (3 teaspoonfuls) of a malt tonic contains 45 mg of niacinamide. How many grains of niacinamide are present in one pound of the tonic if its weight per ml is 1.2?

Answers

1. 20 doses **2.** 6 days **3.** 2 teaspoonful **4.** 4 teaspoonful

5. 0.02 g (20 mg) **6.** 120 mg (1teaspoonful = 5 ml) **7.** (a) 6 mg (b) 4 mg

8. (a) 100 mg (b) 47 mg **9.** 49.44 mg **10.** 55.5 capsules **11.** 10.5 teaspoonful

12. 5.03 g; 265 ml

13. Diphenhydramine-591.36 mg, Ammonium chloride-5.796 g, Sodium citrate- 2395.26 mg, Menthol – 43.68 mg and alcohol-2.625 ml

14. 18 ml; 180 mg **15.** 14; g 80 mg **16.** 17.51 grains

A dispensing pharmacist must remember the doses of important drugs commonly prescribed so as to ensure accuracy in dispensing and avoiding any errors. The doses and uses of commonly prescribed drugs as per Indian Pharmacopoeia are given in the following Table for ready reference.

Table 5.2 : Doses and Uses of Different Drugs

Drug	Dose	Category
Acetazolamide	Initial dose 500 mg, subsequent doses, 250 mg every 6 hours.	Carbonic anhydrase inhibitor used in the treatment of glaucoma
Adrenaline	By s.c. or i.m. injection, 0.2 to 0.5 mg, as a single dose	Sympathomimetic
Adrenaline Bitartareate	By s.c. injection, 0.4 to 1 mg as a single dose	Sympathomimetic
Albendazole	Nematodal infection 400 mg as a single dose and cestodal infection 400 mg daily for three consecutive days	Anthelmintic
Allopurinol	Initial 100 mg daily as a single dose gradually increased to 300 mg daily. Usual maintenance dose 200 to 400 mg daily in divided doses in moderate and severe gout	Gout therapy
Alprazolam	0.25 to 0.50 mg three times daily	Anxiolytic
Aluminium Hydroxide gel	7.5 to 15 ml	Antacid
Dried Aluminium Hydroxide Gel	0.5 to 1 g	Antacid
Amantadine hydrochloride	100 mg daily, increased if necessary to 200 mg daily in divided doses	Antiviral, Antiparkinsonian
Amikacin	By .m. or slow i.v. injection or by infusion upto 1.5 g daily in two divided doses	Antibacterial
Amiloride hydrochloride	Initially 5 to 10 mg daily; maximum 20 mg daily	Diuretic
Aminocaproic acid	Orally and slow i.v. infusion, initially 5 g followed by 1 to 1.25 g every hour until bleeding is under control	Haemostatic; Antifibrinolytic

Table 5.2 : *Contd...*

Aminophyline	Orally 100 to 300 mg; by slow i.v. injection, 250 to 500 mg	Bronchodilator
Amitryptiline hydrochloride	50 to 75 mg daily, in divided doses; maintenance dose, 50 to 100mg daily, in divided doses	Antidepressant
Ammonium Chloride	3 to 6 g daily, in divided doses	Expectorant; diuretic; systemic acidifier
Amodiaquine hydrochloride	Suppressive, the equivalent of 400 mg of amodiaquine weekly. Therapeutic, the equivalent of 400 to 600 mg of amodiaquine daily for three days	Antimalarial
Amoxycillin sodium	By i.m. or i.v. injection, the equivalent of 1 to 3 g of amoxycillin daily in divided doses.	Antibacterial
Amoxycillin Trihydrate	The equivalent of 0.75 to 4.5 g of amoxycillin daily, in divided doses	Antibacterial
Amphotericin B	Orally, upto 200 mg every 6 hr. By slow i.v. injection 0.25 mg//kg body weight daily increased to 1mg/kg daily or 1.5 mg/kg on alternate days	Antifungal
Ampicillin	2 to 6 g daily, in divided doses	Antibacterial
Ampicillin Sodium	By .m. or i.v. injection, the equivalent of 1 to 3 g of ampicillin daily, in divided doses	Antibacterial
Ampicillin Trihydrate	The equivalent of 2 to 6 g ampicillin daily, in divided doses	Antibacterial
Alpha Amylase	200 to 500 mg	Digestive enzyme
Amylobarbitone	As hypnotic, 0.1 to 0.2g. As sedative, upto 0.6 g daily, in divided doses	Hypnotic and sedative
Amylobarbitone Sodium	As hypnotic, 0.1 to 0.2 g. As sedative, upto 0.6 g daily, in divided doses	Hypnotic and sedative
Analgin (Metamizol)	0.5 to 3 g daily, in divided doses	Analgesic
Ascorbic Acid	Prophylatic, 25 to 75mg daily; therapeutic, not less than 250 mg daily, in divided doses	Vitamin (antiscorbutic)

Table 5.2 : *Contd...*

Aspirin (Acetylsalicylic acid)	An analgestic and antipyretic300 to 600 mg four to six times a day; as antirheumatic –1 to 2 g four to six times a day, upto 10 g daily; as antithrombotic, 75 mg daily.	Analgesic; antipyretic, antirheumatic; antithrombotic
Astemizole	For adult 10 mg once daily upto seven days. For children, 5 mg once daily upto 7 days.	Antihistaminic
Atropine Sulphate	Orally, 0.25 to 2 mg daily in single or divided doses; by s.c., i.m. or i.v. injection, 0.4 to 0.6 mg four to six times a day	Anticholinergic; antidote to cholinesterase inhibitors
BCG (Bacillus Calmette-Guerin) Vaccine	Prophylactic, by intracutaneous injection as a single dose 0.1 ml	Active immunizing agent
Belladonna Dry Extract	15 to 60 mg	Anticholinergic
Benzylpenicillin sodium	By i.m or by slow i.v. injection or by infusion, the equivalent of 1.2 to 2.4 g of benzylpenicillin daily in 4 divided doses	Antibacterial
Bephenium Hydroxynaphthoate	5 g, as a single dose	Anthelmintic (hookworms)
Berberine Chloride	0.1g as a single dose	Bitter stomachic, anti bacterial
Betamethasone	0.5 to 5 mg daily, in divided doses	Adrenocortical steroid (anti-inflammatory)
Bethanide Sulphate	Initial dose, 10 to 20 mg daily, in divided doses	Antihypertensive
Bisacodyl	Orally, 5 to10 mg daily	Laxative
Bismuth subcarbonate	1 to 4 g	Antacid
Bleomycin sulphate	By injection, the equivalent of 15 to 30 units of bleomycin weekly, in divided doses.	Antineoplastic antibiotic
Bromhexine hydrochloride	8 to 16mg three to four times daily	Expectorant
Busulphan	2 to 4 mg daily; maintenance dose, 0.5 to 2.0 mg daily	Antineoplastic (Cytotoxic)
Caffeine	300 to 600 mg	CNS stimulant

Calcium Amino salicylate	10 to 20g daily, in divided doses	Antibacterial (tuberculostatic)
Calcium Carbonate	1 to 5 g	Antacid
Calcium Chloride	Orally, 1 to 2 g; by slow i.v. injection 5 to 10 ml of 10% w/v solution.	Calcium replenisher
Calcium folinate	Upto 120 mg in divided doses over 12 to 24 hr by i.m. or i.v. injection or infusion	Antidote to folate antagonists
Calcium Gluconate	By i.m. or i.v. injection, 1 to 2 g; orally upto 15 g daily, in divided doses.	Calcium replenisher
Calcium Lactate	Upto 8 g daily, in divided doses.	Calcium replenisher
Calcium Levulinate	By i.m. or i.v. injection 1 g once a day.	Calcium replenisher
Calcium Pantothenate	10 to 100 mg daily, in divided doses	Vitamin B (enzyme co-factor)
Dibasic Calcium Phosphate	1 to 5 g	Calcium Supplement
Captopril	Initially, 12.5 to 50 mg twice; usual maintenance dose, 25 mg twice daily; maximum, 50 mg twice daily.	Antihypertensive
Carbamazepine	200 mg daily, increasing to 1.2 g daily, in divided doses, as per the needs of the patient	Anticonvulsant
Carbenicillin sodium	By i.v. injection, the equivalent of 12 to 30 g of carbenecillin daily in divided doses.	Antibacterial
Carbenoxolone sodium	300 mg daily, in divided doses for 1 week; subsequently, upto 150 mg daily, in divided doses	Ulcer-healing drug in gastric ulcer
Carbidopa	10 to 25 mg in combination with Levodopa	Antiparkinsonian with Levodopa
Castor Oil	5 to 15 ml	Laxative
Cefadroxil	0.5 to 2.0 g daily, in divided doses.	Antibacterial
Cefazolin sodium	By i.m. or i.v. injection or infusion 1 to 4 g daily, in divided doses.	Antibacterial
Cefotaxime sodium	By i.m. or i.v. injection, the equivalent of 1 to 2 g of cefataxime every 8 to 12 hr.	Antibacterial

Table 5.2 : *Contd...*

Ceftazidime	By i.m. or slow i.v. injection or i.v. infusion, 1 to 2 g, every 8 to 12 hr.	Antibacterial
Cefuroxime sodium	Orally, 250 mg twice daily; by i.m. or i.v. injection or i.v. infusion 0.75 to 1.5 g every 6 to 8 hr.	Antibacterial
Cephalexin	1 to 4 g daily, in divided doses	Antibacterial
Cephaloridine	By i.m., i.v. or deep s.c. injection, 1 to 4 g daily in divided doses.	Antibacterial
Chloral Hydrate	0.3 to 2 g	Hypnotic & sedative
Chlorambucil	0.10 to 0.20 mg/kg of body weight daily for 4 to 8 weeks	Cytotoxic
Chloramphenicol	For an adult, 1.5 to 3g daily, in divided doses; for a child, 25 to 50mg/kg body weight daily, in divided doses	Antibacterial
Chloramphenicol Palmitae	For an adult, the equivalent of 1.5 to 3.0 g daily, in divided doses; for a child, the equivalent of 25 to 50 mg/kg of body weight daily, in divided doses	Antibacterial
Chloramphenical Sodium Succinate	By i.v. injection, the equivalent of 3 to 4 g of chloramphenicol daily, in divided doses	Antibacterial
Chlordiazepoxide	10 to 100 mg daily, in divided doses	Anxiolytic
Chloroquine Phosphate	In treatment of malaria; suppressive, 500 mg weekly, therapeutic, initial dose 1g subsequent doses, 500 mg daily In treatment of amoebiasis 500mg 3 times a day for 2 week, than 750 mg 2 times a week for several months	Antimalarial, antiprotozoal
Chloroquine Sulphate	In treatment of malaria; suppressive, 400mg weekly; therapeutic, 400mg to 1.2g daily In treatment of amoebiasis; 400 to 800mg daily in divided doses	Antimalarial, antiamoebic
Chlorpheniramine Maleate	Orally, 4 to 16 mg daily, in divided doses. By s.c. or i.m. injection, 10 to 20 mg; maximum 40 mg in 24 hr.	Antihistaminic

Table 5.2 : *Contd...*

Chlorpromazine hydrochloride	Orally, 75 to 300 mg daily, in divided doses; by i.m. injection, 25 to 50 mg. As antiemetic, orally, 10 to 25 mg every four hr; by i.m. injection 25 to 50 mg every 3 to 4 hr.	Antipsychotic; antiemetic
Chlorpropamide	100 to 500 mg daily	Antidiabetic (Hypoglycemic)
Chlorthalidone	50 to 200 mg daily	Diuretic
Cholera Vaccine	Over 10 years Prophylactic. By s.c. injection, initial dose 0.5 ml; second dose, 1.0 ml after an interval of 4 to 6 weeks. For children 2 to 10 years, initial dose 0.3 ml; second dose, 0.3 ml after an interval of 4 to 6 weeks. For 1 to2 years, initial dose, 0.2 ml; second dose 0.2 ml.	Active immunizing agents
Cimetidine	Oral, 200 mg increasing to 400 mg when necessary, 3 times a day, and 400 mg at night; by i.v. injection, 200 mg every 4 to 6 hr. Oral and parenteral dose should not exceed 2 g daily	H_2- receptor antagonist
Ciprofloxacin	Orally, 250 to 750 mg twice daily; by i.v. infusion. 100 mg to 200 mg twice daily.	Antibacterial
Cisplatin	By i.v. infusion, 15 to 20 mg per sq. m. of body surface daily for 5 days	Cytotoxic
Clofazimine	For leprosy, previously untreated patients, 100 mg 3 times weekly; For sulphone-resistant patients 100 mg 6 times weekly. For suppression of lepra reactions, 200 mg daily	antibacterial (Antileprotic)
Clofibrate	Upto 2 g daily, in divided doses	Antihyperlipedemic
Clonidine hydrochloride	Orally 0.50 to 0.10 mg three times daily increased gradually according to the needs and response of the patient maximum daily dose 1.2 mg.	Antihypertensive
Cloxacillin Sodium	The equivalent of 500 mg of cloxacillin every 6 hr, at least 30 minutes before food: by i.m. injection; 250mg every 4 to 6 hr	Antibacterial

Table 5.2 : *Contd...*

Codeine phosphate	30 to 60 mg every 4 hr when necessary, to a maximum of 200 mg daily.	Analgesic; antidiarrhoeal; cough suppressant
Colchicine	Initial dose, 1 mg; subsequent doses, 0.5 mg every 2 hr	Gout suppressant
Cortisone Acetate	Orally, 25 to 37.5 mg daily, in divided doses; by i.m. injection 50 to 400 mg daily in single or divided doses.	Adrenocortical steroid (anti-inflammatory)
Cyanocobalamin	In treatment of megaloblastic anemia by i.m. injection, 1 to 2 mg, in divided doses, in the first week. Subsequent doses, 0.25 mg weekly until the blood count is normal, maintenance dose, 0.25 mg every 3 or 4 weeks	B group vitamin; haematopoietic
Cyclizine hydrochloride	25 to 50 mg	Antiemetic
Cyclophosphamide	Orally or by i.v. injection 100 to 150 mg daily	Antineoplastic immunosuppressive
Cycloserine	0.50 to 1.0 g daily, in divided doses	Antibacterial (tuberculostatic)
Cyproheptadine hydrochloride	4 to 20 mg daily, in divided doses	Antihistaminic
Danazol	200 to 800 mg daily, in divided doses	Antigonadotrophin
Dapsone	100 mg daily	Antileprotic
Dehydroemetine hydrochloride	By deep i.m. injection, 60 to 90 mg daily	Antiamoebic
Demethylchlortetracycline hydrochloride	0.6 to 1.8 g daily, in divided doses	Antibacterial
Desoxycortisone Acetate	By i.m. injection, 2 to 5 mg daily	Adrenocortical steroid (Salt regulating)
Dexamethasone	0.5 to 10 mg daily, in divided doses	Adrenocortical steroid (anti-inflammatory)
Dexamethasone Sodium Phosphate	By i.v. or i.m. injection, the equivalent of 12 to 32 mg of dexamethasone phosphate, in treatment of acute adrenal in sufficiently	Adrenocortical steroid (anti-inflammatory)

Table 5.2 : *Contd...*

Diazepam	In anxiety, 2 mg thrice daily, increased if necessary to 15 to 30 mg daily, in divided doses	Anxiolytic; Anticonvulsant, sedative
Diclofenac sodium	Orally or by i.m. injection, 25 to 75 mg	Analgesic; anti-inflammatory
Diethylcarbamazine Citrate	150 to 500 mg daily	antifilarial, anthelmintic
Digitoxin	Initial dose, 1 to 1.5mg, divided over 24 to 48 hr; maintenance dose, 0.05 to 0.2 mg daily	Cardiotonic (Cardiac glycoside)
Digoxin	Initial dose, 1 to 1.5 mg maintenance dose, 0.25 mg once or twice daily. By i.v. injection, initial dose, 0.5 to 1 mg	Cardiotonic (Cardiac glycoside)
Di-iodohydroxyquinoline	1 to 2 g daily, in divided doses	Antiamoebic
Diloxanide Furoate	1.5 g daily, in divided doses	Antiamoebic
Diltiazem hydrochloride	Initially, 30 to 60 mg trice daily; maximum, 480 mg daily	Antianginal; calcium-channel blocker
Dimenhydrinate	25 to 100 mg	Antiemetic
Dimercaprol	By i.m. injection, 2 to 3 mg/kg body weight every 4 hr during first day and subsequently in accordance with the needs of the patient	Antidote in heavy metal poisoning, metal complexing agent
Diphendydramine hydrochloride	50 to 200 mg daily, in divided doses	antihistaminic
Diphenoxylate hydrochloride	5 to 30 mg daily, in divided doses	Antidiarrhoeal
Diptheria Antioxin	By s.c. or i.m. injection, prophylactic, 500 to 2000 international units; therapeutic, not less than 10,000 international units	Immunising agent
Diptheria and Tetanus Vaccine (Adsorbed)	By deep i.m. injection, two injections of 0.5 ml, 4 to 6 weeks apart, and a third reinforcing dose of 0.5 ml, 6 to 8 months later	Immunising agent
Diptheria, Tetanus and Pertussis Vaccine (Adsorbed)	By i.m. injection, three injections of 0.5 ml, 4 to 6 weeks apart, and a fourth, reinforcing dose of 0.5 ml, 6 to 8 months later	Active immunising agent

Table 5.2 : *Contd...*

Doxycycline hydrochloride	Initial, the equivalent of 0.2 g of doxycycline; subsequent doses, the equivalent of 0.1g of doxycycline daily	antibacterial
Disulfiram	500 mg as a single dose for 1 to 2 weeks; maintenance dose, 125 to 500 mg daily	Used in the treatment of alcoholism
Doxepin hydrochloride	Initially, the equivalent of 75 mg of doxepin daily, in divided doses; increased gradually to a maximum of 300 mg daily, in divided doses.	Antidepressant
Dydrogesterone	10 mg twice daily	Progestogen
Emetine hydrochloride	By s.c. or i.m. injection, 30 to 60 mg daily	antiamoebic
Enalapril maleate	Initial, 2.5 to 5.0 mg daily; maintenance dose, 10 to 20 mg daily; maximum 40 mg daily	Antihypertensive; angiotension-converting enzyme inhibitor
Ephedrine	15 to 60 mg	Sympathomimetic; brochodilator
Ergocalciferol	In prevention of rickets, not more than 20 g (800 Units) daily, allowance being made for Vitamin D obtained from other sources. In treatment of rickets and osteomalacia, 0,125 to 1.25 mg (5000 to 50,000 Units) daily. In treatment of hypoparathyroidism, 1.25 to 5 mg (50,000 to 200,000 Units) daily	Vitamin D (antirachitic)
Ergometrine Maleate	By i.m. injection, 0.25 to 1 mg; by i.v. injection, 0.1 to 0.5 mg	Oxytocic (Uterine stimulant)
Ergotamine Tartrate	1 to 2 mg; by s.c. or i.m. injection, 0.25 to 0.50 mg.	Sympatholytic; antimigraine drug
Erythromycin	1 to 2 g daily, in divided doses	Antibacterial
Erythromycin Estolate	The equivalent of 1 to 2 g of erythromycin daily, in divided doses for not more than 10 days	Antibacterial
Erythromycin Stearate	The equivalent of 1 to 2g of erythromycin daily, in divided doses for not more than 10 days	Antibacterial

Table 5.2 : *Contd...*

Ethacrynic Acid	50 to 200 mg daily, in divided doses	Diuretic
Ethambutol hydrochloride	15 to 25 mg/kg body weight daily, for 2 months, followed by 25mg/kg body weight daily	Antitubercular
Ethionamide	0.5 to 1 g daily, in divided doses	Antitubercular
Ethosuximide	500 mg daily, in divided doses increasing to 2 g, as necessary; for a child, 50 to 125 mg twice daily, increasing to 250 mg three to four times daily, as necessay	Anticonvulsant
Ehtyloestrenol	2 to 4 mg daily	Anabolic steroid
Ethylmorphine hydrochloride	6 to 30 mg	Narcotic analgesic
Fenfluramine hydrochloride	Initially, 20 mg morning and evening, increasing to a maximum of 80 mg twice daily, in divided doses	Appetite suppressant
Ferrous Fumerate	0.2 to 0.3 gm	Haematinic
Ferrous Gluconate	Prophylactic, 600 mg daily. Therapeutic, 1.2 to 1.8 g daily, in divided doses	Haematinic
Ferrous Sulphate	0.2 to 0.3g	Haematinic
Dried Ferrous Sulphate	Prophylactic, 200 mg daily; therapeutic, 400 to 600 mg daily, in divided doses	Haematinic
Fluorouracil	By i.v. injection, 3 mg/kg daily for 4 days followed by 6 mg/kg on alternate days, to a maximum of 800 mg daily	Cytotoxic
Fluphenazine hydrochloride	1 to 2 mg daily in single or divided doses (in anxiety states). Upto 15mg daily, in divided doses (for treatment of schizophrenia).	Antipsychotic
Folic Acid	In treatment of megaloblastic anaemia associated with folic acid deficiency, 5 to 20 mg daily. In the prophylaxis of megaloblastic anaemia of pregnancy, 0.2 to 0.5 mg daily	Vitamin B (haematopoietic)
Frusemide	Orally, in oedema, 20 to 40 mg daily; in oliguvria, 250 mg 4 to 6 times daily.	Diuretic

Table 5.2 : *Contd...*

Furazolidone	400 mg daily, in divided doses	Antibacterial, antiprotozoal, Antifungal
Gas Gangrene Antioxin (Cedematiens)	By i.v. or i.m. injection, prophylactic, 10,000 International Units; therapeutic, not less than 30,000 International Units	Immunising agant
Gasgangrene Antitoxin (Perfringens)	By i.v. or i.m. injection, prophylactic, 10,000 International Units; therapeutic, not less than 30,000 International Units	Immunising agant
Gas Gangrene antitoxin (Septicum)	By i.v. or i.m. injection, prophylactic, 5,000 International Units; therapeutic, not less than 15,000 International Units	-do-
Mixed Gas-gangrene Antioxin	By i.v. or i.m. injection, prophylactic, 25,000 International Units; thereapeutic, not less than 75,000 International Units	-do-
Gentamycin Sulphate	By i.m. injection, 80 to 240mg of gentamycin (80,000 to 240,000 Units) daily, in divided doses	Antibacterial
Glibanclamide	5 mg daily, adjusted according to response; maximum 15 mg daily, after food	Hypoglycaemic
Glyceryl Trintrate (Nitroglycerin) Tablets	Glyceryl Trinitrate, 0.5 to 1m.g. Usual strengths 0.25mg; 0.3mg; 0.5mg; 0.6mg	Vasodilator (coronary)
Griseofulvin	0.5 to 1 g daily in divided doses	Antifungal
Guanethidine Sulphate	Initial dose, 10 to 20 mg daily; subsequent doses, increasing daily at weekly intervals to a maximum of 300 mg daily, in accordance with the needs of the patient	Antihypertensive
Guaiphenesin	For an adult 200 to 400 mg every hr	Expectorant
Heloperidol	Orally, 1.5 to 20 mg daily, in divided doses; by i.m. or i.v. injection, 2 to 10 mg.	Antipsychotic
Heparin Sodium	For treatment, by i.v. injection, 20,000 to 50,000 units daily, For prophylaxis by s.c. injection, 10,000 to 15,000 units daily, in divided doses	Anticoagulant

Table 5.2 : *Contd...*

Hepatitis B virus vaccine	Single dose of liquid vaccine containing not less than 20 μg of surface antigen per adult dose. The primary immunization schedule employs 3 intramuscular injections at monthly intervals. To maintain good immunity, a booster dose is recommended every 5 years following primary immunization.	Active immunizing agent
Hydrallazine hydrochloride	Oral, 10 mg 4 times a day, gradually increased upto 50 mg 4 times a day, by i.v. or i.m. injection, 20 to 40 mg, repeated as necessary.	Antihypertensive
Hydrochlorothiazide	25 to 100 mg	Diuretic
Hydrocortisone	In treatment of adrenocortical insufficiency, 10 to 40mg daily	Adrenocortical steroid (anti-inflammatory)
Hydroxycobalamin	In treatment of megaloblastic anaemia, by i.m. injection, 1 to 2 mg, in divided doses, in the first week; subsequent doses, 250 g weekly until the blood count is normal; maintenance dose, 1mg every two months	Vitamin B_{12} (haematopoietic)
Hydroxyethyithe ophyline	100 to 300mg by mouth or by i.v. or i.m. injection	Smooth muscle relaxant (bronchiolar)
Ibuproten	0.6 to 1.2 g daily, in divided doses after food	Analgesic and anti-inflammatory
Imipramine hydrochloride	50 to 150 mg daily, in divided doses	Antidepressant
Indomethacin	Orally, 50 to 200 mg daily, in divided doses, with food	Anti-inflammatory and analgesic
Insulin	By s.c., i.m. or i.v. injection, or i.v. infusion, in accordance with the needs of the patient	Hypoglycaemic
Iron and Ammonium Citrate	1 to 3 g	Haematinic
Iron Dextran injection	By deep i.m. injection, 1 to 2ml daily	Haematinic

Table 5.2 : *Contd...*

Isoniazid	300 mg daily or upto 1 g twice weekly	Antibacterial (tubeculostatic)
Isoprenaline hydrochloride	By subcutaneous or i.m. injection, 200 g: by i.v. injection, 10 to 20 g; 2mg by infusion in Dextrose injection according to the needed of the patient	Adrenergic (bronchodilator)
Isoprenaline Sulphate	5 to 20 mg daily	Adrenergic (bronchodilator and cardiac stimulant)
Diluted Isosorbide Dinitrate	20 to 300mg of isosorbide dintrate daily, in divided doses	Anti-anginal (Vasodilator)
Isoxsuprine hydrochloride	Oral, 10 to 20 mg, 3 or 4 times daily; by i.m. injection, 5 to 10mg 3 times daily	Peripheral vasodilator (uterine relaxant)
Ispaghula Husk	3 to 5 g	Laxative
Kanamycin sulphate	By i.m. injection, the equivalent of 0.5 to 1 g (500,000 to 1,000,000 units) to kanamycin base daily in divided doses	Antibacterial
Ketoprofen	100 to 200 mg daily, in 2 to 4 divided doses, with food.	Anti-inflammatory; analgesic
Light Kaolin	15 to 75 g	Adsorbent (in treatment of diarrhoea)
Lanatoside C Laptazol	For rapid digitalisation, 1 to 1.5mg in single or divided doses. For maintenance 0.25 to 0.75 mg daily 50 to100mg	Cardiotonic CNS stimulant
Levodopa	Initial, 125 to 500 mg daily, in divided doses, after meals, increasing gradually in accordance with he needs if the patient, maintenance dose 2.5 to 8 g daily	Antiparkinsonian
Lignocaine hydrochloride	As local anaesthetic, upto 200mg or 500 mg as a single dose, when given with adrenaline. For treatment of cardiac arrhythmias, by intravenous injection, 50 to 100 mg	Local anesthetic; cardiac depressant

Table 5.2 : *Contd...*

Lincomycin hydrochloride	The equivalent of 1.5 g of lincomycin, in divided doses, 30 minutes before food. By i.m. injection, the equivalent of 0.6 to 1.2 g of lincomycin daily, in 2 doses. By i.v. infusion, the equivalent of 600 mg of lincomycin every 8 hr	Antibacterial
Lithium Carbonate	0.25 to 1.6 g daily, in divided doses	Antidepressant
Lomustine	120 to 130 mg per sq. m. body-surface every 6 to 8 weeks	Cytotoxic
Magaldrate	800 mg to 1.6 g	Antacid
Lynestrenol	2.5 to 15 mg daily	Progestin
Milk of Magnesia	As an antacid, 5 to 10ml; as a laxative, 15 to 30ml	Laxative; antacid
Heavy Magnesium Carbonate	As an antacid, 0.3 to 0.6 g; as a laxative, 2 to 4g	Osmotic laxative; antacid
Light Magnesium Carbonate	As antacid, 300 to 600 mg; as laxative, 2 to 4 g	Osmotic laxative; antacid
Heavy Magnesium Oxide	As gastric antacid, 0.3 to 0.6g; as a laxative, 2 to 4g	Antacid, laxative
Light Magnesium Oxide	As gastric antacid, 0.3 to 0.6g; as a laxative, 2 to 4g	Antacid, laxative
Magnesium Sulphate	2 to 16 g	Cathartic
Magnesium Trislicate	0.5 to 2g repeated in accordance with the needs of the patient	Antacid
Massies Vaccine Live	Pediatric, by s.c. injetion, 0.5 ml of reconstituted vaccine	Active immunising agent
Mebendazole	For threadworm infestation, 100 mg as a single dose; for other infestations, 100 mg twice daily for tow days	Antihypetensive
Mecamylamine hydrochloride	Initial dose, 5mg daily, in divided doses; subsequent doses, in accordance with the needs of the patients.	Antihypertensive
Meclizine hydrochloride	25 to 50 mg	Antihistaminic; anti-emetic
Megestrol acetate	40 to 320 mg daily, in divided doses	Progestogen

Table 5.2 : *Contd...*

Mephenesin	By i.v. infusion 0.1 to 1g	Skeletal muscle relaxant
Meprobamate	0.4 to 1.2g daily, in divided doses	Sedative
Mepyramine Meleate	0.3 to 0.6g daily, in divided doses. By i.m. or i.v. injection, 25 to 50mg	Antihistaminic (H_1 receptor antagonist)
Mestranol	0.05 to 0.15mg daily, usually in conjunction with a progestogen	Estrogen
Metformin hydrochloride	0.5 to 2.0 g daily, in divided doses	Oral hypoglycaemic
Methadone hydrochloride	Oral, 5 to 10mg. By s.c. injection, 5 to 10mg	Narcotic analgesic; narcotic abstinence syndrome suppressant
Methandienone	Adults, 5 to 10 mg daily; children, 0.5 to 10mg daily	Anabolic steroid, weak androgen
Methotrexate	5 to 100mg at suitable intervals	Antineoplastic; antipsoriatic
Methylamphytamine hydrochloride	2.5 to 10mg. By i.m. or i.v. injection, 10 to 30 mg	Adrenergic; central stimulant
Methyldopa	The equivalent of 0.5 to 3g of anhydrous methyldopa, daily, in divided doses	Antihypertensive
Mehylrgometrine Meleate	By s.c., i.m., or .v. injection, 0.1 to 0.2 mg	Uterine stimulant; oxytocic
Metoprolol tartrate	100 to 450 mg daily, in divided doses; the initial dose should not exceed 100 mg daily	Bet-adrenoceptor antagonist
Metronidazole	For trichomoniasis, 200 mg 3 times daily, for 7 days. For amoebiasis, 400mg 3 times daily, for 5 to 10 days. For girardiasis, 2g daily for 3 successive days for adults 1g for children and 400mg daily for infants	Antiamoebic; antitrichomonal; anit-giardial
Mianserin hydrochloride	30 to 90 mg daily, in divided doses	Antidepressant
Morphine hydrochloride	10 to 20 mg	Narcotic, analgesic
Morphine Sulphate	10 to 20 mg	Narcotic, analgesic
Nalidixic Acid	2 to 4 g daily, in four divided doses	Antibacterial
Nalorphine	By i.v. injection, 5 mg, repeated	Antidote for narcotic

Table 5.2 : *Contd...*

hydrochloride	twice at 3 minutes intervals if necessary	analgesics
Neomycin Sulphate	For systemic use, the equivalent of 0.7 to 2.0 g of neomycin base daily in divided doses	Antibacterial (topical and systemic)
Neostigmine Bromide	15 to 30 mg, 3 to 6 times a day	Chlonergic
Niclosamide	2 g as a single dose after a light breakfast followed by a purgative 2 hr later	Anthelmintic (teniacide)
Nicotinamide	Prophylatic, 15 to 30mg daily; therapeutic, 50 to 250mg daily. By i.v. injection, 50 to 250mg daily	B-group vitamins;
Nicoumalone	Initial dose, first day, 8 to 12 mg, second day, 4 to 8 mg; maintenance dose, 1 to 8 mg daily.	Anticoagulant
Nifedipine	Initial dose, up to 30 mg daily, in divided doses	Coronary vasodilator, antianginal
Nicotinic Acid	Prophylactic, 15 to 30 mg daily; therapeutic, 50 to 250 mg daily	B-group vitamin; vasodilator
Nikethamide	By s.c., i.m., or i.v. injection, 0.25 to 2 g 50 to 150 mg 4 times daily	Respiratory stimulant Antibacterial (urinary)
Nitrazepam	5 to 10 mg daily, at a bed time	Hypnotic; sedative
Nitrofurantoin	50 to 150 mg four times daily	Antibacterial
Noradrenaline Acid Tartrate	By intravenous infusion, 2 to 20 g per minute, according to the blood pressure of the patient	Adrenergic (vasopressor)
Norethisterone	5 to 20mg daily, in single or divided doses	Progestin
Noscapine	15 to 30mg	Antitussive
Novobiocin Sodium	The equivalent of 1 to 2g of novobiocin daily, in divided doses	Antibacterial
Nystatin	In treatment of alimentary moniliasis, 1 to 2 million units daily in divided doses	Antifungal
Omeprazole	20 to 40 mg daily; For Zollinger-Ellison syndrome, initially 60 mg once daily; usual range, 20 to 120 mg daily.	Antiulcerative

Table 5.2 : *Contd...*

Oestradiol Benzoate	By i.m. injection, 1 to 5 mg daily	Oestrogenic hormone
Oestradiol Dipropionate	By i.m. injection, initial 1 to 5 mg every 1 to 2 weeks, maintenance, 1 to 2.5 mg every 10 days to 2 week	Oestrogenic hormone
Opium	25 to 200 mg	Hypnotic, sedative; narcotic; analgesic
Oxyphenbutazone	200 to 400 mg daily, in divided doses	Anti-inflammatory; analgesic
Oxyphenonium Br	5 to 10mg	Anticholinergic
Oxytracycline	1 to 2 g daily, in divided doses	Antibacterial
Oxytracycline hydrochloride	1 to 2 g daily, in divided doses. By i.v. infusion, in a concentration 0.1% w/v, 1 to 2 g daily	Antibacterial
Pancreatin	0.50 to 1.0 g	Digestive enzyme
Papain	120 to 600 mg	Proteolytic enzyme
Paracetamol	0.5 to 1 g; up to 4 g daily, in divided doses	Analgesic; antipyretic
Paraldehyde	By i.m. injection, 2 to 8 ml. By rectal injection, 15 to 30ml suitably diluted	Hypnotic; sedative; anticonvulsant
Paramethadione	0.9g daily, in divided doses, increasing to 1.8g in accordance with the needs of the patient	Anticonvulsant
Benzylpenicillin	By i.m. or i.v. injection 500,000 to 1,000,000 units daily, in divided doses	Antibacterial
Pentobarbitone Sodium	0.1 to 0.2g	Hypnotic; sedative; narcotic; analgesic
Pepsin	0.3 to 1 g	Proteolytic enzyme
Phenformin hydrochloride	25 to 100 mg. By s.c. or im. injection, 25 to 100 mg; by i.v. injection 25 to 50 mg	Analgesic
Phenformin hydrochloride	50 to 200 mg daily, in divided doses	Oral hypoglycaemic agent
Phenindamine Tartrate	75 to 150 mg daily, in divided doses	Antihistaminic
Phenindamine Maleate	25 to 50 mg daily, in divided doses	Antihistaminic

Table 5.2 : *Contd...*

Phenobarbitone	Upto 350 mg daily, in divided doses	Hypnotic; sedative; anti-convulsant
Phenobarbitone Sodium	Upto 350 mg daily, in divided doses. By i.v., i.m. or s.c. injection, 50 to 200 mg	Hypnotic; sedative
Phenoxymethyl penicillin Potassium	The equivalent of 0.5 to 1.5g of phenoxymethylpenicillin daily, in divided doses	Antibacterial
Phenylbutazone	100 to 600 mg daily, in divided doses	Anti-inflammatory analgesic
Phenylephrine hydrochloride	By s.c. or i.m. injection, 5mg; by i.v. injection, 0.5mg	Adrenergic (vasopressor)
Phenytoin Sodium	50 mg daily, increasing to 400mg; by i.m. or slow i.v. injection, up to 250 mg in accordance with the needs of the patient	Anticonvulsant
Phthalylsulphathiazole	5 to 10 mg daily, in divided doses	Antibacterial (intestinal)
Physostigmine Salicylate	0.6 to 1.2 mg	Anticholinesterase
Piperazine Citrate	For threadworms 0.6 to 4.5 g daily in divided doses. For roundworms, up to 5 g in a single dose according to the age of the patient	Anthelmintic
Piroxicam	10 to 20 mg daily	Analgesic, Antiinflammatory; antipyretic
Plague Vaccine	By s.c. injection, 1ml (first dose); 1 ml (second dose) after an interval of 7 to 10 days. A single dose of 3 ml may be given in emergency	Active immunizing agent
Potassium Bromide	0.3 to 1.2 g	Sedative; anticonvulsant
Potassium Chloride	1 to 2 g	Electrolyte replenisher
Potassium Citrate	4 to 10 g	Systemic alkaliniser
Potassium Iodide	As expectorant, 250 to 500mg. In pre-operative treatment of thyrotoxicosis, 30 to 60mg	Antifungal; expectorant; source of iodine
Prednisolone	Upto 30 mg daily, in divided doses	Adrencocortical steroid (anti-inflammatory)

Table 5.2 : *Contd...*

Prednisolone Acetate	Upto 30 mg daily, in divided doses	Adrencocortical steroid
Prednisone	Upto 30 mg daily, in divided doses	Adrencocortical steroid
Prednisone Acetate	Upto 30 mg daily, in divided doses	Adrencocortical steroid
Primaquine Phosphate	The equivalent of 15 mg of primaquine base, once a day for 14 days	Antimalarial
Primidone	0.5 to 2g daily, in divided doses	Anticonvulsant
Procaine hydrochloride	Epidural, 25ml of a 1.5% solution. Infiltration, upto 200ml of a 0.25 to 0.5% solution. Peripheral nerve block, upto 25ml of a 2% solution. Spinal, 1 to 3ml of a 3.3 to 5% solution	Local anaesthetic
Procaine Penicillin	By intramuscular injection, 0.3 to 0.9g daily	Antibacterial
Proguanil hydrochloride	As suppressant of malaria, 0.1 to 0.3g daily	Antimalarial
Promethazine hydrochloride	20 to 50mg daily, in single or divided doses	Antihistaminic; anti-emetic
Propranolol hydrochloride	20mg to 2g daily, in divided doses, the initial daily dose should not exceed 40mg; by slow i.v. injection 3 to 10mg	Adrenergic, receptor antagonist (anti-hypertensive, anti-anginal; anti-arrhythmic)
Propylthiouracil	300 to 450 mg daily, in divided doses	Antithyroid
Propyphenazone	1.5 to 3.0 g daily, in divided doses	Analgesic, antipyretic
Pyrazinamide	Upto 35 mg/kg body weight daily, in divided doses	Tuberculostatic
Pyridoxine hydrochloride	Prophylactic, 2 mg daily; therapeutic, 10 to 150 mg 1 to 3 times daily	B-group vitamin
Pyrimethamine	Suppressive, 25 mg once a week; therapeutic, 25 to 50 mg once a day for 2 days	Antimalarial

Table 5.2 : *Contd...*

Quindine Sulphate	In prophylaxis of cardiac arrhythmias 0.2g 3 or 4 times daily. In treatment of atrial fibrillation, 0.2 to 04g every 2 to 4 hr to a total dose of 3g daily	Cardiac depressant (anti-arrhythmic)
Quinine Bisulphate	In suppression of malaria, 0.3 to 0.6g daily. In treatment of malaria, 1.2 to 2g daily, in divided doses	Antimalarial
Quinine Sulphate	In suppression of malaria, 0.3 to 0.6g daily. In treatment of malaria, 1.2 to 2g daily, in divided doses	Antimalarial
Quiniodochlor	0.75 to 1.5 g daily, in divided doses	Antiprotozoal; topical and intestinal antiseptic
Rabies Vaccine	By s.c. injection, 1 to 2 ml daily, for 7 to 14 days according to the site and severity of the bit and the risk of exposure to infection	Specific immunizing agent
Ranitidine hydrochloride	Orally, the equivalent of 300 to 600 mg of ranitidine daily, in divided doses	Histamine H_2-receptor antagonist
Reserpine	In psychiatric states, 1 to 5mg daily, in divided doses. In treatment of hypertension, 0.5 mg daily	Antihypertensive
Riboflavine	Prophylactic, 1 to 4mg daily; therapeutic, 5 to 10mg daily	B-group vitamin
Rifampicin	450 to 600mg	Antibacterial
Salbutamol Sulphate	The equivalent of 6 to 16mg of salbutamol daily, in divided doses	Adrenergic (bronchodilator)
Scopolamine Hydrobromide	By s.c. injection, 300 to 600g	Anticholinergic
Smallpox Vaccine (Freeze-Dried)	For prophylaxis of smallpox, about 0.02 ml applied to the skin and inoculated by scarification or pressure	Immunizing agent

Table 5.2 : *Contd...*

Sodium Acid Phosphate	2 to 4 g	Urinary acidifier
Sodium Aminosalicylate	10 to 15 g daily, in divided doses	Antibacterial (tuberculostatic)
Sodium Antimony Gluconate	By i.m. or i.v. injection, 0.6 to 2.0 g daily, for 10 to 30 days	Systemic leishmaniacidal
Sodium Ascorbate	The equivalent of up to 1g of ascorbic acid daily	Vitamin C
Sodium Bicarbonate	1 to 4 g	Electrolyte replenisher; systemic alkaliser
Sodium Citrate	1 to 10 g	Systemic alkaliser
Sodium Lactate Injection	By i.v. infusion, as a 1/6 molar solution, at the rate of 5ml or less per minute	Fluid and electrolyte replenisher
Sodium Salicylate	0.6 to 2 g. In treatment of acute rheumatism, 5 to 10g daily, in divided doses	Analgesic, antipyretic
Sodium Thiosulphate	By i.v. or i.m. injection, 25g	Antidote to cyanide poisoning
Snake venom antiserum	Usually 20 to 50 ml, injected i.v. as soon as possible	Passive immunizing agent
Streptomycin Sulphate	By i.m. injection, the equivalent of 0.5 to 1g of streptomycin base daily, or at longer intervals. As an intestinal antiseptic, the equivalent of 0.5 g of streptomycin base every 8 hr	Antibacterial (tuberculostatic)
Succinysulphathiazol e	10 to 20 g daily, in divided doses	Antibacterial
Sulphadiazine	Initial dose 3 g; subsequent doses, upto 4g daily, in divided doses	Antibacterial
Sodium fusidate	1.5 g daily, in divided doses	Antibacterial
Sodium salicylate	0.50 to 2.0 g with food; in the treatment of acute rheumatism, 5 to 10 g daily, in divided dose	Ant-inflammatory; analgesic
Spironolactone	100 to 200 mg daily, in divided doses	Diuretic
Sulphadimethoxine	Initial dose, 1 to 2 g; subsequent dose, 500mg daily	Antibacterial
Sulphadimidine	Initial dose 3 g; subsequently upto 6 g daily, in divided doses.	Antibacterial

Table 5.2 : *Contd...*

Streptomycin sulphate	By i.m. injection, the equivalent of 500 mg to 1.0 g streptomycin daily, or at longer period	Antitubercular
Sulphadimidine Sodium	By intramuscular or i.v. injection, 1 to 2 g	Antibacterial
Sulphadoxine	Initial, 2 g by mouth; subsequent doses, 1 to 1.5 g weekly. By deep i.m. or slow i.v. injection 2.5 g initially, followed by 1.5 g after 4days	Antibacterial
Sulphamethizole	100 to 200 mg every 4 to 6 hr	Antibacterial
Sulphamethoxazole	Initial, 2g, then 1g 2 or 3 times daily	Antibacterial
Sulphaphenazole	Initial dose, 1g, every 12 hr, for 2 days; subsequent doses, 500mg every 12 hr for 3 to 5 days	Antibacterial
Testosterone Propionate	By i.m. injection, 5 to 25mg, once or twice weekly	Androgen
Tetanus Antitoxin	By s.c. or i.m. injection, prophylactic, not less than 1500 International Units; therapeutic, not less than 50,000 International Units	Immunizing agent
Tatanus Vaccine (adsorbed)	By deep i.m. injection, two injections of 0.5 ml at an interval of 4 to 6 weeks, followed by a third reinforcing dose of 0.5ml, 6 to 8 months later	Active immunizing agent
Tetracycline	1 to 3g daily, in divided doses	Antibacterial
Tetracycline hydrochloride	For adults, 1 to 3g daily, in divided doses; for children 10 to 30mg/kg body weight daily, in divided doses	Antibacterial; anti-amoebic
Thiabendazole	1.5g, twice daily for 2 or 3 days, in treatment of nematode infestation	Anthelmintic

Table 5.2 : *Contd...*

Thiacetazone	0.15g, daily	Tuberculostatic
Thiamine hydrochloride	Prophylactic, 2 to 5mg once a day; therapeutic, 25 to 100mg daily	Vitamin B_1 (enzyme co-factor)
Thiamine Mononitrate	---do---	Vitamin B_1
Thiopentone Sodium	By i.v. injection, 0.1 to 0.5g; by rectal injection, 40mg/kg body weight. Maximum dose, 2g	Anticonvulsant; general anaesthetic
Thyroid	30 to 250mg daily	Thyroid hormone
Thyroxine Sodium	0.05 to 0.3mg daily	Thyroid hormone
Tolbutamide	0.5 to 1.5g daily, in divided doses	Antidiabetic
Triamcinolone	4 top 12mg, 1 to 4 times daily	Anti-inflammatory
Triamterene	150 to 250mg daily, in divided doses	Diuretic
Trifluoperazine hydrochloride	Oral, the equivalent of 2 to 30 mg of trifluoperazine daily, in divided doses; by i.m. injection, the equivalent of 1 to 2 mg of trifluoperazine every 4 to 6 hr as required	Antipsychotic agent
Trifluopromazine hydrochloride	Oral, the equivalent of 30 to 150mg of trifluopromazine daily. By intramuscular injection, the equivalent of 5 to 10mg of trifluopromazine repeated every 4 hr, if necessary. By i.v. injection, the equivalent of 1 to 3mg of trifluopromazine repeated every 4 hr, if necessary.	Antipsychotic agent
Troxidone	For adults, 1 to 2g daily, in divided doses; for children, 0.25 to 0.5g daily in divided doses	Anticonvulsant

Table 5.2 : *Contd...*

Tubocurarine hydrochloride	By i.m. or i.v. injection, 0.1 to 0.3mg/ kg body weight, not exceeding 25mg, then 0.025 to 0.1mg/kg repeated as necessary	Skeltal muscle relaxant
Typhoid Vaccine	Prophylactic, by s.c. injection, 0.5ml as initial dose; second dose of 1ml after an interval of 4 to 6 weeks	Active immunising agent
Typhus Vaccine	Prophylactic, by s.c. injection, 0.25 to 1ml	Active immunising agent
Urea	5 to 15g	Diuretic
Vitamin A	Prophylactic, 5000 Units of Vitamin A activity, daily; therapeutic, 10,000 to 200,000 Units of Vitamin A activity daily	Antixerophthalmic Vitamin
Yellow Fever Vaccine	Prophylactic, by s.c. injection, not less than 1000 LD_{50} doses	Active immunising agent

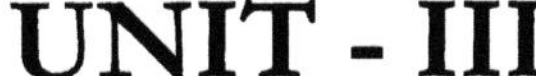
UNIT - III

CHAPTER 6

MIXTURES

Liquid dosage forms are very popular for internal administration because of the following reasons for their popularity.

1. They are more rapidly effective as compare to pills, capsule, tablets because which require previous disintegration in the body before absorption can begin.
2. Some substances can only be administered in liquid form e.g. castor oil, liquid paraffin.
3. Some substances are very effective if administered in a diffused form. For example, light Kaolin is used to adsorb toxic substances in the gut, the great surface area of the fine powder giving maximum adsorbent effect.
4. Some substances may cause pain if administered in the dry state as a powder or tablet., e.g. potassium iodide and bromide.

A Mixture is a liquid medicine for internal use, of which multiple doses are contained in a container / bottle with or without dispenser or marked cap for administration of mixture readily in proper dose.

Mixtures are immediately formulated for long life because they are mainly prescribed for acute conditions such as cough, indigestion, diarrhoea, constipation and rheumatism, for which a short period of treatment is often adequate. The most of BPC mixtures must be freshly prepared because deterioration is likely if they are stored longer than a few weeks under temperate room conditions. Therefore, they are not made more than a few days before issue and the patient is warned to discarded unused part of mixture after a specified date. There is no official recommendation, but a month from the date of issue is most appropriate for use. Some mixtures are not stable and must be freshly prepared, i.e. not more than 24 hours before issue such as Gentian Mixture, Alkaline, Phenobarbitone BPC etc. The expiry date of such preparation is two days after the date on which the last dose should have been taken. If a dose less than, or not a multiple of 5 ml is prescribed, the mixture must be diluted with suitable diluents so that the patient can measure the dose in 5 ml one spoonfuls easily and accurately. Immediate dilution is recommended because dilution of the preparation may reduce the stability before issue. It should be carried out not more than two weeks supply should be dispensed unless otherwise indicated in the monograph. On the label expiry date should be stated fortnight from the date of issue.

FORMULATION

Vehicles

The vehicle is the medium in which the excipients of a mixtures/ formulation are dissolved or dispersed. For oral liquid medicines it may be generally used such as -

1. Water

Many ingredients are very soluble in aqueous. In the formulation of mixtures, potable water or freshly boiled and cooled Purified Water may be used.

Potable water is water freshly drawn from the public mains and suitable for drinking. It must be direct from the mains because water from a local storage tank may be heavily contaminated with microorganisms and other types of contamination.

Freshly Boiled and Cooled Purified Water is used for the preparation of mixture when-

a. the only source of mains water is a local storage tank, or
b. the potable water is not suitable for a particular preparation. For example, mixtures containing ferrous sulphate are discolored by certain tap waters, especially those exhibiting temporary hardness. It must be freshly boiled and cooled to destroy vegetative bacteria of which stored purified water may have a high content.

The additional cost of purified water is not recoverable for NHS prescriptions unless-

(i) Purified Water is specified on the prescription, or
(ii) The use of potable water would cause unwanted modification in the preparation and the pharmacist endorses the prescription to this effect, or
(iii) The local Executive Council has decided that the available source of tap water is not suitable for dispensing.

2. An Aromatic Water

Aromatic waters are used mainly for their flavouring properties although some are mildly therapeutic and/or preservative in action. In the past, they are prepared by diluting a concentrated preparation with suitable volume of aromatic water from the concentrate immediately before dispensing the mixture. But this procedure is not used because other ingredients occupy a large volume, a significant quantity of vehicle is displaced with consequent reduction of preservative activity (for chloroform water) or flavour (in other instances). Now a day specified volume of aromatic water is used.

Table 6.1 Aromatic waters used in Mixtures

Name	Concentrated Preparation	Dilution parts by volume		Application
		Concentrate	Water	
Anise(aniseed) Water	Concentrated Anise Water	1	39	Flavour Carminative Mild expectorant
Camphor Water	Concentrated Camphor Water	1	39	Flavour Carminative Mild expectorant
Caraway Water	Concentrated Caraway Water	1	39	Flavour Carminative
Chloroform Water	Double strength Chloroform Water	1	1	Preservative Flavour
Cinnamon Water	Concentrated Cinnamon Water	1	39	Flavour Carminative
Dill Water	Concentrated Dill Water	1	39	Flavour Carminative (particularly for infants in gripe waters
Peppermint Water	Concentrated Peppermint Emulsion or Concentrated Peppermint Water	1	39	Flavour Carminative Weak preservative

3. A medicament

Occasionally a vehicle with definite therapeutic activity is given such as –

a. Compound Gentian Infusion - a bitter that stimulates the appetite

b. Orange Peel Infusion - bitter and carminative

c. Senega Infusion – expectorant and also used as Infusions

The infusion are generally prepared by diluting 1 part of the corresponding concentrated infusion with 9 parts of water but, as with aromatic waters, and for the same reason, it is not unusual to find in an official formula a quantity of concentrated infusion that does not correspond to this ratio. The diluted preparations of fresh infusions should be used within 12 hours. In concentrated waters made from essential oils (anise, caraway, cinnamon, dill and peppermint) the oil is dissolved in a high concentration of alcohol. Hence, on dilution with water, part of the oil is precipitated and, although the dispersion is very fine. On the label an instruction to shake the bottle is desirable. It was also found that the turbidity may develop when a concentrated infusion is diluted. The direction to shake is desirable before use. As a result of these precipitations, many mixtures are very fine suspensions rather than true solutions.

Chemical Stabilisers

Only antoxidants and reducing agents are used. The adult and pediatric mixtures of ferrous sulphate contain 0.1 percent ascorbic acid to prevent oxidation of ferrous to ferric ion because ferric salts are relatively ineffective at promoting haemoglobin formation.

Mixtures containing sodium salicylate is slightly darken during storage due to atmospheric oxidation. This is removed by adding 0.1 percent sodium metabisulphate.

Colours : No special colouririg agents are added but some mixtures are coloured because of medicaments and additives colours.

Flavours : Following flavoring agents are used in the preparation of mixtures such as –

- Aromatic waters is very popular as flavoring agent ex. Anise water
- Syrup and/or glycerol-for sweetening children's preparations.
- Liquorice Liquid Extract-for disguising the taste of saline ingredients, such as ammonium salts and alkali iodides in cough mixtures.
- Lemon Spirit- to wrap the taste of alkaline citrates.
- The metallic and astringent tastes of iron salts in children's mixtures disguise by Orange Syrup and Compound Orange Spirit.

Preservatives : Antimicrobial agents are necessary in mixture because mixtures are prepared by diluted vegetable extracts and flavouring agents provide favourable media for the growth of bacteria and, particularly, fungi. The two most useful compounds are used as preservative in mixtures.

1. Chloroform : It is generally added in the form of double-strength chloroform waterv(0·25 per cent v/v) and is a very good preservative of products containing vegetable extracts. It is widely used in mixtures due sweetening properties.
2. Benzoic Acid : It is used 0·1 per cent w/v as preservative because this compound is due to the un dissociated acid and, therefore, it is effective in acid preparations of pH 5 or below, but not in neutral or alkaline solutions. [It is only slightly and slowly soluble in water. A stock solution, containing 5 per cent of benzoic acid and 75 per cent of propylene glycol in water, is used for dispensing].

CLASSIFICATION OF MIXTURE

Mixtures are classified according to the nature of substance used in the preparation of mixtures. On the basis of substance, they are six types.

A. Simple Mixtures containing Soluble Substances only
B. Mixtures containing Diffusible Solids.
C. Mixtures containing Indiffusible Solids.
D. Mixtures containing Precipitate-forming Liquids.
E. Mixtures containing Slightly-soluble Liquids.
F. Miscellaneous Mixtures.

A. Simple Mixtures containing Soluble Substances only

Some substances are readily soluble in aqueous medium without reducing the particle size of the powder. List of some substances are given in Table 6.1. Some substances are not soluble without reducing the size upto fine particles. The list of these substance is given in Table 6.2.

Method of preparation of Simple Mixtures

The method of preparation is divided in five stage.

Stage 1 : Dissolve the solids in about three-quarters of the vehicle without reduced particle size (Table 6.2) and if used Table 6.3 substance reduced the particle size prior to add vehicle and mixed properly. The volume occupied by the other ingredients will rarely exceed the remaining one-quarter, but, if it should, the quantity of vehicle used must be reduced accordingly. Solution is hastened by using as much of the solvent as convenient.

Stage 2 : Examine the solution critically in proper light. Strain the solution through a plug of cotton-wool placed in a funnel if particles of foreign matter are visible and adjusted the volume by vehicle.

Stage 3 : Add any liquid ingredients as given in Table 6.4. After measuring each, rinse the vessel used with a little of the aqueous vehicle, and add to the contents of the measure. These are highly volatile liquids hence need to take precaution and minimize loss.

Stage 4 : Prescribed volume was produce by the prescribed vehicle. Adjustment to volume should be made in a graduated measure, because of the frequent discrepancy between the reputed and actual capacity of dispensing bottles.

Stage 5 : Transfer the mixture to the bottle and cork properly. Clean the container with soft cloth and to remove finger-marks. Put the label, wrap the bottle and address it.

Table 6.2 Readily soluble substance without powdering in the preparation of Mixture

Ammonium Bicarbonate	Ephedrine Hydro-chloride	Potassium Acetate	Sodium Citrate
Ammonium Bromide	Hexamine Homatropine	Potassium Iodide	Sodium Iodide
Ammonium Chloride	Hydrobromide Hyoscine	Potassium Bicarbonate	Sodium Nitrite
Atropine Sulphate	Ammonium Citrate	Potassium Citrate	Sodium Salicylate
Caffeine and Sodium Iodide	Lithium Citrate	Potassium Bromide	Urea
Calcium Chloride	Magnesium Sulphate	Permanganate Quinine	Strontium Bromide
Chloral Hydrate	Morphine Hydrochloride	Bisulphate Quinine	Sodium Sulphate
Citric Acid	Morphine Tartrate	Dihydrochloride Sodium	Strychnine Hydrochloride
Cocaine Hydrochloride	Acid Phosphate	Sodium Bicarbonate	Tannic Acid
Dextrose Mono-hydrate	Sodium Benzoate	Sodium Bromide	Zinc Sulphate

Table 6.3 Soluble after finely powdered in aqueous vehicle

Alum	Boric Acid	Ferrous Sulphate	Potassium Nitrate
Amidopyrin	Caffeine Citrate	Mercuric Chloride	Quinine Hydrochloride
Borax	Calcium Lactate	Potassium Chlorate	Sodium Phosphate

Table 6.4 Liquid Volatile Substances

Tincture of Chloroform	Ethereal Tincture of Lobelia B.P.C
Morphine B.P.C.	Aromatic Spirit of Ammonia B.P.C.
Ether	Compound Spirit of Orange B.P.C

Containers for Mixtures

Preferencely plain bottles should be used for mixtures. Moulded graduations on large bottles may be sufficiently accurate for ordinary mixtures. For small amount the line divisions numerous, accurate dosage cannot be obtained from the graduations-these being Moulded equidistant, regardless of the varying internal diameter of the bottle. Similarly, the measurement of doses in the domestic teaspoon or tablespoon may admit variation in size and capacity. It is therefore desirable for the patient to use a graduated medicine glass. Although the words 'teaspoonful' and ·tablespoonful' are used on such measures, they are based upon one-eighth and one-half of an ounce respectively.

In all children's mixtures, in all cases for proper dose accuracy it is necessary to call attention to the dose by underlining it and b) prefixing the word 'measured,' i. e. a measured teaspoonful. Some times mixture is not expressed in teaspoonfuls or table-spoonfuls, and in such cases it is necessary to place a narrow strip of gummed paper at the back of the bottle, and to mark thereon the level of each dose. The label should indicate the dose, e.g. one-sixth part, etc. The bottle selected should then be fitted with a cork. Unsuitable corks may be returned to stock for later use in other container. The ideal fit should leave about two-thirds of the cork projecting from the neck of the bottle, to ensure easy removal.

Exercise 1: Formula

Potassium bromide

Tincture Nux Vomica

Chloroform water

Procedure : Potassium bromide is soluble salt hence apply method for simple mixture of formulation as mentioned above. Final maintain the prescribed volume of mixture and dispensed in a suitable container with proper label.

Exercise 2: Formula

Sodium bicarbonate

Nux Vomica Tincture

Compound Gentian Infusion

Procedure : Sodium bicarbonate is soluble in water. The method of preparation is same as described in simple mixture. The concentrated infusion is eight time stronger than ordinary infusions. It is essential to mentioned dilution instruction on the label. I volume of infusion added to 7 volumes of purified water gives the ordinary strength of infusion.

B. Mixtures containing Diffusible Solids

Diffusible solids are substance which do not dissolve in water, but may be mixed therewith, so that, upon shaking, the powder is uniformly diffused throughout the liquid for sufficient time to ensure uniform distribution in each dose.

These are mainly two types –

a. Insoluble substance (Table – 6.5)
b. Slightly soluble (Table -6.6)

Substance which is slightly soluble listed in Table -6.1 because in the proportion usually prescribed, they may not completely dissolve in the vehicle. This partial solubility is, for convenience, ignored, and the substances are classified as diffusible solids, although in some ratio they may entirely dissolve. The most of substances dissolve more freely in hot water than in cold, but when the water is cooled to room temperature it may slightly come out in a crystalline form while initially dissolved substance. This must be carefully handled during the measuring of dose because of the impossibility of evenly re-diffusing the substance and also crystals are unpleasant in the mouth. For maintaining the dose accuracy any part of the substance which does not completely dissolve will be present as a fine diffusible powder in the vehicle..

Method for Diffusible Solids

Stage 1 : Powdered the substance if not already in fine powder, using a mortar; add any soluble substances, and mix properly. Add three-quarters of the vehicle into the mortar containing the powder, and triturate to form a smooth cream; then gradually add the remainder part of the vehicle. The presence of air in the interstices of many powders, particularly those of vegetable origin, causes some of the powder to float on the water. For removing this type of problem, make a smooth cream first, by adding only a small quantity of vehicle and then finally diluted.

Stage 2 : Examine the contents in the mortar

a. if only one or two foreign particles are visible, remove them with a glass rod.
b. if particles of foreign matter are visible, passed the mixture through muslin and rinse the mortar with a small amount of vehicle.

Stage 3 -5 : Same as in method for simple mixture.

Table 6.5 Diffusible Substances

Aromatic Chalk Powder	'Magnesium Carbonate Light or Heavy	'Magnesium Oxide, Light or Heavy
Bismuth Carbonate	'Light Kaolin	Magnesium Trisilicate
Bismuth Subnitrate	Compound Rhubarb Powder	Phenolphthalein
Compound Bismuth Powder	Compound Magnesium Trisilicate Powder	Quinine Sulphate
Compound Kaolin Powder	Compound Liquorice Powder	Rhubarb, powdered

Table 6.6 Substance prescribed in a quantity than Dissolve

Borax	**Caffeine citrate**	**Potassium chloride**
Boric acid	Calcium lactate	

Exercise 3: Formula

Magnesium sulphate

Magnesium carbonate

Peppermint water

Procedure : Magnesium sulphate and carbonate is diffusible solids. Dispense the formula as per diffusible solids mentioned above. Calculate exact quantity measurable and excess amount discarded accordingly.

C. Mixtures containing Indiffusible Solids.

A solid is regarded as indiffusible when it will not remain evenly distributed in the vehicle long enough to ensure uniformity of the measured dose. The vehicle must, required to increased the viscosity using suspending agent for uniform distribution of indiffusible substance. The quantity of suspending agent required depends upon the volume of the mixture. The best two suspending agents are general used for preparation of mixture.

1. Compound Tragacanth Powder (2 percent)
2. Tragacanth mucilage ($1/4^{th}$ volume of the mixture)

Note : Tragacanth Mucilage is prepared with Chloroform Water to avoid replacement of some of the medicinally-active vehicle by the mucilage.

Method for Indiffusible Solids

(a) *Using Compound Tragacanth Powder*

Stage 1 : Indiffusible substance finely powdered in a mortar, add any soluble or diffusible solids and the Compound Tragacanth Powder and mix intimately. Form a smooth cream using small amount (three-quarters) of the vehicle with triturate the powders and then add the remainder of the vehicle measured out.

Stage 2: Examine the contents of the mortar properly. If any particles of foreign matter are visible, pass through the a piece of muslin and rinse the mortar with little amount of vehicle. If only one or two foreign particles are visible, remove them with a glass rod and omit to pass through the muslin.

Stage 3 -5 : Same as in method for simple mixture.

(b) *Using Tragacanth mucilage*

Stage 1 : Indiffusible substance finely powdered in a mortar, add any soluble or diffusible solids and mix intimately. Triturate the material with the Tragacanth Mucilage to form a smooth cream, and then gradually dilute with half the vehicle. The product will thus measure about three-quarters of the finished volume.

Stage 2 : Same as above

Stage 3 -5 : Same as in method for simple mixture.

Table 6.7 Substance which required suspending agent (Indiffubile substance)

Acetylsalicylic Acid	Chlorbutol	Quinidine Sulphate
Barbitone	Jalap Resin	Quinine Salicylate
Benzoic Acid	Phenacetin	Salicylic Acid
Bismuth Oxychloride	Phenobarbitone	Salol
Bismuth Salicylate	Podophyllum Resin	Succinylsulphathiazole
Calomel	Prepared Chalk	Sulphadimidine

Exercise 4: Formula

Phenacitin

Caffeine

Syrup

Purified water

Procedure : Phenacitin is Indiffusible substance (Table 6.7). For dispensing of this formula is required some suspending agent. The vehicle is water and either compound Tragacanth powder or Tragacanth mucilage may be used.

D. Mixtures containing Precipitate-forming Liquids

Several resins are not only insoluble in water but they are formed indiffuble masses in the presence of salts. Some liquid preparations, given Table 6.8 , contain resinous matter, and, when mixed with water, the resin is precipitated and may adhere to the sides of the bottle, or form a clotted precipitate which will not re-diffuse upon shaking. For solving this problem, it is necessary in mixtures of this type to add Compound Tragacanth Powder or Tragacanth Mucilage, in the same proportion/concentration as given under the category of indlffusible powders.

Table 6.8 Resinous Tincture yield an indiffusible precipitate with aqueous

Ammoniated solution of Quinine	Tincture of Benzoin	Tincture of Myrrh
Compound Benzoin	Tincture of Lobelia	Tincture of Tolu

Method for Precipitate forming Liquid

(a) *Using Compound Tragacanth Powder*

This method is very suitable for diffusible or Indiffusible solids are also present in the mixture. This method must be used when the vehicle is medicinally useful.

Stage 1 : Powdered in the mortar indiffusible, diffusible and Compound Tragacanth Powder. Mix thoroughly with three-quarters of the vehicle, and triturate the powders with sufficient to room a smooth cream. G gradually add the remainder or the vehicle measured out. Measure the precipitate forming liquid and in the centre of the cream and stirring rapidly all time. Add if any other soluble ingredients and stir until dissolved. For stabilizing this preparation, resin particle converted in colloidal state and protective them with protective colloid.

Phase 2 : Examine the contents of the mortar properly. If any particles of foreign matter are visible, pass through the a piece of muslin and rinse the mortar with little amount of vehicle. If only one or two foreign particles are visible, remove them with a glass rod and omit to pass through the muslin.

Stage 3 -5 : Same as in method for simple mixture.

(b) *Using Tragacanth mucilage*

This method is more quick than the other, and may be used when insoluble solids are absent, and the vehicle is water, or chloroform water.

Note : Tragacanth Mucilage is prepared with chloroform water.

Stage 1 : Mix the Tragacanth Mucilage with an equal volume of the aqueous vehicle. Measure the precipitate forming liquid in a dry measure, and pour slowly into the centre of the mixture, with constant stirring. It is important to precipitate the resin and stabilize the colloidal particles of it with Tragacanth Mucilage before adding soluble solids.

Stage 2 : Use one-quarter of the aqueous vehicle for dissolving solids. Strain if necessary, and add to the above mixture, which will now form about three-quarters of the final volume (Stage 1).

Stage 3 -5 : Same as in method for simple mixture.

Exercise 5: Formula

Potassium Iodide

Tincture of Lobelia

Staramonium Tincture

Chloroform water

Procedure : Tincture of Lobelia is resinous tincture (Table 6.8) and vehicle is water. In this preparation there is no insoluble solids. Dispense the formula as given in above.

E. Mixtures containing Slightly-soluble Liquids

The slightly soluble solids are frequently prescribed in excess of their solubility, and that the undissolved portion is diffusible provided. It is in the form of a fine powder. The insoluble portion of slightly-soluble liquid on the other hand, is not readily diffusible, and a suspending agent is therefore necessary. Compound Tragacanth Powder and Tragacanth Mucilage are used for this purpose. They are used in same in the proportions directed for indiffusible solids.

Table 6.9 Slightly soluble Liquid prescribed in excess of solubility

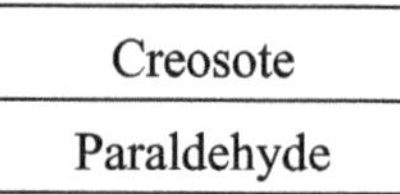

Creosote
Paraldehyde

Method for Mixture containing slightly soluble Liquid

(a) ***Using Compound Tragacanth Powder***

This method is convenient when insoluble solids are absent, and the vehicle is not medicinally active.

Stage 1 : put the slightly-soluble liquid in a bottle, add the mucilage and shake vigorously.

Stage 2 : Dissolve any soluble ingredients in half the aqueous vehicle, filter if necessary and add it gradually to the contents of the bottle, shaking thoroughly after each addition. If soluble solids are absent, use half the aqueous vehicle in the same way. Transfer the liquid from the bottle to a measure.

Stage 3 -5 : Same as in method for simple mixture.

(b) ***Using Tragacanth mucilage***

This method is necessary when insoluble solids are present, or when the vehicle is medicinally active.

Stage 1 : Finely powder the insoluble solids in a mortar, add any soluble solids and the Compounds Tragacant. Powder and mix intimately. If there are no solids. Place the Compound Tragacanth Powder in a mortar. Measure out three-quarters of the aqueous vehicle. Add sufficient to form a smooth cream; then add the slightly-soluble liquid, and mix thoroughly. Gradually add the remainder of the measured-out quantity of aqueous vehicle.

Phase 2 : Examine the contents of the mortar properly. If any particles of foreign matter are visible, pass through the a piece of muslin and rinse the mortar with little amount of vehicle. If only one or two foreign particles are visible, remove them with a glass rod and omit to pass through the muslin.

Stage 3 -5 : Same as in method for simple mixture.

Exercise 6: Formula

Paraldehyde

Syrup

Liquid Glycyrrhiza Extract

Purified water

Procedure : Follow the method of preparation as discussed in the above the same category. The Paraldehyde is given in Table 6.9.

F. Miscellaneous Mixtures

1. Mixtures containing Small Doses of potent Medicaments

The single doses of many substances is a small fraction of a grain, and the total quantity prescribed may not be weighable directly.

Formula

Hyoscine Hydrobromide	gr 1/150
Chloroform water .	ad 3 ii

There are 12 doses of gr 1/150 = 12/150 = 2/25 of a grain of Hyoscine Hydrobromide. This amount is not possible to weight. The procedure in these situation is as follows -

Dissolve the smallest weighable quantity greater than that required (i.e. the nearest 1/2 grain above-minimum 1 *grain)* in a volume of the aqueous vehicle which will ensure that the portion of the solution to be used can be measured simply and accurately.

The smallest weighable quantity above 2/25 of a grain is 1 grain.

i. Dissolve 1 grain in 12.5 ml of solvent, it means it 1 ml is equivalent to 2/25 grain.
ii. This is for 12 dose concentrated preparation.
iii. Its 1 ml diluted with 59 ml means total is = 60 ml / 12 = 5 ml

After final dilution total volume 60 ml suitable for 12 dose (each dose 5 ml) and each dose contains Hyoscine Hydrobromide 1/150 grain.

Note : a much larger volume of vehicle (chloroform water) must be used as a solvent for the potent drug (Hyoscine Hydrobromide).

2. Use of Official Solutions to obtain Small Doses

The Pharmacopoeia and the British Pharmaceutical Codex include a few solutions of potent substances examples -

Arsenical Solution containing 1.0% w/v arsenic trioxide.

Adrenaline Solution, containing 1.0% w/v of adrenaline.

Strychnine Hydrochloride Solution containing 1.0% w/v of strychnine hydrochloride.

Morphine Hydrochloride Solution containing 1.0% w/v of morphine hydrochloride.

These are suitable in appropriate cases where fractions of a grain are required.

3. **Calcium Lactate Mixtures**

The solubility of Calcium Lactate is officially given as 1 in 20 and it varies 1 in 12.9 to 1 in 26.5 according to the method of manufacture. Hence, about 30 grains of one sample may dissolve in an ounce, and only 16 grains of another. This is the reason the mixture sometimes it may be clear, and sometimes there may be a diffused powder. Some commercial specimens have the objectionable odour of sour milk to an undesirable extent.

The Odour is not so apparent and solubility is also good if freshly made. It may be prescribed in the Calcium carbonate and lactic acid are allowed to interact, to form this product. Lactic Acid BP contains lactic acid and lactide, together equaling not less than 87.5 percent w/w of real lactic acid. The reaction and the quantity can be found from the equation –

$$2HC_2H_5O_3 + CaCO_3 + 4H_2O = Ca(C_2H_5O_3)_2, 5H_2O + CO_2$$

2 x 90	100	308
Lactic acid	Calcium carbonate	Calcium lactate

The weight per ml of the official acid is 1.20 and contain the equivalent of 87.5 percent w/w of real acid. Theere for the quantity of official acid needed for 100 G of Calcium Lactate BP.

4. **Other forms of Mixtures**

Drops : These may be remedies given in their original form without dilution, perhaps because of decomposition In aqueous media. Hence such liquids are properly prescribed either alone, or with alcoholic liquids, Compound Cardamom Tincture being often used fat this purpose. Special attention must be given to the labelling of these preparations, as there is a considerable difference between 'drops' and 'minims.' The following table shows the number of drops in 60 minims of some important vehicles. (Detail given in solution).

Table 6.10 Number of Drops in 60 Minims

Vehicle	No. of Drops in 60 minims
Alcohol	170
Belladona Tincture	150
Chloroform	292
Nux Vomica Tincture	163
Spirit of Camphor	169
Opium Tincture	152
Distilled Water	70

Linctuses : These preparations are usually containing medicaments for a local action on the mucous membrane of the throat. The vehicle is some mucilaginous, syrupy, or viscous substance, and, to ensure prolonged action. They are sipped or swallowed slowly without dilution. (Detail given in solution).

Elixirs : These are sweet aromatic preparations, often containing a proportion of alcohol: they are mostly simple solutions or admixtures. (Detail given in solution).

CHAPTER 7

SOLUTIONS

Liquid dosage forms commonly encountered in pharmaceutical practice are either monophasic or biphasic. Monophasic systems are characterized by the presence of a single homogeneous phase *e.g.* solutions, waters, tinctures etc., whereas biphasic liquid dosage fonns consist of two distinct phases *e.g.* emulsions and suspensions.

A solution may be defined as a monophasic system of two or more substances. The components of a solution are so intimately mixed with each other that a physically homogeneous system results. Many solutions are classified separately.

- Syrups are aqueous solutions containing sugar
- Elixirs are sweetened hydroalcoholic solutions
- Spirits are solutions of aromatic materials in alcohol and
- Aromatic waters are the solutions of aromatic materials in water.

Solutions may be solid, liquid or gaseous but liquid solutions constitute the most important category from pharmaceutical viewpoint. A solution consisting of only two substances is referred to as a binary solution and the components are known as the solvent and the solute. The component present in the greater amount in a solution is designated as solvent and the component present in the lesser amount is the solute. When a solid is dissolved in a liquid, the liquid is generally taken as the solvent and the solid as the solute: irrespective of the relative amounts of the components. In a true solution *e.g.* a syrup, the particles of the solute dispersed in the solvent are so small that they consist of molecules or ions. Thus a true solution is regarded as a molecular dispersion. A colloidal solution or dispersion *e.g.* silver protein in water or methylcellulose in water, consists of the particles ranging in size from 0.1 μm to 1 μm and may be detected with the help of an ultra microscope.

Problems Involved in Preparation and Stability of Liquids

1. **Solubility :** Most of the modem therapeutic agents are poorly soluble in water and hence the techniques for enhancing solubility described earlier are employed.

2. **Stability :** Some drugs are unstable in the form of aqueous preparations. Thus the finished product may not be stable with reference to the chemical composition of the active ingredient(s), viscosity, 'clarity, colour etc. Liquid preparations may also be liable to microbial growth. Use of suitable preservatives or preservation methods are helpful in maintaining the stability.

3. **Sterility :** Parenteral liquids and liquids for ophthalmic use must be sterile and the sterility should be maintained throughout the period over which the preparation is being used. Preparations can be made sterile by employing the well known sterilization techniques. Incorporation of preservatives is also helpful in preventing the *in-use* microbial contamination in sterilized preparations.

4. **Organoleptic characteristics :** Liquid preparations must be pharmaceutically elegant so that they are acceptable to the patients. Hence the preparations must satisfy the requirements of taste, appearance, colour, flavour etc. Organoleptic additives like sweeteners, colorants and flavorants are employed in order to impart patient acceptance to a preparation.

5. **Viscosity :** This is particularly important in case of viscous preparations like syrups. Throat paints must be viscous enough for effective action. Viscous preparations must be easily pourable from the containers. Viscolizers and thixotropic agents are generally useful in imparting desired viscosity to a preparation.

6. **Specific gravity and tonicity:** Adjustment of tonicity is generally required in all parenteral and ophthalmic solutions. Adjustment of specific gravity is occasionally necessary in some preparations of intraspinal fluids. Isobaric solutions have same specific gravity. Hypobaric and hyperbaric solutions respectively have lower or higher specific gravity as compared to a fluid under consideration.

In pharmaceutical practice solutions are defined as liquid preparations containing one or more chemical substances usually dissolved in water. Solutes are usually nonvolatile. Solutions are used for specific therapeutic effect of solute either internally or externally. They vary widely in composition, method of preparation, strength, and potency, mode of administration, use and dosage.

I. INTERNAL LIQUID PREPARATIONS

(A) Monophasic liquid preparations

(a) Syrups (b) Elixirs (c) Solutions (d) Linctuses

(B) Biphasic liquid preparations

(a) Suspension (Mixture) (b) Emulsion

II. EXTERNAL LIQUID PREPARATIONS

(A) Applied on the skin

(a) Lotions (b) Liniments (c) Throat paints (d) Collodions

(B) Instilled into body cavities

(a) Douches (b) Enemas (c) Ear Drops d) Nasal Drops (e) Nasal Sprays

(f) Inhalations

(C) Used in the mouth

(a) Gargles (b) Mouthwashes

Advantages of Solutions

1. Easy to swallow than solid dosage form like tablet and capsules.
2. Suitable for more paediatric preparation.
3. Drug in solution form is immediately available for absorption.
4. A solution is a homogeneous system and therefore the drug remains uniformly distributed throughout the preparation.
5. Drugs that can irritate and damage the gastric mucosa if localized in specific area, Its irritation is reduced by administration in solution form.

Disadvantages of Solutions

1. In convenient to transport and store because they are bulky.
2. Whole product is lost immediately if any breakage in the container.
3. The stability of most of substances in aqueous solution is lesser than solid dosage form.
4. Shelf life of solution is shorter than solid preparation.
5. Suitable media for the microbial contamination and may therefore require the suitable preservatives.
6. Dose inaccuracy compared to solid dosage form.
7. Bitter unpleasant substances are not suitable for solutions and needs to add sweetening and flavoring agent to make them more palatable.

Formulation of Solution

Following additives are generally required for the preparation of solution.

1. Solvents : a. Aqueous b. Non-aqueous (fixed oil, alcohol, polyhydric alcohol, dimethyl-sulphoxide, ethyl ether, liquid paraffin, etc.)
2. Buffers : Carbonates, citrates, gluconates, lactates, phosphate, tartrate, borates, etc.

3. Colors : water soluble dye amaranth.
4. Density modifiers
5. Flavors and perfumes

Taste of product	Flavor
Salty	Apricot, butterscotch, liquorice, peach, vanilla
Bitter	Anise, chocolate, mint, wild cherry
Sweet	Vanilla fruits, etc.
Sour	Citrus fruits, raspberry, etc

6. Isotonicity modifiers
7. Preservatives
8. Antioxidants and reducing agents

Containers : Narrow mouth, screw capped colorless plain bottle.

Methods of Preparation

1. **Simple dissolution:** Simple solutions are prepared by dissolving the solute in a suitable solvent with or without heating. Examples include Adrenaline Hydrochloride Solution, Morphine Hydrochloride Solution, Calcium Hydroxide Solution etc.
2. **Solution by chemical reaction :** Solutions of this type are prepared by reacting two or more solutes with each other in a suitable solvent *e.g.* Aluminium Subacetate Solution.
3. **Solution by extraction :** These preparations are classified as extractives *e.g.* liquid extracts and tinctures.

Some important solutions are discussed below.

1. Cresol with soap solution (Lysol)

Cresol is a mixture of o, m and p-cresol. It acts as disinfectant. The solubility of cresol in water is only about 3% whereas the quantity of cresol present in this preparation is 50%. For dissolving this high proportion of cresol, solubilising agent is required. Fatty acids containing vegetable oil react with hydroxide and form soap. This soap acts as solubilising agent. The reaction between vegetable oil and potassium hydroxide is known as saponification. The cresol is mixed only after completion of the reaction between vegetable oil and potassium hydroxide. The reaction between vegetable oil and potassium hydroxide can be enhanced by adding small amount of ethyl alcohol. Cresol is a phenolic compound and caustic in nature, therefore, it should be handled carefully.

Cresol	50.0 ml
Vegetable oil	18.0 g
Potassium hydroxide	4.20 g
Purified water, sufficient to produce	100.0 ml

Procedure

1. Dissolve potassium hydroxide in 25 ml of purified water.
2. Add vegetable oil and heat on a water-bath and mix thoroughly.
3. Continue heating until a small portion dissolves in water without separation of oily drops.
4. Add cresol and mix thoroughly.
5. Add sufficient purified water to produce the required volume.

Category : Disinfectant **Storage :** Preserve in a narrow mouthed bottle

Uses : Disinfectant

2. Aqueous iodine solution (Lugol's solution)

Iodine	5.0 g
Potassium iodide	10.0 g
Purified water	100.0 ml

Procedure

1. Dissolve potassium iodide and iodine in 10 of purified water.
2. Add sufficient purified water to produce 100 ml.

Category : Source of Iodine **Dose :** 0.3 to 1.0 ml

Storage : Preserve aqueous Iodine solution in a well-closed container. It should be resistant to iodine.

Uses : Source of iodine

3. Strong Iodine solution

Iodine	10.0 g
Potassium iodide	6.0 g
Purified water	10.0 ml
Ethanol, sufficient to produce	100.0 ml

Procedure

1. Dissolve potassium iodide and iodine in purified water.
2. Add sufficient ethanol to produce 100 ml.

Category : Antiseptic

Storage : Preserve strong Iodine solution in a well-closed container. The material of the container should be resistant to iodine.

4. Weak Iodine solution (Iodine Tincture)

Iodine	2.0 g
Potassium iodide	2.5 g
Purified water	10.0 ml
Ethanol, sufficient to produce	100.0 ml

Procedure

1. Dissolve potassium iodide and iodine in purified water.
2. Add sufficient ethanol to produce 100 ml.

Category : Antiseptic **Dose :** 0.3 to 2.0 ml

Storage : Preserve strong Iodine solution in a well-closed container. The material of the container should be resistant to iodine.

5. Strong lead subacetate solution

Lead mono oxide and lead acetate react together and form a number of basic lead acetates. The basic lead acetate is formed by the following reaction.

$$(CH_3COO)_2Pb + PbO \rightarrow (CH_3COO)_2Pb.Pb(OH)_2$$

This basic acetate of lead is soluble in water. Highly alkaline solution of acetate of lead $(CH_3COO)_2Pb.Pb(OH)_2$ is poorly soluble.

Filtration should be conducted as quickly as possible and preferably performed in to a bottle in such a manner that the filtrate should not expose to carbon dioxide any longer than required because carbon dioxide of atmosphere precipitates the basic lead acetate and convert insoluble basic lead carbonate. For the same reason, the preparation is stored in small bottles which well filled and well closed.

Lead acetate	25.0 g
Lead monoxide, in powder	17.5 g
Purified water, sufficient to produce	100.0 ml

Procedure

1. Dissolve lead acetate in 75 ml of purified water.
2. Add lead monoxide.
3. Set a side for forty-eight hours.

4. Shaking, occasionally filter and pass through the filter.
5. Add sufficient purified water to produce 100 ml.

Category : Soothing astringent

Storage : Preserve in a well-filled and well closed container.

6. Strong ammonia acetate solution

Strong solution of ammonium contains 57.5% w/v of ammonium acetate and it is prepared by reacting glacial acetic acid with ammonium bicarbonate and strong solution of ammonia.

$$NH_4HCO_3 + CH_3COOH \rightarrow (CH_3COO)\,NH_4 + H_2O + CO_2$$

$$NH_4OH + CH_3COOH \rightarrow (CH_3COO)\,NH_4 + H_2O$$

It is not possible to prepare the solution by reacting glacial acetic acid with ammonium bicarbonate alone because the reaction between these substances ceases before the formation of required amount of ammonium acetate. In this reaction the formation of ammonium acetate is enhanced and concentration of acetate ions increases and ionization of acetic acid decreases.

$$CH_3COOH \longleftrightarrow CH_3COO^- + H^+$$

$$NH_4HCO_3 \longleftrightarrow HCO_3^- + NH_4^+$$

$$H_4^+ + CH_3COO^- \longleftrightarrow CH_3COO\,NH_4$$

$$CH_3COO\,NH_4 \longleftrightarrow NH_4^+ + CH_3COO^-$$

Glacial acetic acid can not be replaced with acetic acid because glacial acetic acid is 99% pure while acetic acid is only 33% pure. This preparation can be prepared using ammonia strong solution alone because 453 g of glacial acetic acid is neutralized with about 1000 ml. Ammonium hydroxide is used to neutralize the unreacted acid and to make the preparation alkaline with pH range 7.6 to 8.1. The pH is adjusted by using two indicators like bromothymol blue and thymol blue.

Glacial acetic acid	45.3 g
Ammonium bicarbonate	47.0 g
Ammonia solution strong	10.0 g
Purified water, sufficient to produce	100.0 ml

Procedure

1. Mix the glacial acetic acid with about 35 ml of purified water.
2. Add the ammonium bicarbonate in small amount at a time until it is all dissolved.
3. Add sufficient of the ammonia solution until one drop of the resulting solution, diluted with ten drops of water.

4. Add one drop of solution of bromothymolblue, gives a full blue color and shows a full yellow color with one drop of solution of thymol blue.
5. Add sufficient purified water to produce the required volume.

Category : Diaphoretic **Dose :** 1 to 4 ml

Storage : Preserve in a well closed lead-free glass containers. **Uses :** Diaphoretic

7. Chloroxylenol solution

Chloroxylenol	5.00 g
Potassium hydroxide	1.36 g
Oleic acid	0.75 ml
Castor oil	6.30 g
Terpineol	10.0 ml
Ethanol (96%)	20.0 ml
Purified water, sufficient to produce	100.0 ml

Procedure

1. Dissolve potassium hydroxide in small amount of purified water.
2. Add a solution of the castor oil in 63 ml of ethanol.
3. Mix and allow to stand for one hour or until a small portion of the mixture remains clear when diluted with nineteen times its volume of purified water and then add oleic acid.
4. Mix the terpineol with a solution of the chloroxylenol in the remainder of the ethanol and pour into the soap solution.
5. Add sufficient purified water to produce the required volume 100 ml.

Category : Topical antiseptic **Storage :** Preserve in a well-closed container.

Uses : It is used as topical antiseptic in the treatment of minor burns, acne, eczema, psoriasis, seborrhea, diaper rash and in the treatment of athlete's foot.

8. Compound sodium chloride solution (Ringer's solution)

It is an isotonic solution of Sodium chloride, potassium chloride, and calcium chloride. It is used as fluid and electrolyte replenisher to irrigate the tissues during experiments on animals. Ringer's injection has the same composition except water for injection in place of purified water, when it is used during cardiopulmonary bypass heart surgery.

Sodium chloride	8.6 g
Potassium chloride	0.3 g
Calcium chloride hydrated	0.33 g
Purified water, sufficient to produce	100.0 ml

Procedure

1. Dissolve sodium chloride, potassium chloride, and calcium chloride hydrated in a sufficient quantity of recently boiled purified water.
2. Add purified water to make up the volume.

Category : Fluid and electrolyte replenisher

Storage : Preserve in a well closed-container. Always freshly prepared solution is used.

Uses : Fluid and electrolyte replenisher

Some important liquid preparations considered in the category of solutions :

a. Syrups b. Elixirs c. Spirits d. Linctuses e. Collodions f. Douches

g. Enemas h. Ear Drops i. Nasal Drops j. Gargles h. Mouthwashes

(a) SYRUPS

Syrups are concentrated oral solutions of sugar or nearly saturated solutions of sucrose in water or other aqueous liquids. Syrups containing 85% *w/v* or 66.7% *w/w* sucrose will retard the growth of microorganisms. It is important to note that sucrose concentration should not reach the saturation point as a saturated solution may lead to crystallization of a small amount of sucrose due to change of physical condition viz. temperature. Dilute solution of sucrose provides an excellent nutritional source for yeast, moulds and other microorganisms. When heat is employed for the preparation of syrups, a small portion of sucrose changes to dextrose and levulose. This phenomenon is called as inversion. Sucrose solution is optically active and rotates polarized light to right while on heating optical activity decreases, rotates the light to left due to formation of other compounds (dextrose ad levulose). The rate of inversion is enhanced by the presence of acids and hydrogen ions, which act as catalyst.

Syrups are mainly of three types :

Simple syrup : It contains sucrose in purified water alone or in combination of other polyols such as glycerin or sorbitol. These substances are added in syrups to reduce the crystallization of sucrose or enhance the solubility of excipients. (e.g. simple syrup etc.)

Medicated syrups : It contains some added medicinal substances in the syrups and used for therapeutic purpose (e.g. ephedrine sulphate syrup, chlorphineramine maleate syrup)

Flavored syrup : It contains various aromatic or pleasantly flavored substances but are non-medicated and generally used as vehicle or as a flavoring agent or for preservation. (e.g. cherry syrups, tolu balsam syrup, cocoa syrup etc.)

Methods of Preparation

Preparation of syrup depends on the physical and chemical characteristics of the substance employed for its preparation. Four methods are commonly used for preparation of syrups.

1. Agitation without heat : This method is used for the preparation of syrups containing volatile substances. In this process active substance is added in solution and agitated in a glass-stoppered bottle. Closing of bottle is necessary to protect the syrup form contamination and loss of solution during the process. For preparation of large quantities, glass lined tank with mechanical agitators is employed. This method is used for the preparation of wide variety of syrups. Cough syrups are commonly prepared by this process. (e.g. codeine syrup, ephedrine sulfate syrup etc.)

2. Solution with heat : This process is generally preferred as it is simple and less time consuming method, particularly if the constituents are not effected by heat and are non volatile in nature. In this process sucrose is added in the aqueous solution and heated till the sucrose is dissolved completely. Adding remaining amount of distilled water makes up volume of the solution. If the syrups containing any substances which are coagulated, it can be separated subsequently by straining. The concentration of the syrup is measured using saccharometer if the specific gravity of the solution is known. Excessive heating of syrup is not suitable because more inversion of sucrose occurs with the increase in temperature. Syrups cannot be sterilized in autoclave without caramelization. This solution is converted in yellowish to brown color due to formation of caramel by the effect of heat on sucrose.

3. Addition of a medicated liquid : This method is put to use in those cases in which tinctures, fluid extracts or other medicated substances in liquid form are added to syrup to medicate it. In this process some time precipitation takes place due to the presence of resinous and oily substances. It is necessary to take care that medicated substance should not get precipitated in this process.

4. Percolation : In this process, purified water or an aqueous solution is allowed to pass through a bed of crystalline sucrose. A pledget of cotton is put in the neck of the percolator and purified water or aqueous solution is added in the percolator containing sucrose. The flow rate is controlled by the stopcock and maintained such that drops appear in rapid succession. If required, a small portion of liquid is re-passed through the percolator to dissolve the sugar completely in the liquid or aqueous solvent.

Preservatives

Syrup should be kept at low temperature, about 25°C is suitable for preservation. Following preservatives are used to prevent bacterial and mould growth viz. methylparaben, sodium benzoate, benzoic acid, glycerin etc.

Label and storage Syrup should be kept in well-closed containers and stored at temperature below 30°C. Bottle should be completely filled, carefully stoppered and stored in cool dark place.

1. **Simple syrup**

Sucrose	66.7 g
Purified water, sufficient to produce	100.0 g

or

Sucrose	85.0 g
Purified water, sufficient to produce	100.0 ml

2. **Invert syrup**

Sucrose	66.7 g
Purified water, sufficient to produce	100.0 g
Hydrochloric acid	qs

Sodium carbonate solution as neutralizing agent

Method of Dispensing: Prepare syrup of sucrose 66.7% w/w in purified water and add hydrochloric acid slowly with continuous stirring. Neutralize the solution using sodium carbonate solution. Identify inversion of simple syrup to invert syrup by measuring optical activity of syrup.

3. **Tolu Syrup**

Tolu balsam	1.25 g
Sucrose	66.0 g
Purified water, sufficient to produce	100.0 g

Method of Dispensing : Boil 400 ml of purified water in dish or tared vessel. Add weighed amount of tolu balsam in boiled water. Cover the vessel partially and boil the contents for 30 min. with frequently stirring. Add purified water to make the contents of the vessel about to 360 g. Cool it and filter the solution. Add sucrose in the solution and warm it on a water bath to dissolve sucrose completely. Add sufficient purified water to make 1000 g of the solution.

(b) ELIXIRS

Elixirs are clear, liquid, flavored hydroalcoholic preparation intended for oral use. They contain one or more medicaments, pleasantly flavored, usually attractive color containing high proportion of alcohol or sucrose or suitable polyhydric alcohols together with suitable additives (including antimicrobial agents). The alcoholic contents in elixir vary from 5% to 40%. In general they are more stable than mixture as sufficient alcohol is added to maintain the drug in solution. Most of the elixirs become turbid when moderately diluted by aqueous fluids.

Elixirs are mainly of two types

1. **Non-medicated elixir :** They are used purely as diluting agents or solvents for drugs containing approximately 25 percent alcohol, e.g. simple elixir, Iso-alcoholic elixir or low alcohol elixir (containing 8-10% alcohol), High alcoholic elixir (containing 75-78% alcohol)
2. **Medicated elixirs :** Elixirs containing therapeutically active compounds are known as medicated elixirs. e.g. Phenobarbital elixir USP, Dexamethasone elixir USP, Chlorpheniramine Maleate elixir USP, Diphenhydramine Hydrochloride elixir USP, Piprazine Citrate elixir, Terpin Hydrate elixir etc.

   The elixir is used as a vehicle for other drugs in many commercially available cough syrups viz. dextromethorphan hydrobromide, codeine phosphate, pyrilamine maleate, ammonium chloride, creosote, chloroform, and a wide variety of other drugs with expectorant and anti-tussive properties.

   Some proprietary elixirs (phenethicillin and phenoxymethyl penicillin) are available in the market in granule or powder form because active ingredients are unstable in solution. They are dispersed by adding measured amount of water or at a specified point in bottle and shaken until solution is complete. The preparation is labeled so as to be stored in cool place and used within one week.

FORMULATION

Generally elixirs contain following ingredients.

Vehicles : About 10% to 20% of alcohol is used for keeping oils, vegetable extracts, tannin etc. in solution form. Faint opalescence from flavoring agents containing essential oils and light precipitants from vegetable extracts are not considered acceptable in elixirs. Glycerol and propylene glycol are used as solvents.

Stabilizers : In neomycin elixir, citric acid is used to adjust pH 4.0 to 5.0 to minimize the darkening that occurs on storage. Disodium edetate should be used to sequester heavy metals that catalyse decomposition of the antibiotics.

Colouring agents : Elixirs are attractive preparations containing following dyes.

Colouring agent	Color	Elixir
Amaranth	Magnetic red	Paediatric paracetamol, Paediatric streptomycin Ephedrine, Isoniazid, Neomycin, Phenobarbitone Piperazine citrate
Compound tartrazine	Saffron	
Green S, tartrazine	Green	

Flavouring agents : Sweetening agents and fruit flavors are used in many medicinal preparations e.g. Black currant syrup in chloral elixir, Concentrated raspberry juice with inverted syrup in paracetamol elixir, Lemon spirit with invert syrup in ephedrine elixir, compound orange spirits with glycerol in phenobarbital elixir.

Preservatives : In elixir, fermentation and mold growth are inhibited when it contains more than 20% of alcohol, propylene glycol or glycerol. Syrup containing saturated solution of sucrose is also inhibitory to many microorganisms because of high osmotic pressure. The commonly used preservatives are double strength chloroform, spirit, and benzoic acid and methyl ester of p-hydroxy benzoic acid.

METHOD OF PREPARATION

Elixirs are prepared by dissolving the ingredients with agitation / or by admixture of two or more liquid components in the suitable solvent. Usually, the alcohol soluble substances are dissolved in alcohol and water soluble in water separately. As a rule, the aqueous solution is always added to alcoholic solution. The aqueous solution is then added to the alcoholic solution with constant stirring and make up the volume with the solvent or vehicle specified in the formulation. At this stage the product may not be clear due to the separation of some of the flavouring agents because the alcoholic strength is reduced. In such case the elixir is allowed to stand for some time to ensure the saturation of the hydroalcoholic solvent and permit the oil globules to coalesce. Talc (upto 3%) can be used to absorb the excess of oils and assist in their removal from solution. Filtration gives a bright clear product.

CONTAINER

It should be dispensed in narrow mouthed, screw capped, colorless plain bottle.

1. Low Alcohol Elixir

Formula :	Compound orange spirit	1.0 ml
	Alcohol	10.0 ml
	Glycerin	20.0 ml
	Sucrose	32.0 ml
	Purified water, sufficient to produce	100.0 ml

Method of Dispensing : Mix the alcohol, glycerin and 50.0 ml of purified water and add measured amount of compound orange spirit with agitation. Allow to stand for 24 hours, Filter this solvent mixture through filter papers and dissolve the weighed amount of sucrose in the filtrate by agitation or percolation and finally add the solvent mixture to make volume to100 ml.

2. High Alcohol Elixir

Formula :

Compound orange spirit	: 0.40 ml
Saccharin	: 0.30 ml
Glycerin	: 20.0 ml
Alcohol, sufficient to produce	: 100.0 ml

Method of Dispensing : Dissolve the compound orange spirit and the saccharin in 70.0 ml of alcohol and add glycerin. Add sufficient amount of alcohol to produce 100.0 ml and mix properly. Filter the mixture and preserve in suitable container.

3. Paediatric Paracetamol Elixir

Formula :

Paracetamol	: 2.4 ml
Ethanol (96%)	: 10.0 ml
Propylene glycol	: 10.0 ml
Concentrated raspberry juice	: 2.5 ml
Chloroform spirit	: 2.0 ml
Invert syrup	: 27.5 ml
Amaranth solution	: 0.2 ml
Glycerin, sufficient to produce	: 100.0 ml

Method of Dispensing : Mix ethanol (96%), propylene glycol and chloroform spirit and make a mixture. Dissolve paracetamol and shake it, add other additives and sufficient amount of glycerin to produce 100 ml.

4. Piperazine Citrate Elixir

Formula :

Piperazine citrate	: 18.0 ml
Chloroform spirit	: 0.5 ml
Glycerin	: 10.0 ml
Orange oil	: 0.025 ml
Syrup	: 50.0 ml
Purified water, sufficient to produce	: 100.0 ml

Method of Dispensing : Dissolve piperazine citrate in required amount of the purified water and add other additives to produce 100.0 ml with water.

(c) SPIRITS

Spirits are alcoholic or hydroalcoholic solution of volatile substances and contain 50% to 90% of alcohol. The high alcoholic contents maintain water-insoluble oils in solution. If water is added to a spirit the oil acts separated. Some spirits are used as flavoring agents e.g. compound orange spirit, cardamum spirits etc. and some spirits are used as medicinal agents e.g. aromatic ammonia spirit. Spirits are prepared by dissolving the volatile substances in ethanol 90 percent except aromatic ammonia spirit, prepared by distillation method.

Containers

Spirit should be kept in well-closed containers of glass or other suitable materials and should be stored at temperature not exceeding 25°C to reduce loss of evaporation.

Labelling

Comply with the general requirements for labeling.

1. **Compound orange spirit**

   It is an alcoholic solution of oils which permits uniform introduction of small proportion of oils and also preserves orange and lemon oils from rapid oxidation. These oils should be brought in small quantities by the pharmacist and the spirit is most satisfactorily made from oils taken from bottles not previously opened. This will insure that delicacy of flavor which should always be characteristic of elixirs.

Terpeneless lemon oil	1.3 ml
Terpeneless orange oil	2.5 ml
Anise oil	4.25 ml
Corinader oil	6.25 ml
Ethanol (90%), sufficient to produce	1000.0 ml

Procedure

1. Measure terpeneless lemon oil, terpeneless orange oil, anise oil and coriander oil accurately and mix with ethanol (90%).
2. Make up the volume using ethanol (90%).
3. Mix it by shaking and store in a well-closed container.

Category : Flavoring agent and carminative **Weight per ml :** 0.8280 to 0.8410 g.

Storage : Lemon spirit should be kept in a well-filled container and protected from light.

Uses : Flavoring agent and carminative.

2. Surgical spirit

Methyl salicylate	0.5 ml
Diethyl phthalate	2.0 ml
Castor oil	2.5 ml
Industrial methylated spirit, Sufficient to produce	100.0 ml

Procedure

1. Mix measured quantity of methyl salicylate, diethyl phthalate, castor oil, and industrial methylated spirit.
2. Add sufficient industrial methylated spirit to produce 100 ml and mix.

Category : Surgical dressing

Storage : Preserve in a well closed container and put label on the container as Caution : 'This preparation is inflammable. Keep away from a naked flame'.

Uses : Surgical dressing

3. Aromatic spirit ammonia (Spirit of Sal Volatile)

Generally the spirits are prepared by solution method but aromatic ammonia spirit is prepared by distillation method, because the oil of Nutmeg contains non-volatile resinous matter due to which the preparation changes to dark color on storage. Different distillation parts are collected separately. First part of distillate contains a major part of alcohol, volatile oils and a small proportion of water. This part contains volatile oils hence can not be subjected to heat. The second portion of distillate contains a major part of water, a little quantity of alcohol and volatile oil. Second portion of distillate is heated with ammonium bicarbonate to converts it into ammonium carbonate, completely process is performed in a closed vessel to prevent the evaporation of carbon dioxide which is produced during heating. The conversion of ammonium bicarbonate to ammonium carbonate is necessary before mixing it with reverse distillate because ammonium bicarbonate is insoluble in alcohol. Freshly prepared ammonium carbonate is used because ammonium carbonate on storage partially changes into ammonium bicarbonate. Due to this reason the bottles are well filled and due to presence of volatile ingredients it is stored in a cool place well-closed container.

Nutmeg oil	0.3 ml
Lemon oil	0.5 ml
Ammonium bicarbonate	2.5 g
Strong ammonia solution	67.5 ml
Ethanol (90%)	75.0 ml
Purified water, sufficient to produce	100.0 ml

Procedure

1. Take a mixture of lemon oil, nutmeg oil, ethanol and 37.5 ml of purified water in a distillation assembly.
2. Collect 87.5 ml of first distillate in separate container.
3. Second distillate of about 5.5 ml collected in separate flask.
4. Add the ammonium bicarbonate and strong ammonia solution in second distillate by heating on a water-bath to 60° C in a sealed bottle of not less 50 ml capacity.
5. Shake the mixture occasionally until solution is formed.
6. Cool and filter through absorbent cotton.
7. Mix the filtrate with the first distillate.
8. Add sufficient purified water to produce 100.0 ml and mix properly.

Category : Stimulant **Dose :** 1 to 4.0 ml

Storage : Preserve in a well-closed container and keep in cool place.

Uses : Stimulant

4. Chloroform spirit

Chloroform is used as analgesic, anaesthetic and muscle relaxant. It is less as anaesthetic as some times it is poisonous due to formation of phosgene gas during the storage in the presence of light. Chloroform spirit is used as carminative, flavoring agent, sweetening agent and preservative. When it is exposed to light or air, oxidation takes place. If the alcohol is added in small proportion it retards the oxidation. It should be stored in a well-closed, completely filled container due to volatile nature as well as for retarding oxidation.

Chloroform	5.0 ml
Ethanol (90%), sufficient to produce	100.0 ml

Procedure

1. Mix chloroform with ethanol (99%) and shake it.
2. Add sufficient ethanol to produce 100.0 ml of spirit and mix

Category : Pharmaceutical aid **Dose :** 0.3 to 1.0 ml

Storage : Preserve in a air tight container and store in cool place.

Uses : Sweetening agent, carminative and preservative

(d) LINCTUSES

Linctuses are solutions of one or more medicaments, usually containing large amounts of sucrose, and sometimes glycerin as a sweetening agent, and also have a demulcent effect on the mucous membrane of the throat. The vehicle syrup has soothing effect on the sore mucous membrane of the throat. Linctuses are usually intended for use in the treatment of cough, being sipped and swallowed slowly without the addition of water. For local and prolonged action, they should be administered undiluted and sipped and swallowed slowly. The usual dose of linctuses is 5.0 ml.

Dilution of Linctuses : If a dose is prescribed which is less than or not a multiple of 5 ml, the linctus should be suitably diluted to achieve a dose-volume that is a multiple of 5.0 ml, using the specified diluent. They are diluted by syrup except codeine linctus. It is diluted by chloroform water. For this purpose chloroform water must be freshly prepared. Diluted linctuses should be used within two weeks of preparation, or any other period as may be specified. They contain following substances.

1. Vehicles : Syrup, tolu syrup, invert syrup, glycerin, chloroform water, sorbitol etc.
2. Stabilizers : Syrups
3. Coloring agents : Compound tartrazine solution, coal tar dyes, etc.
4. Flavoring agents : Tolu syrup, fruit flavored syrup, lemon syrup, blackcurrent syrup.
5. Preservatives : Benzoic acid, chloroform spirits, cinnamic acid, tolu syrup etc.

1. Codeine Linctus

Formula :	Codeine phosphate	: 0.3 g
	Benzoic acid	: 2.0 ml
	Compound tartrazine solution	: 1.0 ml
	Chloroform spirit	: 2.0 ml
	Lemon syrup	: 20.0 ml
	Purified water	: 2.0 ml
	Syrup, sufficient to produce	: 100.0 ml

Method of Dispensing: Dissolve the codeine phosphate in purified water and other additives to produce 100 ml.

2. Simple Linctus

Formula :

Concentrated anise water	: 1.0 ml
Amaranth solution	: 1.5 ml
Citric acid monohydrate	: 2.5 g
Chloroform spirit	: 6.0 ml
Syrup, sufficient to produce	: 100.0 ml

Method of Dispensing : Separately dissolve the citric acid monohydrate in chloroform spirit and mix amaranth solution, concentrated anise water and add sufficient quantity of syrup.

(e) COLLODIONS

Collodions are liquid preparations for external use, containing pyroxylin in a mixture of ethyl ether and ethanol. They are applied to skin by a soft brush or other suitable applicator or rod. The volatile vehicle ether and ethanol have evaporated, leave a film of pyroxylin on the skin surface. The collodions are mainly two types –

a. Medicated : Official medicated collodoin, salicylic acid contains 10% *w/v* of salicylic acid in flexible collodion USP and is used as kerotolytic agent used in the treatment of corns and warts

b. Non-medicated : for protection of small cuts and scratches

Flexibility of collodion is made by addition of castor oil and camphor. Collodion has been used to reduce or eliminate the side effects of fluorouracil treatment of solar keratoses. In salicylic acid preparation, polyacrylic base is used as vehicle. Pyroxylin is a nitrated cellulose obtained by treating defatted cotton with a mixture of nitric acid and sulphuric acids and its principal constituent is cellulose tetranitrate.. It is high inflammable. It is kept moist with industrial methylated spirit and stored, loosely packed in well-closed containers, protected from light.

Container : Collodions are stored in small, wide mouth, scre-capped coloured, fluted glass vial with a brush or applicator within the container or supplied separately.

Label : 'For External use Only'; 'Store in a Cool Place'; 'Highly Inflammable, keep away from naked flames'

1. Pyroxylin collodion

Formula :

Pyroxyllin	: 4.0 g
Ether	: 75.0 ml
Ethanol	: 25.0 ml
To make about	: 100.0 ml

Method : Procedure : Add the ethanol and ether to the pyroxylin container and closed the container. Shake the mixture occasionally until the pyroxylin is dissolved. Allow to stand for a few days while impurities settle, decant the supernatant liquid because the solution is highly inflammable. Store the preparation in well-closed container with suitable label.

External Liquid Preparations Instilled into body cavities

(f) DOUCHES

A douche is an aqueous solution directed against a part or into a cavity of the body. Douches are most frequently dispensed in the form of a powder with directions for dissolving in a specified quantity of warm water. If powder or tablets are employed for this purpose, they must be completely soluble in water to produce a clear solution.

Tablets are prepared by simple process but the lubricants and diluents must be soluble in water. For preparation of tablets, boric acid is used as lubricant and sodium chloride is used as a diluent.

Tablets deteriorate on exposure to moist air and should be stored in air tight conatainers. Douches are not official preparation. Some preparations contain alum, zinc sulphate, boric acid, phenol, sodium borate. Some compendia have reported a few substances such as benzylkonium chloride to be used in various douches and compound sodium borate solution in nasal or pharyngeal douche.

Douches are mainly used as

1. Antiseptic (e.g. chlorhexidine, chloroxylenol, lactic acid, mercuric chloride, potassium permanganate etc.)
2. Astringent (e.g. alum, tannic acid, zinc sulphate, etc.)
3. Cleaning (e.g. sodium chloride, boric acid, saponated cresol, etc)
4. Soothing action

CLASSIFICATION OF DOUCHES

1. Eye douches : It is used to remove foreign particles and discharges from the eyes use allowed to run from the inner to the outer cornea of the eye.
2. Nasal douches : It is used to cleanse nose by using bulb syringes.
3. Pharyngeal douches : It is used in infection of throat for an operation.
4. Vaginal douches : It is used for irrigation of the vagina by using 8-10 oz capacity bulb syringes with a large vulcanite or rubber spray tube.
5. Rectum douches : It is meant for irrigation of rectum using rectal syringe of the bulb type with a long narrow nozzle.

Container : It is dispensed in colored fluted bottles or single use plastic packs with rectal nozzles for enema.

Labeling : Comply with the general requirement of the label and additional information should be mentioned clearly on the label -'For external use only', 'For nasal use Only' or 'For vaginal use Only' or 'For rectal use Only'

1. **Potassium Permanganate Douche**

   Formula : Potassium permanganate : 0.1 g

   Purified water, sufficient to produce : 100 ml

Method : Triturate weighed amount of potassium permanganate with purified water in a pestle mortar. Allow undissolved crystals to settle and pour the supernatant into a conical flask. Filter through a clean sintered glass filter and make up the volume through filter.

2. **Astringent Douche**

   Formula : Alum : 0.1 g

   Zinc sulphate : 0.5 g

   Liquefied phenol : 0.6 ml

   Glycerin : 12.5 ml

   Purified water, sufficient to produce : 100.0 ml

Method: Mixed weighed amount of alum with purified water, add zinc sulphate and dissolve and gradually add liquefied phenol and glycerin and shake.

(g) ENEMAS

Enemas are aqueous or oily solutions or suspension that are employed to evacuate the bowel, to influence the general system by absorption or to affect locally the seat of disease or introduced into the rectum for cleansing, therapeutic or diagnostic purpose. Cleansing preparations are used to evacuate feces in constipation before an operation. Enemas are usually given at body temperature in quantities of 1 to 2 pt injected slowly with a syringe. If they have to be retained in the intestine they should not be used in larger quantities than 6 fl. ounces for an adult. Sodium chloride, sodium bicarbonate, sodium monohydrogen phosphate and sodium dihydrogen phosphate are used in enemas.

The enemas act in following ways :

- Large volume enemas (about 0.5 to 1.0 liter) e.g. water, soap and turpentine enemas or other type of enemas stimulate peristalsis.
- Small volume enemas (about 100 to 500 ml) like olive and arachis oil enemas act by lubricating impacted feces.

Therapeutic enemas may be used as :

- Anthelmintic : Quassia enema for thread worms
- Sedatives : Chloral hydrate, paraldehyde enemas.
- Anti-inflammatory agent : Corticosteroids for ulcerative colitis
- Stimulating enemas
- Nutritive : When absorption by mouth is impaired, enemas are useful e.g.
- X-ray examination : Barium sulphate suspension is used for X-ray examination of the lower bowel.

Containers : Large volume enemas are administered from a douche can and should be warmed to body temperature before use. Some commercially available small volume enemas are in disposable polyethylene or polyvinyl chloride bags sealed with a rectal nozzle.

Labelling : Special labeling requirements for enemas are 1) To be warmed to body temperature before use, 2) 'Not to be taken orally', 3) 'For rectal use only'

Storage : The enema should be stored in a cool place in complete darkness and an expiry date of only two days after issue is advisable.

1. Chloral Hydrate Enema

Formula :	Chloral hydrate	: 2.0 g
	Mucilage of starch, sufficient to produce	: 100.0 ml

Method : Dissolve weighed quantity of chloral hydrate in mucilage of starch and add sufficient to produce 100 ml.

2. Phosphate Enema

Formula :	Sodium acid phosphate	: 160 g
	Sodium phosphate	: 60.0 g
	Purified water, sufficient to produce	: 100.0 ml

Method : Mix sodium acid phosphate and sodium phosphate and powder in a pestle and mortar. Dissolve this mixture in purified water and make up volume to produce 100 ml.

(h) EAR DROPS

Ear drops are liquid preparation or suspension or emulsion or solution of drug(s) in water, diluted alcohol, glycerin or polyethylene glycol intended for instillation into the ear. Aqueous solutions are not suitable because the secretions in ear are mainly fatty and aqueous solutions do not easily mix with them. Eye drops are generally safe for the ears even if there is a hole in the eardrum. The ingredients of ear drops are different depending on the purpose, 15 ml to be dispensed unless otherwise directed.

Ear drops range from liquids designed to soften ear wax, to medicines made to cure bacterial infections, to medicines against fungus. Many kinds of eye drops can be used in the ear but the opposite is *not* true. Ear drops are too harsh for the eyes.

Ear drops fall into two major practical categories

1. Those that are gentle enough to be safe in the part of ear behind the ear drum,
2. Those that are not safe for ear drum.

How to Use Ear Drops

1. Warm the ear drop bottle by holding it in your hands for a few minutes. Shake the
2. bottle well.
3. Unscrew the cap of the bottle and draw some liquid into the dropper.
4. Either lie on your side or tilt your head over so that the ear which needs the drops is facing upwards.
5. Gently pull your earlobe upwards, away from your neck, and squeeze the correct number of drops into the ear.
6. Keep your head tilted for about five minutes so that the drops can spread into the ear.
7. Straighten your head and wipe away any extra liquid with a clean tissue.
8. Replace the cap on the bottle.
9. Store your ear drops in a cool, dark place.
10. You must use your ear drops for the full length of the treatment course, even if your ear feels better. If you stop too soon, your ear problems may return.
11. While using your ear drops, try not to get water in your ear. Be careful when washing your hair and do not go for swimming until the course is finished.
12. When you have finished your course of treatment, throw any leftover drops away, or return them to your pharmacist for disposal.
13. Don't mix-up! Eyes drops or ear drops? Ear drops never go in the eye, but some eye products can be used safely in the ear.

Containers : Ear drops should be supplied in containers of glass or suitable plastic which are fitted with an integral dropper or with a cap of suitable materials incorporating a suitable dropper tube and rubber or plastic teat. Alternatively, such cap assembly is supplied separately.

Labeling : Comply with the general requirements for labeling on the ear drops container. It should clearly state that the prescription is intended 'for external use only'.

1. Aluminium Acetate Ear Drops

Formula : Aluminium sulphate : 4.5 g
Acetate acid : 5.0 ml
Tartaric acid : 0.9 g
Calcium carbonate : 2.0 g
Purified water : 15.0 ml

Method : Weigh required amount of aluminium sulphate and dissolve in 10.0 ml of purified water, add acetic acid and then calcium carbonate. Add remaining amount of purified water and mix properly. Allow to stand for not less than twenty-four hours in a cool place and stir occasionally. Filter the solution after twenty-four hours. Add tartaric acid in the filtrate and mix.

2. Hydrogen Peroxide Ear Drops

Formula : Hydrogen peroxide solution (6.0%) : 3.75 ml
Purified water, sufficient to produce : 15.0 ml

Method : Mix measured amount of hydrogen peroxide solution with purified water and filter the solution.

3. Boric Acid Ear Drops

Boric acid is produced from native borax or from the other borates by reacting with hydrochloric acid or sulphuric acid. It is colorless scales of a somewhat pearly luster or crystals but more commonly a white powder slightly unctuous to the touch. It is odorless and stable in air and volatilizes with steam. It is slightly soluble in water hence in this preparation denatured spirit is used as it enhances the solubility of boric acid in purified water. It is a very weak germicide. It is nonirritating hence suitable for application to delicate structures such as cornea of the eye.

Formula : Boric acid 0.1 g
Specially denatured spirit 3.0 ml
Purified water, sufficient to produce 15.0 ml

Method : Weighed quantity of boric acid is to be dissolved in denatured spirit and add purified water to make sufficient volume. Filter to remove impurities, if any and dispense in a suitable container.

(i) NASAL DROPS

Nasal drops are aqueous or liquid paraffin solutions meant for instillation into the nostrils. Nasal drops often contain vasoconstrictor drugs to relieve nasal congestion. Oily solutions are not preferred since the oil may retard the ciliary action of the mucosa and may even cause lipoid pneumonia if drop of the oil enter the trachea. A vehicle for formulating nasal drops should have- i) pH between 5.5 and 7.5, ii.) buffering capacity, iii) tonicity equivalent to normal saline, and iv) viscosity not exceeding the normal viscosity of nasal mucosa.

Nasal drops are dispensed in 10 to 25 ml quantities in colored fluted bottles fitted with a screw cap and dropper. Commercially available products are supplied in plastic, squeeze-type containers.

External Liquid Preparations Used in the mouth

(j) GARGLES

Gargles are aqueous solutions used for treating the pharynx and nasopharynx by forcing air from lungs through the gargle that is held in the throat. Gargles are generally dispensed in concentrated form. They must be diluted with water prior to use. Gargles are pleasantly flavored and medicated than mouthwashes. Many mouthwashes are used as gargles, either as such or diluted with purified warm water. Gargles generally contain following substances viz. antibiotics (e.g. benzocaine), antiseptics (e.g. borax), anti-inflammatory (e.g. clove oil), anti-fungal (e.g. phenol, thymol etc.), analgesic (e.g. potassium permanganate), astringents (e.g. benzalkonium chloride, potassium chlorate), alkalinizing agents (e.g. cresote), deodorants (e.g. sodium bicarbonate), local anesthetics (e.g. eugenol).

Container : Narrow mouthed, screw capped, colorless fluted bottles.

1. Phenol Glycerin Gargles

Formula :	Phenol glycerin	: 5.0 ml
	Amaranth solution	: 1.0 ml
	Purified water, sufficient to produce	: 100.0 ml

Method : Prepare phenol glycerin using phenol and glycerin. Mix phenol glycerin with purified water and add amaranth solution. Add sufficient purified water to produce 100 ml.

2. Potassium Permanganate Gargles.

Formula :	Potassium permanganate	: 25.0 mg
	Purified water, sufficient to produce	: 100.0 ml

Method : Grind weighed amount of potassium permanganate with water. Remove undissolved permanganate by filtration and add sufficient amount of purified water to produce 100 ml.

(k) MOUTHWASHES

A mouthwash is an aqueous solution which is most often used for its deodorant, refreshing or antiseptic effect. It may contain alcohol, glycerin, synthetic sweeteners, surface-active agent, flavoring and coloring agents. Mouthwashes generally contain following substances.

1. Antibacterial agents : alkaline phenol, hydrogen peroxide, buffered sodium perborate, thymol glycerin.
2. Astringents : zinc sulphate, zinc chloride, etc.

Container : Narrow mouthed screw capped colored fluted bottle.

Labeling : Comply with the general requirements for labeling. In addition the label on the container states - 'Not to be Swallowed in large amount', and 'Store in cool place'.

1. Compound Sodium Chloride Mouthwash.

Formula :	Sodium bicarbonate	: 1.0 g
	Sodium chloride	: 1.5 g
	Concentrated peppermint emulsion	: 2.5 ml
	Double strength chloroform water	: 50.0 ml
	Purified water qs	: 100.0 ml

Method: Dissolve sodium bicarbonate and sodium chloride in purified water, add concentrated peppermint emulsion and mix. Add double strength chloroform water.

2. Mouthwash.

Formula :	Cetylpyridinium chloride	: 0.10 g
	Citric acid	: 0.10 g
	Sweetener (sodium saccharin)	: 0.04 g
	Flavor oils (peppermint, eucalyptus, and clove oils)	: 0.15 ml
	Polyoxyethylene (20) sorbitan monostearate,	: 0.3 g
	Ethanol	: 10.0 ml
	Sorbitol solution	: 20.0 g
	Purified water, sufficient to produce	: 100.0 ml

Method of Dispensing : Dissolve cetylpyridinium chloride, citric acid, and sodium saccharin in a sufficient amount of the water and add ethanol. Mix polyoxyethylene (20) sorbitan monostearate and flavor oils and add slowly hydroalcoholic solution with stirring, sorbitol and mix. Add sufficient amount of purified water to produce 100 ml.

CHAPTER 8

EMULSION

Emulsions are biphasic systems consisting of two immiscible liquids, one of which (the dispersed phase) is finely subdivided and uniformly dispersed as droplets throughout the other phase is known as dispersion medium. The dispersed phase is also called as the internal phase and the dispersion medium as external phase. These immiscible liquids are made miscible by adding a third substance known as emulsifying agent. They stabilize the system by forming a thin film around the globules of the dispersed phase.

In other words an emulsion may, therefore be defined as a disperse system consisting of heterogeneous system consisting of at least one immiscible liquid dispersed in another in the form of droplets whose diameter in general exceed 0.1µm. Such systems posses a minimal stability because the droplets quickly coalesce and the two liquids get separated. The stability of the emulsion is increased by adding another substance known as emulsifying agent or emulsifier. The liquid droplets, generally known as the emulsion phase or emulsion globules or dispersed phase or internal phase or the interrupted phase while the liquid in which they are dispersed is known as the continuous phase or the dispersion medium or the external phase.

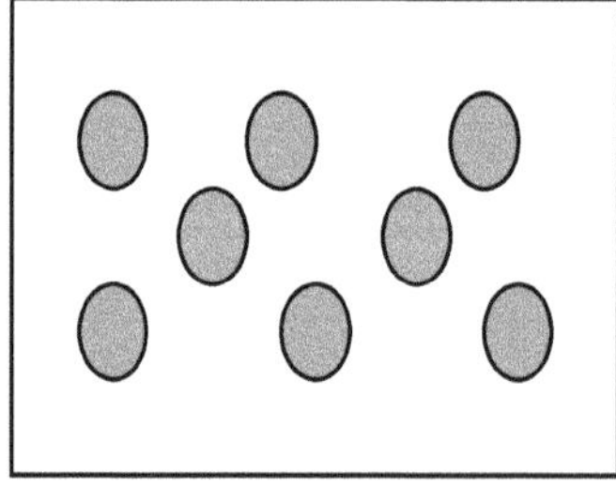

Oil-in-water emulsion (*o/w*)

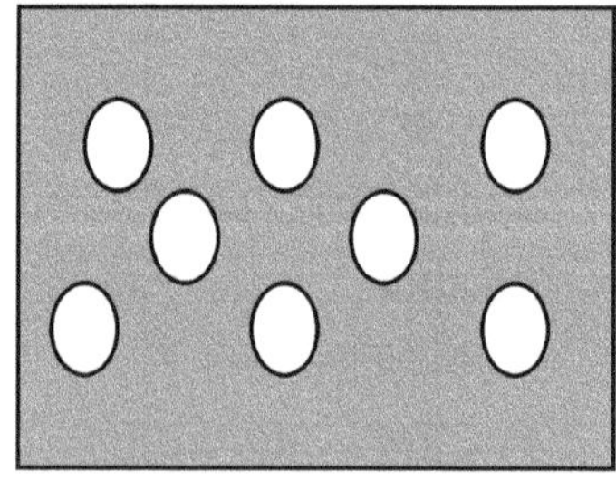

water-in-oil emulsion (*w/o*)

Advantages

- Suitable to mask the bitter taste and odor of drug and making more palatable dosage form e.g. castor oil, cod-liver oil etc.

- Some nutrients like carbohydrates, fats and vitamins can all be emulsified and can be administered to bed ridden patients as sterile intravenous emulsions.
- Used to prolong the release of the drug thereby providing sustained release action.
- Emulsions provide protection to drugs which are susceptible to oxidation or hydrolysis.
- Intravenous emulsions are useful for diagnosis and parenteral nutrition.
- Suitable to formulate externally used products like lotions, creams, liniments etc.

PURPOSE OF EMULSION

- It increases stability of many drugs, which are unstable in aqueous solution.
- It improves the taste of objectionable medicinal agents and makes them more acceptable form.
- It improves appearance of those materials which are generally intended for topical application.
- It improves penetration and spreading ability.
- It enhances the rate and extent of absorption through alimentary canal.
- It can be used as diagnostic agent e.g. radiopaque emulsion in X-ray examination.
- It improves solubility of many drugs, which have limited solubility in aqueous phase.
- It can prolong drug action.

EMULSION TYPES

(a) Water-in-oil (*w/o*) emulsion (Dispersed phase – water, Continuous phase – oil)

(b) Oil-in water (*o/w*) emulsion (Dispersed phase – oil, Continuous phase – water)

(c) Multiple emulsion (Water-in-oil-in-water (*w/o/w*), Oil-in water-in oil (*o/w/o*))

(d) Miscellaneous: Globule size or the disperse phase size of emulsion can vary enormously but are commonly in the range of 0.25-25μm diameter.

On the basis of size emulsions are mainly of three types

(i) Coarse emulsion : globule size more than 25.0 μm.

(ii) Fine emulsion : globule size less than 5.0 μm.

(iii) Microemulsion or miceller emulsion: globule size range of 10-75 nm, such emulsions appear transparent to the human eye in daylight.

Oil-in-water (*o/w*) emulsion

In this emulsion oil is the dispersed phase (internal phase) and aqueous is the dispersion medium (external phase). These emulsions are used mainly for internal/oral use to mask the bitter or disagreeable taste and odor of drugs. External preparations of these emulsions are used for formulating non-greasy lotions, creams and liniments. Moreover easy assimilation of oil in the body takes place as oil is present in a finely dispersed state.

Cosmetic products prepared using *o/w* emulsions can easily be removed from the surface of the skin e.g. castor oil emulsion, foundation creams, vanishing creams.

Water in oil (*w/o*) emulsions

In this emulsion water is the dispersed phase (internal phase) and oil is the dispersion medium (external phase). These emulsions are mainly used for external preparations e.g. lotions and creams as the external layer of oil forms an occlusive film and prevents the evaporation of moisture from the surface of the skin. They are also effective as cleansing cream as they solubilize the oil soluble dirt from the surface e.g. Cold creams.

Multiple Emulsions

In this emulsion, oil in water (*o/w*) or water in oil emulsion (*w/o*) is dispersed in another liquid medium. Thus, oil-in-water-in-oil (*o/w/o*) emulsion consists of very small droplets of oil dispersed in the water globules of water in oil emulsion and water-in-oil-in-water (*w/o/w*) emulsion consists of droplets of water dispersed in the oily phase of oil in water emulsion. Multiple emulsions are primarily used for formulating sustained release dosage forms as the drug entrapped in the innermost layer has to pass through the other two phases before being released for absorption.

Table 8.1 Differences between *o/w* and *w/o* emulsions

Oil in water emulsion (*o/w*)	Water in oil emulsion (*w/o*)
In this type of emulsion, water is the continuous phase (dispersion medium) and oil is the dispersed phase	While in this type of emulsion oil is the dispersion medium and water is the dispersed phase
Generally non greasy and easily removable from the skin surface	More greasy and not washable with water
This type of emulsions is generally meant for internal use as bitter taste of oils can be masked.	This type of emulsions is generally meant for external use like creams.
Externally applied emulsion e.g. vanishing cream provide cooling effect	Externally applied emulsion prevent evaporation of moisture from the surface of skin e.g. cold cream
Water soluble drugs are more quickly released from *o/w* emulsions	Oil soluble drugs are more quickly released from *w/o* emulsions
Show a positive conductivity test, as water is the external phase, which is a good conductor of electricity.	Do not give a positive conductivity test, as oil is the external phase, which is a poor conductor of electricity.

Routes of administration of emulsions

(a) Oral Emulsions

Generally *o/w* emulsions are used for oral administration of drugs or substance because oil is more readily absorbed in a fine state of subdivision through the gastro intestinal tract and secondly the preparation becomes more palatable when water forms the continuous phase. From manufacturing point of view, oil is enveloped in a thin film of emulgent, which masks the bitter and oily taste of the drug like liquid paraffin. Orally, emulsions are also used to enhance the absorption of the oil soluble drugs like vitamins A,D, E and K.

Example 01: Liquid Paraffin Emulsion

Rx

Liquid Paraffin	50 ml
Methyl cellulose	2.0 g
Vanillin	50 mg
Chloroform	0.25 ml
Benzoic acid solution	2.0 ml
Saccharin sodium	50 mg
Purified Water q.s	100 ml

Method of Preparation : Triturate the weighed quantity of liquid paraffin and chloroform with methyl cellulose in mortar and pestle, creamy emulsion is formed. Add and mix other additices and add sufficient purified water with contineous stirring.

Uses: Laxative and acts as an emollient purgative in chronic constipation especially during pregnancy and geriatric patient.

Example 02 : Castor oil Emulsion

Rx

Castor oil	16 ml
Gum acacia	q.s
Water	80 ml

Method of Preparation : Triturate the weighed quantity of castor oil and cinnamon water with gum acacia in morter and pestle. Add remaining quantity of cinnamon water and mix properly.

Use: Purgative

Example 03 : Cod-Liver oil Emulsion

Rx

Cod-liver oil	50 ml
Acacia powder	12.5 ml
Tragacanth powder	0.75 g
Benzaldehyde Spirit	0.25 ml
Saccharin sodium	0.01 g
Chloroform	0.25 ml
Water, to	100 ml

Method of Preparation : Mix two gums and prepare the primary emulsion by the dry gum method and add cod-liver oil. Add and mix other additives with constant stirring and make up the volume.

Uses : Source of vitamin A and D. It is used as dietary supplement in infants and children to prevent the occurance of rickets and to improve nutrition in undernourished children and patients with rickets.

(b) External Emulsions

Both types of emulsions are used for external purpose but *w/o* emulsions are more commonly used for this purpose. Emulsions find maximum use in topical preparations, both for therapeutic and cosmetic use. Therapeutically they are used as carrier for a drug. In cosmetic industry *o/w* emulsions have been used for formulation of make up foundation lotions, moisturing lotions, and hand lotions. Cold cream *w/o* is used when oily layers are desired to prevent moisture loss from the surface of skin, for barrier action and for cleansing action.

Example 01 : Antiseptic cream

Rx

Cetrimide	1g
Cetostearyl alcohol	10 g
White soft paraffin	10 g
Liquid paraffin	29 g
Purified water	50 g

Method of Preparation : Dissolve cetostearyl alcohol in the liquid paraffin with gentle heat in a beaker and in another beaker dissolve cetrimide in purified water. Add warm oily phase into aqueous phase with stirring until cold.

Uses : Antiseptic cream for the treatment of wounds, cuts and burns.

Example 02 : Cold Cream

Rx

Liquid paraffin	20 g
Hard paraffin	4.5 g
Lanette wax	3.5 g
Glycerine	4.5 g
Water	17.5 g
Propyl paraben	0.1 g

Method of preparation : Melt all oily substance in a beaker and dissolve aqueous substances in another beaker. Add aqueous solution to the mixture of oily phase with continuous and rapid stirring until it hascongealed.

Uses: Skin protective and skin smoothner.

(c) Rectal Emulsions:

Enemas are formulated as *o/w* types of emulsions for various purposes.

EMULSIFYING AGENTS

These are the substances added to an emulsion to prevent the coalescence of the globules of the dispersed phase. They are also known as emulgents or emulsifiers. These agents have both a hydrophilic and a lipophilic part in their chemical structure. All emulsifying agents concentrate at and are adsorbed onto the oil/water interface to provide a protective barrier around the dispersed droplets. In addition to this protective barrier, emulsifiers stabilize the emulsion by reducing the interfacial tension of the system. Some agents enhance stability by imparting a charge on the droplet surface thus reducing the physical contact between the droplets and decreasing the potential for coalescence.

The effectiveness of an emulsifying agent depends on the following factors viz.

- Chemical structure
- Concentration
- Solubility
- pH
- Physical properties
- Electrostatic effect

Emulsifiers act in three ways -

(1) Formation of a protective barrier

(2) Reduction of interfacial tension

(3) Decreasing the potential for coalescence by forming an electrical double layer

CLASSIFICATION

I. HYDROCOLLOIDS

A. Natural products

(i) Tree exudate : gum arabic (acacia), gum ghatti, karaya gum, tragacanth
(ii) Sea weeds : agar, carrageenan, alginate etc.
(iii) Seed extracts : locust bean, guar gum etc.
(iv) Steroid containing substance : beeswax, woolfat, wool alcohol
(v) Animal substances : gelatin, casein etc.
(vi) Mineral substances : bentonite, veegum

B. Inorganic : Colloidal alumia, milk of magnesia, mag. oxide, magnesium trisilicate

C. Semisynthetic : methyl cellulose, carboxy methyl cellulose, hydroxy methyl cellulose, microcystalline cellulose.

D. Synthetic : carbopol, colloidal silicone dioxide.

II. SURFACTANTS

A. *Anionic*

(i) Carboxylic acid : soap, actylates, polypeptide condensates
(ii) Sulfuric acid esters : sulfated monoglycerides, alkyl sulfates
(iii) Alkyl and alkyl-aryl sulfonates : dodecylbenzene sulfonates
(iv) Phosphoric acid esters : trioleyl phosphate
(v) Substituted alkyl amides : sarcosinates, taurates
(vi) Hemiesters : sulfosuccinates

B. *Cationic*

(i) Amines : alkoxyalkylamines,
(ii) Quaternaries : benzylkonium chloride

C. *Nonionic*

(i) Polyalkoxyethers : polyoxyethylene alkyl/aryl ethers, polyoxyethylene polyoxypropylene, block polymers.
(ii) Polyalkoxyesters : polyoxyethylene fatty acid esters, polyoxyethylene sorbiton acid esters
(iii) Polyalkoxyamide fatty acid esters : sorbitan esters, glyceryl esters, sucrose esters
(iv) Fatty alcohols : lauryl alcohol.

Selection of Emulsifying Agents using HLB method

In 1949 William C. Griffin developed a system to assist making systematic decisions about the amounts and types of surfactants needed in stable products. The system is called the HLB (hydrophile-lipophile balance) system and has an arbitrary scale of 1 - 18. HLB numbers are experimentally determined for the different emulsifiers in laboratory.

An emulsifier having a low HLB number indicates that the number of hydrophilic groups present in the molecule is less and it has a lipophillic character. For example, spans generally have low HLB number and they are oil soluble. Because of their oil soluble character, spans cause the oil phase to predominate and form a *w/o* emulsion.

A higher HLB number indicates that the emulsifier has a large number of hydrophilic groups on the molecule and therefore is more hydrophilic in character. Tweens have higher HLB numbers and they are also water soluble. Because of their water soluble character, tweens will cause the water phase to predominate and form an *o/w* emulsion.

HLB Range	**Application**
0-3	Antifoaming agents
4-6	*w/o* emulsifying agent
7-9	Wetting agents
8-18	*o/w* emulsifying agent
13-15	Detergents
10-18	Solubilizing agents

HLB values of some common emulsifying agents are given below.

Emulsifying agent	**HLB Value**
Oleic acid	1.0
Sorbitan tristearate	2.1
Glyceryl monostearate	3.8
Sorbitan mono-oleate (Span 80)	4.3
Sorbitan monolaurate (Span 20)	8.6
Polyethylene lauryl ether (Brij 30)	9.5
Gelatin (Pharmagel B)	9.8
Methyl Cellulose	10.5
Polyoxyethylene lauryl ether	10.8
Polyoxyethylene monostearate (Myrj 45)	11.1
Triethanlamine oleate	12.0
Polyoxyethylene Sorbitan mono-oleate (Tween 80)	15.0
Polyoxyethylene Sorbitan monolaurate (Tween 20)	16.7
Polyoxyethylene lauryl ether (Brij 35)	16.9
Sodium oleate	18.0
Potassium oleate	20.0
Sodium lauryl sulphate	40

METHODS OF PREPARATION

Preparation of emulsion depends on the scale at which it is produced. In laboratry or on small scale, mortar and pestle can be used but its efficiency is limited. To overcome these problems small electric mixers can be used although care must be exercised to avoid excessive entrapment of air. In large scale production mechanical stirrers are used to provide controlled agitation and shearing stress to produce stable emulsions. e.g.

- Kenwood mixer
- Silverson mixer
- The Q.P. emulsifiers
- Colloid mills
- Standard slurry-type dispersed mixer with vaned-rotor
- Standard paste-type dispersed mixer with clipped rotor
- Two stage homogenizer

Small Scale Preparation

(a) Wet gum method

A primary emulsion can be prepared by various methods. However it depends on the type of ingredients involved. Stable preparation of fixed oil, water and acacia (ratio in parts 4 : 2 : 1) is prepared by the following methods.

- Two parts of water and one part of acacia mixture are triturated in a mortar and pestle until a smooth mucilage is formed.
- Oil is added slowly with continuous trituration until a smooth cream of primary emulsion is formed.
- The mixture should be again triturated for another 5 minutes and then add water to make up the volume with continuous triturating.

(b) Dry gum method

A primary emulsion of fixed oil, water and acacia (ratio in parts 4: 2:1) is prepared by the following methods.

- The oil is mixed with acacia in a dry mortar and pestle until acacia powder is distributed uniformly.
- Purified water is added with rapidly trituration until a primary emulsion is formed.
- Add other additives and remaining quantity of water with continuous trituration to finish the product.

(c) Bottle method

It is a modified dry gum method. The ratio of oil, water and acacia should be 3: 2:1 or 2 :1 :1 is used for the preparation of emulsion as the low viscosity of the volatile oil requires a higher proportion of acacia.

- The oil is mixed with acacia by shaking the bottle uniformly
- Add measured quantity of water and shake until uniform emulsion is formed.

(d) Soap method

Soap is formed by mixing equal volumes of oil and an aqueous solution containing a sufficient amount of alkali. This method is suitable for the formation of an *o/w* or *w/o* emulsion. It is dependent on the formation of soap e.g. olive oil and lime water are mixed during the preparation of calamine lotion to form calcium oleate, an emulsifying agents.

Table 8.2 Proportions of Oil, Water and Gum required for formation of primary emulsion

Type of Oil	Proportions of		
	Oil	Water	Gum
Fixed Oil	4	2	1
Mineral Oil	3	2	1
Volatile Oil	2	2	1

ADDITIVES

(a) Thickening agents : e.g. emulsifying agent

(b) Antimicrobial agents

- Acids and acid derivatives : benzoic acid, sorbic acid, propionic acid, dehydro-acetic acid
- Alcohols : chlorobutanol, phenoxy-2-ethanol
- Aldehydes : Formaldehyde, glutareldehyde
- Phenolics : phenol, cresol, chlorothymol, o-phenylphenol, p-chlorometaxylenol, methyl p-hydroxybenzoate, propyl p-hydroxybenzoate, butyl p-hydroxybenzoate
- Quaternaries : benzethonium chloride, benzalkonium chloride, cetyl pyridinium chloride, cetyltrimethyl ammonium bromide, chlorhexidine and salts
- Mercurials : phenylmercuric acetate, sodium ethylmercurithiosalicylate
- Miscellaneous : 6-acetoxy-2,4-dimethyl-m-dioxane, Imidizolidinyl urea compound

(c) Antioxidant : ascorbic acid, ascorbyl palmitate, butylated hydroxyanisol, butylated hydroxytoluene, gallic acid, 4-hydroxymethyl-2,6-di-tert-butylphenol, L-tocopherol, sulfites.

(d) Organoleptic agent : e.g. coloring agent, flavoring agent, and sweetening agent

EVALUATION OF EMULSIONS

a. Organoleptic properties
b. Particle size or globule size analysis by microscopic method
c. Rate of phase separation by centrifugation
d. Viscosity by viscometer
e. Electrophoretic properties
f. Measurement of dielectric constant
g. Measurement of conductivity
h. Microwaves irradiation

TESTS FOR IDENTIFICATION OF EMULSION TYPE

Final preparation of both emulsions (*o/w* or *w/o*) looks the same in appearance with naked eyes, therefore certain tests are required to differentiate between them. It is also important that at least two tests should be performed to draw a final conclusion.

(1) Dilution test

In this test the emulsion is diluted either with oil or water. If the emulsion is *o/w* type and it is diluted with water, it will remain stable as water is the dispersion medium but if it is diluted with oil, the emulsion will break as oil and water are not miscible with each other. Oil in water emulsion can easily be diluted with an aqueous solvent whereas water in oil emulsion can be diluted with a oily liquid (Shown in Fig. 8.1)

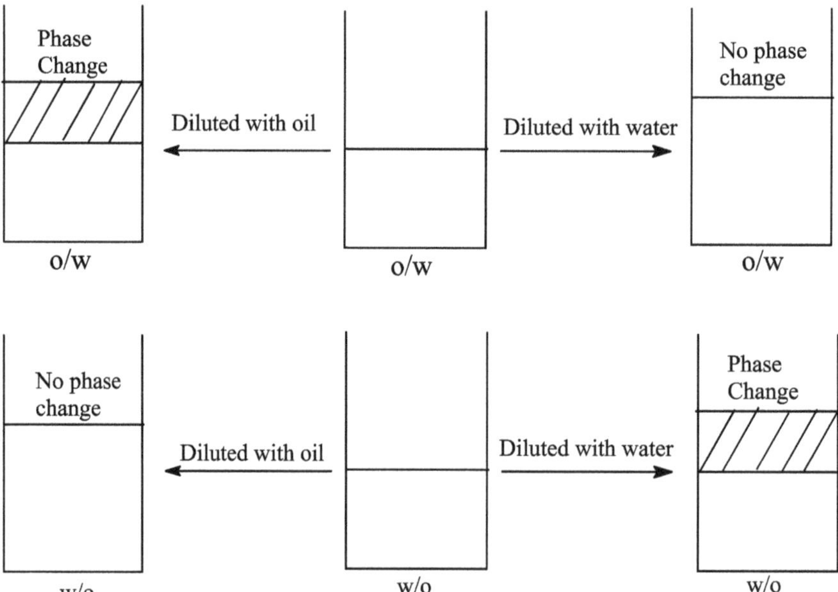

Fig. 8.1 Dilution Test for *o/w* and *w/o* type emulsion

(2) Conductivity Test

The basic principle of this test is that water is a good conductor of electricity. Therefore in case of *o/w* emulion, this test will be positive as water is the external phase. In this test, an assembly is used in which a pair of electrodes connected to an electric bulb is dipped into an emulsion. If the emulsion is o/w type, the electric bulb glows.

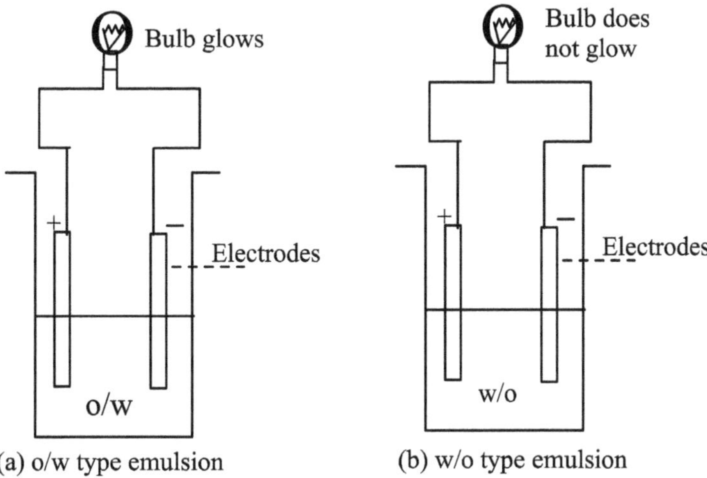

(a) o/w type emulsion (b) w/o type emulsion

Fig. 8.2

(3) Dye Solubility Test

In this test an emulsion is mixed with a water soluble dye (amaranth) and observed under the microscope. If the continuous phase appears red, it means that the emulsion is *o/w* type as water is in the external phase and the dye will dissolve in it to give color. If the scattered globules appear red and continuous phase colorless, then it is *w/o* type. Similarly if an oil soluble dye (Scarlet red C or Sudan III) is added to an emulsion and the continuous phase appears red, then it is *w/o* emulsion.

(4) Cobalt Chloride Test

When a filter paper soaked in cobalt chloride solution is dipped in to an emulsion and dried, it turns from blue to pink, indicating that the emulsion is *o/w* type.

(5) Fluorescence Test

If an emulsion on exposure to ultra-violet radiations shows continuous fluorescence under microscope, then it is *w/o* type and if it shows only spotty fluorescence, then it is *o/w* type.

INSTABILITY OF EMULSION

A stable emulsion is one in which the globules retain their initial character like mean size and size distribution and remain uniformly distributed throughout the continuous phase. During storage of emulsions instability is endorsed by creaming, cracking, reversible aggregation and/or irreversible aggregation etc.

(1) Cracking or coalescence

Coalescence is a growth process during which the emulsified particles join to form large particles. When small droplets are merged and large droplets are formed, it suggests that the emulsion will separate completely and cannot be re-dispersed by shaking. This process is also known as cracking. Any chemical, physical or biological effects that change the nature of the interfacial film of an emulsifying agent may cause cracking. Creaming can be induced by the following methods.

- Addition of an emulsifying agent of opposite type
- Decomposition or precipitation of emulsifying agent
- Addition of a common solvent
- Addition of proper preservatives
- Incorporation of excess of disperse phase

(2) Creaming

Under the influence of gravity suspended particles or globules tend to upward movement, known as creaming while downward movement of particles or droplets is called sedimentation. Creaming or sedimentation depends on the differences in specific gravity between the phases. If creaming take place without any aggregation, the emulsion can be reconstituted by shaking. Process of creaming is explained by Stoke's law.

$$v = \frac{d^2(\rho_1 - \rho_2)g}{18\eta}$$

where,

v = terminal or settling velocity

d = diameter of globules

ρ_1 = density of disperse phase

ρ_2 = density of continuous phase

η = viscosity of dispersion medium

g = acceleration due to gravity

Factors that influence the rate of creaming and sedimentation:

- **Globules size :** Globules of small size have less tendency to cream.
- **Viscosity :** Higher the viscosity of continuous phase, less creaming
- **Density :** Less difference in density of two phases means more stability of emulsion.
- **Temperature :** Lower temperature is more suitable for the better stability of emulsion

(3) Phase inversion

It is known that *w/o* emulsion of benzene in water that was stabilized with sodium stearate will invert to *o/w* emulsions upon heating and reform *w/o* emulsions upon cooling. The temperature at which the inversion occurs depends on the emulsifier concentration and is called Phase Inversion Temperature (PIT). An *o/w* emulsion stabilized by a non-ionic polyoxyethylene-derived surfactant contains oil-swollen miscelles of the surfactant as well as emulsifying oil.

CONTAINERS

Emulsion should be supplied in wide mouthed bottles

STORAGE

Emulsion should be kept at temperature not exceeding 20°. They should not be allowed to freeze.

LABELING

Comply with general requirements for labeling, in addition the label should indicate following information : quantity of emulsifying agent, preservative, "Shake well before use", and "Keep in cool place".

EXAMPLES

Example 01 : Prepare and dispense Liquid Paraffin Emulsion

Rx

Liquid paraffin	50.0 ml
Indian gum in powder	12.5 g
Tragacanth in powder	0.5 g
Sodium benzoate	0.5 g
Vanillin	10.05 g
Glycerin	12,5 ml
Chloroform	0.25 ml
Purified water, sufficient to produce	100.0 ml

Method of Dispensing : Triturate the weighed quantity of liquid paraffin and chloroform with the Indian gum, tragacanth the vanillin in mortar and pestle and triturate until a creamy emulsion is formed. Dissolve sodium benzoate in small quantity of purified water and add other additives with continuous stirring.

Use : laxative

Example 02 : To and prepare and dispense castor oil emulsion

Rx

Castor oil	37.5 ml
Acacia in powder	10.0 g
Cinnamon water, sufficient to produce	100.0 ml

Method of Dispensing : Triturate the weighed quantity of castor oil and the cinnamon water with acacia in mortar and pestle. Add remaining quantity of cinnamon water to produce 100 ml.

Use : Laxative

Example 03 : Prepare and dispense Concentrated Peppermint Emulsion

Rx

Peppermint oil	2.0 ml
Polysorbate-20	0.10 ml
Double strength chloroform water	50.0 ml
Purified water, sufficient to make	100.0 ml

Method of Dispensing : Mix peppermint oil with the polysorbate-20 by shaking and add gradually to double strength chloroform water. Add sufficient purified water to produce 100 ml with shaking.

Use : Carminative

Table 8.3 Some Marketed Emulsion Products

Generic Name	Company	Active Ingredients	Indications
Cremaffin	Abott. Lab.	Liquid paraffin and milk of magnesia	Stool softner
Ivelip (10%)	Baxter India Pvt. Ltd.	Intravenous fat emulsion. Not to exceed 3g/kg body weight per day	Caloric agent, Total parenteral nutrition
RESTASIS	Allergan India Pvt. Ltd.	Cyclosporine 0.05%	Keratoconjuctivitis
Estrasorb	Ranbaxy Research Lab.	Each g contain 2.5 mg Estradiol hemihydrate	Vasomotor symptoms in menopausal women
Diprivan	Astra Zeneca	1% Propofol Injection	General anesthesia
Lipfudin 10% Fat Emulsion	Braun India Pvt. Ltd	Intravenous fat emulsion	Total parenteral nutrition (TPN)

CHAPTER 9

POWDERS

Powder is a term generally applied to solid substances in small particle size. The particles may be crystalline or amorphous or a resultant of larger particles rendered to a fine state of subdivision. In the context of dispensing, powders is a class of solid preparations meant for internal or external use containing one or more drugs intimately mixed with each other in a fine state of subdivision. If necessary, an inert diluent may be added to the potent medicament. Small proportions of volatile constituents- solids or essential oils may also be present.

Historically, powders are the oldest form of presenting a medication. It is perhaps the simplest too, where comparatively little processing and manipulation are involved because most of the basic drugs are marketed in powder form. Powders are dispensed in bulk or as individual doses. In the former case, the patient uses sufficient quantity at a time as directed from the bulk supplied to him. Powders for internal use are dispensed both in bulk as well as in individual doses; however external powders are generally dispensed in bulk excepting sterile powders, which may be dispensed in separate packets. The packet after opening should be used immediately and another sterile packet is opened when required next time. Sometimes, powders for internal use are not dispensed in fine state of subdivision but are rendered to a granular form by moistening, passing the mass through a sieve and drying. This form of medication is called **granules**. The granules are free-flowing and convenient to handle and are generally dispensed in bulk form. Before use, the granules which contain ingredients that react to evolve a gas, when added to water, are called **effervescent granules**.

Powders for internal use, in course of time, have been partially replaced by tablets and capsules; however in hospitals powders are still very commonly used.

Advantages of powders:

- Powder form is the most versatile and convenient to prescribe, compound and administer.
- A physician has the option to deviate from the conventional dose of a medicament according to the requirement of the patient.
- Powders are stable and do not enter into reaction in solid state, lesser difficulties are experienced in compounding them together.

- It is possible to reduce them in the desired particle size range and thus facilitate rapid absorption.
- Less incompatibility as compared to liquid dosage form.
- Powders are in the form of small particles; they offer a large surface area and are rapidly dissolved in the gastrointestinal (GI) tract minimizing the problems of local irritation. Drugs that have to be given in bulk can be best administered in powder form by mixing them with foods or drinks.
- Whenever effervescence is desired, accurate quantities of the two reacting powders are mixed with water.
- It is difficult for children and infants to swallow tablets and capsules and under such circumstances drugs may be administered in powder form making them palatable by mixing with milk, fruit juice or honey.
- Manufacturing of powder is economic hence product cost is quite economic as compare to other dosage form.

Disadvantages of Powder

- As compared to other dosage forms, powders are time consuming to compound.
- Volatile, hygroscopic, oxidizing and deliquescent drugs create obvious difficulties when dispensed as powders.
- Dose inaccuracy.

The degree of coarseness or fineness of a powder is differentiated and expressed by reference to the nominal mesh aperture size of the sieves used. The terms used in the classification of powders are –

1. **Coarse powder (10/44) :** A powder all particles of which pass through a 10 no. sieve and not more 40% by weight through 44 no. sieve.
2. **Moderately coarse powder (22/60) :** A powder all particles of which pass through a 22 no. sieve and not more 40% by weight through 44 no. sieve.
3. **Moderately fine powder** (44/85) **:** A powder all particles of which pass through a 44 no. sieve and not more 40% by weight through a 85 no. sieve.
4. **Fine powder (85/120) :** A powder all particles of which pass through a 85 no. sieve and not more 40% by weight through a 120 no. sieve.
5. **Very fine powder (120/350)** : A powder all particles of which pass through a 120 no. sieve and not more 40% by weight through a 350 no. sieve.
6. **Microfine powder (350) :** A powder of which not less than 90% by weight of the particles pass through a no. 350 mesh.
7. **Superfine powder :** A powder of which not less than 90% by number of the particles are less than 10 μm in size.

General compounding methods:

The dispensing process, irrespective of the powder being in bulk or divided doses, for internal or external use or in a granular form, consists of grinding (if necessary), weighing, mixing (to provide homogeneous admixture) and wrapping.

A. Grinding (Milling)

It is presumed that a student is familiar with the process of grinding and its importance particularly the fact that the size of the particles of a drug influences its physico-chemical properties due to increase in its specific surface affecting rate of absorption. The milling operation is usually done by the manufacturer of the drug. However, at the compounding stage a pharmacist may have to grind crystalline substances or particles that tend to form lumps. This can be done with the help of mortar and pestle. This process of size reduction can be performed behind the counter in advance and drugs put on the dispensing shelves duly powdered to save time at the compounding stage. While grinding, excessive pressure need not be applied to the pestle as it leads to sticking of the mortar or to each other. The drug adhering to the pestle or mortar should be scrapped during the operation with the help of spatula. Generally, it is not necessary to sift the powder unless the drug is required to be in smaller size than particular sieve range.

B. Weighing

The pulverized drug is weighed to the required accuracy with the help of a suitable balance as described earlier. A watch glass or a paper with a suitable counterpoise is used for placing the drug while weighing. All ingredients are weighed one after another and kept separately. It may be reemphasized that the drug should be placed either directly from the container on the watch glass or paper or with the help of a spatula. At no stage the drug is to be touched with hands. Similarly the weights should be removed from the box and replaced using forceps. Due care should be exercised to avoid any contact between the weights and the drugs.

C. Mixing

Mixing is an important operation and the quality of mixing determines the even and uniform distribution of each ingredient in the powders and thereby the accuracy of dosage of each drug. Mixing at the dispensing counter is not done by mechanical devices such as blenders or mixers. Four alternative methods are available for hand mixing of the medicaments. These methods are trituration, sifting, tumbling or spatulation. The nature of the finished product is to be borne in mind before deciding upon the method. Sometimes it becomes necessary to dissolve an ingredient in a volatile solvent for even distribution e.g. iodine in alcohol using a glass mortar and pestle.

(i) Trituration

Trituration is the most common method using Wedgwood or porcelain mortar and pestle. A mortar which is large enough to hold all the ingredients leaving sufficient space above is selected for the purpose. While handling substances that are likely to react with porcelain, a glass mortar and pestle are to be used. The ingredients are transferred to the mortar beginning with the one present in smallest quantity and mixed with the pestle with equal proportion of the drug in next higher quantity. This process of mixing is known as **geometric dilution**. Geometrical mixing is suitable when potent substances are to be mixed a large amount of diluent. The potent dug is placed upon an approximately equal volume of the diluent in mortar and mixed by trituration. A second portion of diluent equal in volume to the powder mixture in mortar is added, and trituration is repeated. (e.g. 1g potent drug and 15 g diluent should be mixed in such a way : **1**+1 = 2; 2 + 2 = 4; 4 + 4 = 8; 8 + 8 = 16 where **1** is the quantity of potent drug and other quantities represent diluent). The geometrical dilution is essential to achieve uniform admixture resulting in a homogeneous product. This process of mixing equal quantity of two lots ensures better mixing and is referred to as trituration. If a coloured ingredient is present in the mixture, uniformity in mixing is visually apparent. Homogeneity in colour of the powder indicates even mixing. Sometimes an edible dye in minute quantity dissolved in a volatile solvent is added to provide a tint to the product to ascertain uniform mixing. Dispensing of potent medicaments warrants dilution with an inert solid by trituration to minimize error in dosage.

(ii) Sifting

Sifting is another method used for mixing. It controls the particle size and brings about homogeneity in distribution of each ingredient. Particle agglomerates, if any, get broken by this method. The ingredients after simple mixing are sifted through a sieve with the help of a brush or one may use standard sieves for the purpose. Household sieves of fine grade are good enough for this work.

(iii) Tumbling

Tumbling is an extremely simple and expedient method of mixing. However it is useful for sticky particles only. All the drugs are kept in a wide mouth bottle with a tight-fitting cap; taking care that the bottle is large enough to fill up to not more than half of its height with the medicaments. The bottle is closed and tumbled up and down allowing the particles to fall freely. The process brings about an even randomization of particles of different densities after the bottle is tumbled 8 to 10 times.

(iv) Spatulation

Spatulation or mixing with the help of a spatula is an effective and expedient method when powdered drugs of similar densities are to be mixed. Perfect mixing can be achieved if the particle size range is also similar. The powdered drugs are kept on a tile or a sheet of glazed paper and mixing done with the blade of a spatula.

Most powders are dispensed in divided doses and therefore the mixed ingredients have to be divided in requisite number of doses, each powder representing uniform quantity of each ingredient. This can be achieved by any one of the three methods-

(i) using powder measures e.g. spoons, boxes, cups etc;

(ii) making a block of the mixture and cutting it in desired number of parts and;

(iii) weighing each powder.

The measure method is the least accurate of the three methods because a measure will never hold the same weight of different powders of different compositions due to differences in bulk densities of the ingredients or the mixture. Variation is inherent by this method unless one uses a calibrated measure for the same powder over and over again. Blocking and cutting is a fairly dependable method of dividing powders. The mixed ingredients are transferred to a smooth tile or glazed paper and built to a solid rectangular block with a spatula having a long blade. When the rectangle looks uniform it is cut with a knife or a spatula in as many blocks of equal size as the number of powders required. Thus each block is expected to represent equal weight and uniformity of content of each ingredient. Each block is transferred to a paper in which it is to be wrapped. Since blocking is done by approximation there is likelihood of some error in the uniformity of weight of each power. Wherever accuracy is required each power should be weighed in a balance and then wrapped.

(v) Levigation

Particle size is reduced by adding a suitable nonsolvent known as levigating agent to form a paste and then mixed in mortar with pestle. This method is used to incorporate solids into ointments and suspension to remove gritty feel.

(vi) Pulverization by intervention

Particle size is reduced by adding a suitable material that can be removed easily after pulverization. This method is most suitable for gummy substances.

Calculation in Powder Dispensing

During mixing etc. there is always a chance of loss of some of the powder and therefore on weighing, the last powder is likely to be lesser in weight. This can not be allowed to happen. A pharmacist therefore weighs each medicament for an additional powder over the number to be dispensed. Thus if 10 powders are to be dispensed quantities of each ingredient are weighed for 11 powders. The first ten are dispensed, the last one being rejected. It is a good practice to weigh the extra powder also which should be less in weight. If it is not so, it establishes an error in weighing at some stage. It is often felt that weighing is time consuming but an experienced pharmacist should be able to weigh quickly without any difficulty. Using a powder measure or **blocking** should be avoided when small powders containing potent medicaments are to be dispensed.

D. Wrapping

Bulk powders are dispensed in bulk containers. Divided powders are packed in powder papers. Powder papers are of four types:

1. Vegetable parchment, a thin semi-opaque moisture resistant paper.
2. White bond, an opaque paper with no moisture-resistant properties.
3. Glassine, a glazed, transparent moisture-resistant paper.
4. Waxed, a transparent waterproof paper.

Wrapping or enclosing the powder in a suitable paper is the last stage in dispensing divided powders. Special papers are available for enclosing powders with or without lining. The quality of the paper is important because the wrapper has to provide protection to the contents without cracking at the folds or springing back in its position on folding. It should also be reasonably impervious to atmospheric moisture etc. It should be light in weight and preserve pharmaceutical elegance of the finished wrapping. A water repellent paper is preferable to a paper that absorbs water. Powder papers of special grades are available ready cut in different sizes. Alternatively a pharmacist may cut the sheets in suitable sizes and preserve them or cut to a desired size whenever needed. Hygroscopic materials are best enclosed in double wrapping, the inner wrapping being of waxed or parchment paper or glassine. Powders containing volatile substances are also provided with double wrapping.

Selection of Paper and box

- The shape of the paper is rectangular.
- The size depends on the quantity to be enclosed and on the size of the powder box in which the powders are to be packed.
- The size of the paper should neither be too large nor too small in which case the medicament bulges excessively from the folds or there is a possibility of the powder spilling out in handling.
- A box of suitable dimensions in first selected and it should hold the requisite number of powders with a tight fit.

- The length of the wrapping paper ought to be 40 to 50mm less than double the inside length of the box so that the powder can be conveniently placed in the box after a double fold lengthwise.
- The powders are placed either vertically or horizontally in the box and width of the paper after folding should conform either to the width or depth of the box, after three folds i.e. it ought to be three times as wide as the height or depth of the box as the case may be.

Wrapping in paper

a. The requisite number of papers of the proper size are taken and three to six of them may be folded lengthwise at one time at one of the ends to about 1/7th of the width of the paper.

b. They are kept on the bench with the folded ends away from the pharmacist or towards the pan of the balance if the powders are to be divided by weighing.

c. The papers should be as much in number as the total number of powders to be dispensed. Each paper should slightly overleap the other ususally a little more than the folded portion of the paper.

d. The whole operation of weighing and wrapping should be done over a clean sheet of paper to avoid soiling of the powder wrappers.

e. The proper quantity of the powder to be wrapped is placed in the centre of the paper.

f. The lower edge of the length is brought under the folded edge at the top and creased.

g. The paper is further folded in a manner that the height of the paper after folding is a little more than the powder box.

h. The powder paper in this position is put over powder folder of the proper size (in little smaller than the length of the powder box).

i. The position of the paper ought to be such that folds of equal size are possible on both sides.

j. After the crease mark is made, it is carefully folded back, one fold under the other, so that the final crease is neat.

k. The wrapped powders are then arranged in the powder box placing one after the other with the folds up. Sometimes the powders are enclosed in envelopes of a suitable size.

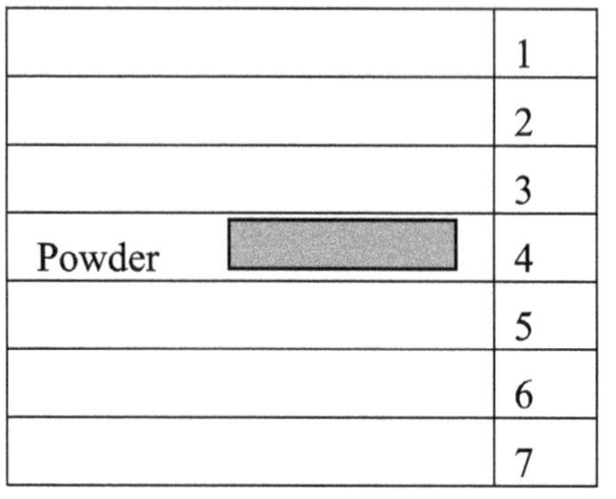

a. Paper equally divided in seven fold

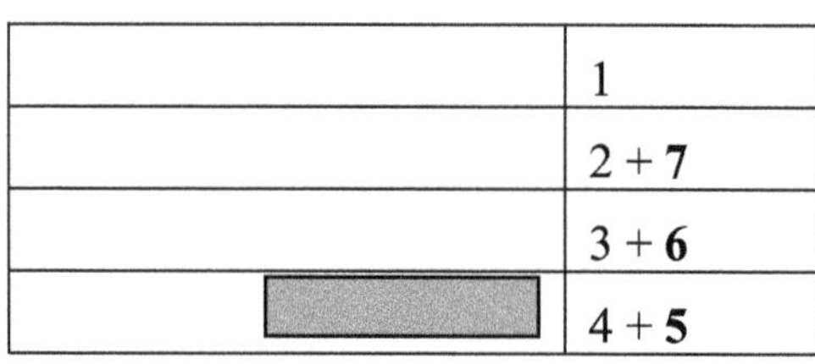

b. In centre on forth fold placed the powder and overlap as given fold number

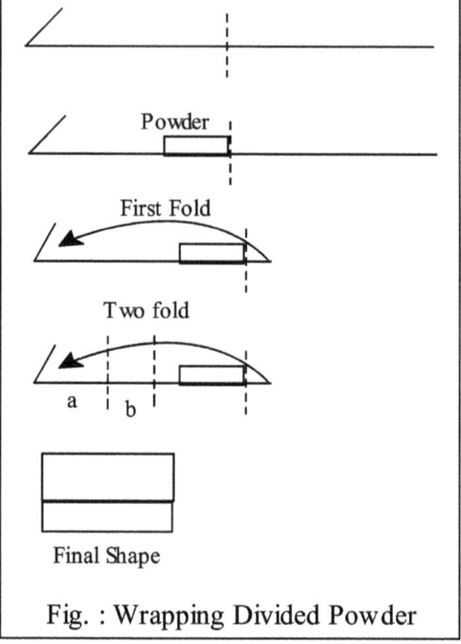

Fig. : Wrapping Divided Powder

	1+2+7
	3 + **6**
	4 + **5**

c. Overlap as given fold number

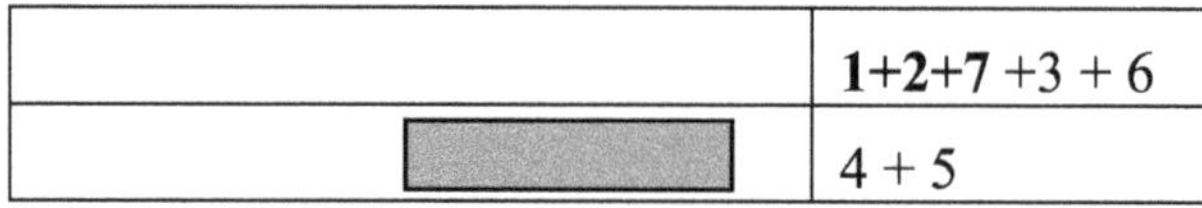

d. Overlap as given fold number

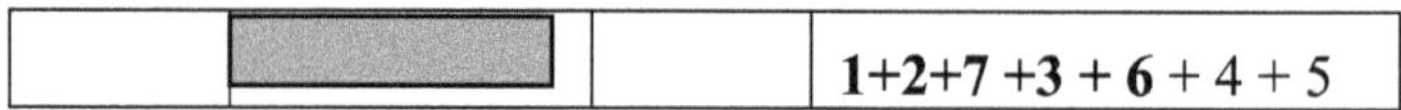

e. Final position of power in the paper rapping in side the box

Fig. 9.1 Powder Rapping in Papers

There is another method of enclosing powders. The drug is placed in a small envelope of a suitable size and sealed. Such envelopes are provided with lining of a water impervious material and made of superior paper. This provides an elegant wrapping to the drug. Bulk powders are usually supplied in cylindrical boxes made of cardboard with a metallic rim both for the upper and lower edges.

Granules are an interesting form of dispensing solid medication. When the dose of a medicament is large it is convenient to present it as granules. Granules are aggregates of particles of the drugs and can be compounded with colours and flavours to make the product attractive and tasteful so that the patient accepts even a large quantity as a single dose. Drugs that are unstable in liquid form can also be dispensed as granules to be mixed with water or another liquid before use. Sometimes the pharmacist himself may mix granules in a liquid before use if there is the possibility of a drug relating its potency till it is consumed. In such cases the pharmacist states in the directions the period after which the medicament should not be administered. Sometimes the granules provide effervescence on mixing with water which yields a sparkling liquid giving it a palatable appearance. Ordinary granules do not require special precautions in compounding. The process includes weighing the ingredients, making due allowance for the loss in granulation; making a cohesive mass with a suitable liquid which evaporates in air or on heating; passing the mass through a suitable sieve; and drying the granules. Effervescent granules however, require special care and the method is described under special procedures for powders and granules in the following text.

Classification of Powders

Powders are subdivided solids which are classified in the BP according to the size of their constituent particles of range from 1.25 μm to 1.7 mm in diameter. Another classification of powders is based on the manner of their dispensing.

1. Bulk powders for external use :
   a. Dusting powders
   b. Snuffs
   c. Dental powder
   d. Insufflations
2. Bulk powders for internal use.
3. Simple and compound powders for internal use.
4. Effervescent granules
5. Cachets

1. Bulk powders for external use

External bulk powders contain non-potent substances for external applications. These powders are dispensed in glass, plastic wide mouth bottles and also in cardboard with specific method of application. Bulk powders for external used are of four types.

a. Dusting powders b. Snuffs c. Douche powders d. Dental powder e. Insufflation

a. Dusting powders

These are used externally for local application not intended for systemic action. The desired characteristics of powders include- a) homogeneity, b) non-irritability, c) free flow, d) good spreadability and covering capability, e) adsorption and absorption capacity, f) very fine state of subdivision, and g) capacity to protect the skin against irritation caused by friction, moisture or chemical irritants.

Dusting powders usually contain substances such as zinc oxide, starch and boric acid or natural mineral substances such as kaolin or talc.

Talc may be contaminated with pathogenic microorganisms such as – *Clostridium tetani* etc. and hence it should be sterilized by dry heat. Dusting powders should not be applied to broken skin. If desired, powders should be micronised or passed through a sieve # 80 or 100. Dusting powders should preferably be dispensed in sifter-top containers. Such containers provide the protection from air, moisture and contamination as well as convenience of application. Currently some foot powders and talcum powders have been marketed as pressure aerosols.

Dusting powders are employed chiefly as lubricants, protectives, absorbents, antiseptics, antipruritics, astringents and antiperspirants.

Rx

Zinc oxide	20 parts
Salicylic acid	2 parts
Starch powder	78 parts

b. Snuffs

These are finely divided solid dosage forms of medicaments dispensed in flat metal boxes with hinged lid. These powders are inhaled into nostrils for decongestion, antiseptic, and bronchodilator action.

c. Douche powders

These powders are intended to be used as antiseptics or cleansing agents for a body cavity; most commonly for vaginal use although they may be formulated for nasal, otic or ophthalmic use also. As douche powder formulation often include aromatic oils, it becomes necessary to pass them through a # 40 or 60 sieve to eliminate agglomeration and to ensure complete mixing. They can be dispensed either in wide mouth glass bottles or in powder boxes but the former are preferred because of protection afforded against air and moisture.

Rx

Zinc sulphate	0.25%
Magnesium sulphate	20.0%
Boric acid	3.0%
Oil of lemon	0.02%
Water	q.s.

d. Dental powders

Dental powders are rarely prescribed. However this class of powders is interesting from the compounding angle. This preparation is a type of dentifrice meant for cleaning the teeth. As such, dental powders contain detergents, abrasives, antiseptics and colouring and flavouring agents incorporated in a suitable base. Generally the base is calcium carbonate. The detergent is in the form of soap and the abrasive action is provided by finely powdered pumice stone. Essential oils are added to provide flavour and freshness to the mouth as well as antiseptic action. Essential oils, if present in smaller quantity, are easily absorbed by calcium carbonate and pumice. This makes the uniform distribution of the oil difficult. Best results are obtained if the oil is triturated in the solids taking considerable care to distribute it uniformly.

e. Insufflation

Insufflations are a class of powders meant for application to the body cavities e.g. ear, nose, vagina etc. The powder has to be extremely fine and must find an entry in the cavity deep enough to bring about its action at the site. It is delivered to the affected part in a stream with the help of a device called an insufflator, which blows the powder to the site. Some of the insufflations contain volatile liquid ingredients which may require uniform distribution in the powder. If these liquid ingredients are present in large quantity, the liquid portion may have to be evaporated. Generally evaporation is brought about slowly in a china dish which is heated on a water bath. The resultant product is re-powdered and sifted through a sieve of a suitable size. However, active volatile liquids present in small portions should not be removed by evaporation but only incorporated by trituration in the powder. The pharmaceutical industry packages the insufflations in pressurized form i.e. aerosols. Aerosols contain the medication in a stout container with a suitable valve, the delivery of the powder being accomplished by a liquefied or compressed gas propellant of very low boiling point. On pressing the actuator of the valve the propellant delivers the medication in a stream.

2. Bulk powders for internal use

Bulk powders contain many doses in a wide-mouth container that is suitable to remove the powder by a teaspoon. The non-potent substances are used in bulk powder form such as antacid, laxative, purgative, constipation, etc.

Rx

Rhubarb powder	25%
Light magnesium carbonate	32.5%
Heavy magnesium carbonate	32.5%
Ginger powder	10.0%

Make a powder.

3. Simple and compound powders for internal use.

These are unit dose powders normally packed in properly folded papers and dispensed in envelopes, metal foil, small heat-sealed plastic bags or other containers.

Usually for the preparation of simple powders, the ingredients are weighed correctly and blended by geometrical mixing in ascending order of weights. The mixture is then either divided into blocks of equal size, numbers of blocks representing the number of powders to be dispensed or each dose is weighed separately and placed on a powder paper. The paper is then folded according to the pharmaceutical art and placed in either an envelope or a powder box.

4. Effervescent granules

This class of preparations can be supplied either by compounding the ingredients as granules or dispensed in the form of salts. The ingredients whether in granular form or present as salts, react in presence of water evolving carbon dioxide gas. For evolution of the gas two constituents are essential, a soluble carbonate such as sodium bicarbonate and an organic acid such as citric or tartaric acid. The preparation can be supplied either as a bulk powder or distributed in individual powders.

There are three alternative methods of dispensing depending upon the nature of prescription.

(i) If the effervescent salts are prescribed to be the dispensed in bulk form, no granulation is necessary. The ingredients are mixed uniformly and directions stated on the label to add the prescribed quantity to water, before use.

(ii) If the effervescent salt is prescribed in divided doses, the ingredients which cause effervescence on mixing with water are enclosed separately in papers of different colour. The patient is advised to take one powder of each colour and add to water, before use. Quantities of the sodium bicarbonate and the organic acid, citric or tartaric, are equimolecular in proportion.

(iii) In the third case the product contains all the ingredients mixed together in a granular form. Preparation of granular products requires pharmaceutical technique. If sodium bicarbonate and citric acid are taken in equimolecular proportion and mixed to make granules, the quantity of water of crystallization liberated from the citric acid is large enough to make the mass wet and carbon dioxide may be liberated during the preparation itself. If one tries to substitute citric acid by tartaric acid, which contains no water of crystallization; it may not be possible to form a mass necessary for granulation. Therefore both citric and tartaric acids are taken in suitable proportions leaving a little acid in surplus than the quantity required to neutralize sodium bicarbonate. This surplus is necessary to give the final preparation an acidic taste that is more palatable. There is a certain loss in weight of such a preparation due to the loss of water in drying the granules and partial loss of carbon dioxide due to its release during preparation. Heating is done on a water bath keeping all the ingredients thoroughly mixed in a porcelain dish. Gentle application of heat liberates the water of crystallization from citric acid and the mass tends to be coherent. Prolonged heating may result in complete evaporation of the released water leaving the product in the form of a dry lump which can not be rendered into granules. The coherent mass is transferred from the porcelain dish to an inverted sieve of suitable aperture size kept over a glazed paper. The mass is pressed through the sieve taking care to change the position of the sieve over the paper to prevent the formation of a lump of the sieved granules. The granules are dried in an oven taking care to regulate the temperature which should be generally kept below 80^0C. The operation requires considerable skill and experience to obtain granules of uniform size and an elegant product. If necessary, the dry granules are passed through a sieve of appropriate size to break larger granules which result due to sticking of the sieved wet granules.

The water of crystallization of the citric acid and the water from the reactions make the material coherent. Loss of weight occurs during granulation due to a) evaporation from the damp mixture, and b) loss of carbon dioxide. The losses constitute approximately one-seventh of the weight of powder used and must be allowed for when calculating the amount to be prepared.

Chemical reaction

$$3\ NaHCO_3 + C_6H_8O_7.H_2O = C_6H_5Na_3O_7 + 3\ CO_2 + 3\ H_2O$$

(Sodium bicarbonate) (Citric acid)

$$2\ NaHCO_3 + C_4H_6O_6 = C_4H_4Na_2O_6 + 2\ CO_2 + 2\ H_2O$$

(Sodium bicarbonate) (Tartaric acid)

5. Cachets

Cachet as a unit dosage form was very popular sometime back. Presently cachets are seldom used and have been replaced by capsules. Cachets, like capsules, can be easily filled and sealed at the dispensing counter. This dosage form holds larger quantity of the medication as compared to capsules. Since the cachets are made of flour and water they are easily damaged in handling. Further this dosage form offers little protection against light and moisture. Due to its size and shape a cachet is difficult to swallow. The process of filling is similar to that of capsules. The drug is placed in one of the two halves of the cachet, the upper half is then placed over it and pressed with the help of a suitable device. The flange of the upper plate is moistened carefully taking care not to wet it, with the help of a dampener. The sealing takes place due to the moisture between the flanges of the upper and the lower half and the pressure over the flanges. About 15 minutes are allowed for drying of the seal. After this time the middle portion of the cachet is slightly pressed to ensure complete sealing. In absence of a machine a pharmacist can improvise and use two bottles the mouths of which are broad enough so that flanges of the plates – upper and lower, when kept over the mouths of the bottles, just rest over them. The drug is transferred to one of the plates resting over the mouth of the bottle kept vertically on the working bench. The flange of the empty half resting over the mouth of another bottle is moistened with the help of a damp camel hair brush. The empty half of the cachet is then placed over the other half in which the medication is kept so that the flanges of the two halves are perfectly superimposed. The second bottle is then inverted and brought over the superimposed cachet and carefully put over the flange and pressed in position without disturbing the resting place of the cachet. This provides a good seal. Cachets can be dry-sealed also. These cachets however are of a different shape where the cap is pressed over the body of the cachet. A protruded stud is also provided to hold the upper and lower halves together. Like capsules, cachets are also expected to remain untouched by hand and one should use gloves while handling them. Since there are inherent losses of the drug in this operation also like that of powders and capsules, the quantities of each ingredient should be weighed for an extra powder over the number to be dispensed. The cachets are dispensed in wide-mouthed bottles of glass or plastic with a perfectly fitting cap. The patient should be instructed to keep the bottle securely closed.

R_x

Phenolphthalein	1 grain
Rhubarb powder	5 grain
Magnesium sulph.	15 grain

M.Ft.cachet. Mitte tales sex.

SPECIAL POWDERS

Ordinarily the powders can be prepared by the general method stated above. However, special procedure may have to be adopted under the following condition:

(a) medicaments liquefying on mixing;

(b) hygroscopic and deliquescent substances;

(c) efflorescent materials;
(d) volatile substances;
(e) liquids;
(f) explosive mixtures and incompatible salts.

(a) Medicaments liquefying on mixing

Some of the drugs which tend to liquefy on mixing include Camphor, Thymol, Menthol, Phenol, Aminopyrine, Chloral hydrate, Acetylsalicylic acid, Antipyrine, Salol and Acetanilide. Mixtures of these drugs liquefy and create problems in compounding. Their mixtures have a melting point below room temperature. Such mixtures are called **eutectic mixtures**. There are two alternatives in overcoming this difficulty. Firstly, one may add an absorbent e.g. talc, calcium phosphate, lactose or starch in sufficient quantity to each ingredient and then mix them. Alternately, one may allow the eutectic mixture to form and add sufficient quantity of the absorbent to the liquid. Second method is that each of the substances is dispensed separately as a powder with directions to take one powder of each one of these at a time. In the former case, there is a chance of the resultant bulk becoming too much should a lot of liquid result on mixing two or more of the eutectic forming substances.

(b) Hygroscopic and deliquescent substances

Substances which absorb moisture from the air are called **hygroscopic.** If the content of water absorbed is so much that the material becomes a liquid it is called a **deliquescent** solid. It is difficult to dispense such substances. However the situation can be partly met by taking the crystalline form without powdering and thus minimizing the surface area available for absorption of water. Secondly, such substances should be dispensed in double wrapping taking due care to provide maximum protection from the air. In highly humid climate one may use aluminium foil or plastic packets for preventing the access of air. Commonly used drugs under this category include Pepsin; Ephedrine sulphate; Hyoscine hydrobromide; Iron and ammonium citrate; Bromide, Iodide and Nitrate of sodium; Potassium citrate; Physostigmine salts; Phenobartibone sodium; Halides of ammonium; and Pilocarpine.

(c) Efflorescent substances

Substances that are crystalline and contain water of crystallization tend to lose it. Such substances are called **efflorescent**. This usually occurs due to change in humidity and solid powder may become pasty in course of time. The only way out is to use the anhydrous salt in place of the crystalline substance. However allowance should be made for the water of crystallization associated with the material while calculating the quantity of the anydrous salt. Efflorescent substances met in dispensing practice include Morphine acetate; Ferrous sulphate; Sodium carbonate; Sodium phosphate; Sodium acetate; Quinine bisulphate, hydrobromide and hydrochloride; Alum; Atropine sulphate; Caffeine; Terpin hydrate; Scopolamine hydrobromide; Cocaine; Codeine phosphate and sulphate; and Citric acid.

d. Volatile substances

Volatilization of substances like menthol, camphor and essential oils may take place on incorporation in powders. This is prevented or minimized by use of double wrapping with an inner waxed paper and outer bond paper cover or by using heat-sealed plastic bags.

e. Liquids

For the incorporation of a relatively small portion of liquid into a powder, the liquid can be triturated with an equal weight of powder followed by the addition of the remaining powder in several portions with trituration.

Large portions of liquids such as tinctures or fluid extracts are evaporated on a water bath to a syrupy consistency to reduce the volume. Addition of lactose during process enhances the rate of evaporation by increasing the evaporating surface. Substitution of a liquid extract by a dry extract, wherever possible, is another alternative.

f. Explosive mixtures and incompatible salts

Trituration of an oxidiging agent such as potassium chloride in a mortar with a reducing agent such as tannic acid may result in a violent explosion. Other potentially explosive materials include potassium dichromate, potassium nitrate, sodium peroxide etc. as oxidizing agents; and sulphur, charcoal and sulfides as reducing agents. Such materials should be mixed by employing minimum force and preferably by tumbling in a jar or on a paper. Alternatively they can be dispensed separately with appropriate directions to the patient.

PRACTICE EXERCISES

$R_{x,}$

Aspirin 600 mg

Send 8 powders. 1 s.o.s.

(Simple individual powder for internal use)

Rx

Sodium bicarbonate	gr v
Heavy mag. oxide	gr ii
Al. hydroxide dried	gr iii

M.ft.pulv.Mitte 10 tales. Mode dicto utenda.

(Compound individual powder for internal use)

Rx

Phenolphthalein 2 mg

Atropine 1 mg

Mitte tales 8.

(Compound individual powder containing small quantity of potent medicament)

Rx

Thymol 10 mg

Menthol

Camphor aa 20 mg

M.ft. pulv. Mittle xv.

(Compound individual powder containing liquefiable substances)

Rx

Calcium lactate 200 mg

One tablespoonful to be taken with water.

(Bulk powder for internal use)

Rx

Sod. bicard. 10 mg

Pot bromide 20 mg

Phenobarbitone sodium 2 mg

D.T.D. # 6

(Compound individual powder containing hygroscopic substances)

Rx

Codeine sulphate 60 mg

Caffeine 20 mg

D.T.D. chart numero 16.

(Compound individual powder containing efflorescent substances)

Rx

Precipitated chalk 80

Soap 10

Pumice	9
Ol. menth. pip.	1
Ol. caryophylli	1

M.ft.dental powder. Mitte 100 gm. Tint suitably.

(Dental powder. Alcoholic solution of an edible dye in small quantity may be used for tinting. Preferred colours are pink or cream.)

Rx

Tr.Benz. Co.	fl dr ii
Starch	oz i

M.ft. insufflatio. Mode Dict. Ut.

(Insufflation containing a liquid which should be slowly evaporated on a water bath after thoroughly mixing with starch)

Rx

Talcum	100 gm
Precipitated chalk	50 gm
Peppermint oil	10 minims

M.ft. Conspergio. Sprinkle when irritation occurs.

(Dusting powder)

Rx

ASA	200 mg
Mag. sulph.	80 mg
Citric acid	100 mg
Sod.bicarb.	200 mg

D.T.D. 8. One every 4 hours with water during effervescence.

(Effervescent powder)

Rx

Rhubarb	gr xxxxv
Sodium bicarbonate	oz i
Citric and tartaric acids	q.s.

Prepare an effervescent powder. Use as directed.

(Effervescent granules may require calculating the quantities of citric and tartaric acids required to neutralize sod.bicarb.)

CHAPTER 10

LOTIONS AND LINIMENTS

(a) LOTIONS

Lotions are usually liquid or liquid suspensions or semi-solid preparations containing one or more medicaments, intended to be applied to the uniform skin *without rubbing*. They are lightly applied on the skin or applied on a suitable dressing and covered with waterproof substance to reduce evaporation. They may be prepared by triturating the ingredients to a smooth paste and then gradually adding the remaining liquid phase. For large quantity preparation of lotion, high-speed mixers or homogenizers produce better quality of lotions. The particles in colloidal dimension are more soothing to inflamed areas and are more effective in contact with infected surfaces. A wide variety of ingredients are employed in the preparation to produce better dispersions that show good cooling, soothing, drying or protective nature of the lotion. Following substances are used in the preparation of lotions.

1. Bentonite : used as a suspending agent.
2. Methylcellulose or sodium carboxymethylcellulose : used to hold the active ingredient in contact with the affected site.
3. Glycerin : keep the skin moist for considerable period of time.
4. Alcohol : used for accentuated action like drying, cooling etc.
5. Miscellaneous : benzocaine, calamine, resorcin, steroids, sulphur, zinc oxide, etc.

Lotions are generally prescribed for the following purpose – anesthetic, antiseptic, astringent, germicide, protective, antihistaminic, screening agent. Microorganisms may grow in certain lotions if no preservative is included in the preparation. Care should be taken to avoid contamination during the preparation of lotion, even if it contains preservative.

Dilution of Lotions : Care should be taken in dilution, particularly to prevent microbial contamination. The appropriate diluent should be used and heating should be avoided during mixing. Diluted lotions should be used within four weeks of their preparation.

Examples

Acriflavine Lotion	Dichloroxylenol Lotion	Salicylic acid Lotion
Boric acid Lotion	Gentian violet Lotion	Thiomersal Lotion
Calamine Lotion	Oily calamine Lotion	Zinc sulphate Lotion
Cetrimide Lotion	Phenolated Lotion	White Lotion
Dichloroxylenol Lotion	Potassium permanganate Lotion	

LABELLING

Comply with the general requirements for labeling. In addition the label on the container states - 'Shake Well Before Use' and 'For External Use Only'

Example 1: Prepare and dispense Calamine Lotion

Rx

Calamine	15.0 g
Zinc oxide	5.0 g
Bentonite	3.0 g
Sodium citrate	0.5 ml
Liquefied phenol	0.5 ml
Glycerin	5.0 ml
Rose water, sufficient to produce	100.0 ml

Method of Dispensing : Prepare sodium citrate solution in 70 ml rose water. Triturate calamine, zinc oxide, and bentonite with citrate solution and add other additives and make sufficient volume with rose water.

Example 2 : Prepare and dispense Boric Acid Lotion

Rx

Chlorinated lime	1.25 g
Boric acid	1.25 g
Purified water, sufficient to produce	100.0 ml

Method of Dispensing : Mix chlorinated lime and boric acid and dissolve in purified water to produce 100 ml.

Example 3 : Prepare and dispense gentian violet lotion

Rx

Gentian violet	1.0g
Ethanol (95%)	10.0 ml
Purified water, sufficient to produce	100.0 ml

Method of Dispensing : Dissolve gentian violet in ethanol (95%) and add sufficient purified water to produce 100 ml.

Example 4 : Prepare and dispense oily calamine lotion

Rx

Calamine	5.0 g
Oleic acid	0.5 ml
Wool fat	1.0 g
Arachis oil	50.0 ml
Calcium hydroxide solution qs	100.0 ml

Method of Dispensing : Melt oleic acid, wool fat and arachis oil in a container, trituratethe calamine with the mixture and transfer to a suitable container. Add calcium hydroxide solution sufficient to produce 100 ml and shake vigorously.

Containers : Narrow mouthed, fluted bottle or container distinguished from types used for orally-administered preparations.

(b) LINIMENTS

Liniments are solution or mixture of various substances in oil, alcoholic solution of soap or emulsions or occasionally semi-solid preparations intended for external application and should be labeled accordingly. They are applied with rubbing or massaged into the skin as counter irritating or stimulating agents to the effected area and because of this were known as embrocations.

Dental liniments, which are no longer official, are solutions of active substances and are applied onto the gums by rubbing. Liniments are usually applied *with friction* and rubbing of the skin, the oil or soap base proving for ease of application and massage. Alcoholic liniments are used generally for their rubifacient, counter irritant, mildly astringent and show penetrating effects. These types of liniments easily penetrate to the skin than those with oil base.

The oily liniments are slow in their action but are more useful when massaged. The function of liniment depends on the additives but most of liniments may function solely as protective coating on the affected area. Liniment should not be applied to the broken or bruised skin because they would be very irritating especially if alcohol is used as solvent.

They may contain following substances : a) analgesic, b) antimicrobial, c) rubefacient, d) counter irritant, e) stimulants, and f) soothing agents.

Although alcohol is primarily used as solvent, it enhances the penetration of the medicaments into the skin and has counter irritant or rubefacient action. Counter irritants are used to mask pain from fibrositis, sciatica, nuralgia and similar complaints by producing warmth, tingling and numbness. When rubbed onto the skin, they also cause redness and hence are called as rubefacients. Cottonseed oil and arachis oil are less irritant than alcohol and spread more easily on the skin.

Two types of vehicle are used for the preparation of liniments i) alcohol e.g. soap liniment and aconite liniment, and ii) oils e.g. camphor liniment and methyl salicylate liniment.

LABELLING

It should comply with the general requirements for labeling. In addition the label on the container should indicate - For External Use Only, Shake Well Before Use, Not To Be Applied to Wounds or Broken Skin, Store in Cool Place, Inflammable.

CONTAINER

Narrow mouthed screw capped colored bottles can be used for dispensing liniments.

Examples 1: Prepare and dispense **W**hite Liniment

Rx

Oleic acid	85.0 ml
Turpentine oil	25.0 ml
Dilute ammonia solution	45.0 ml
Ammonium chloride	12.5 g
Purified water	625.0 ml

Method of Dispensing : Mix the oleic acid with the measured quantity of turpentine oil. Mix dilute ammonia solution with 45 ml of purified water and warm it. Add warm diluted ammonia solution to the oily solution and shake to form an emulsion.

Examples 2 : Prepare and dispense Camphor Liniment (Syn. - Camphorated oil)

Rx

Camphor	20.0 g
Arachis oil	80.0 g

Method of Dispensing : Mix weighed amount of camphor in arachis oil in a closed vessel.

Examples 3 : Prepare and dispense Soap Liniment

Rx

Soft soap	1.0 g
Camphor	4.0 g
Lemon grass oil	1.5 ml
Purified water	17.0 ml
Alcohol (90.0%), sufficient to produce	100.0 ml

Method of Dispensing : Dissolve the weighed quantity of soft soap, camphor and lemon grass oil in alcohol. Add purified water and remaining amount of alcohol to make up the volume and mix. Keep aside for a week and filter to remove the undissolved substance.

Example 4 : Prepare and dispense Turpentine Liniment

Rx

Soft soap	5.0 g
Camphor	5.0 g
Turpentine oil	65.0 ml
Purified water, sufficient to produce	100.0 ml

Method of Dispensing : Mix the soft soap with small amount of purified water (10 ml). Make solution of camphor in fresh rectified turpentine oil. Gradually add camphor solution to the soap mixture with trituration until a thick creamy emulsion is formed. Add sufficient amount of purified water to make up the volume and mix.

Example 5 : Prepare and dispense Calamine Liniment

Rx

Calamine	5.0 g
Wool fat	1.0 g
Oleic acid	0.5 ml
Arachis oil	50.0 ml
Calcium hydroxide solution	100.0 ml

Method of Dispensing : Melt weighed amount of wool fat, oleic acid and arachis oil. Triturate calamine with the melted oil. Add calcium hydroxide solution and shake it. Transfer it to a suitable container and shake vigorously.

CHAPTER 11

SUSPENSIONS

A pharmaceutical suspension may be defined as a dispersion in which finely divided solid particles are suspended in a liquid medium. Dispersed solid particles are known as internal phase and dispersion medium is known as continuous phase/external phase. Particles smaller than 0.1 to 0.2 μm are generally considered to be colloidal. A solid in liquid dispersion in which the particles are above colloidal size (upto 1000 μm) is termed as coarse suspension. In other words suspensions are heterogeneous (biphasic) system consisting of two phases. The continuous phase or external phase is generally a liquid or semisolid and the dispersed or internal phase is made up of particulate matter that is essentially insoluble in but dispersed throughout the continuous phase.

Ideal Suspension

- The suspension must remain sufficiently homogeneous for at least the period between shaking the container and removing the required dose from the container.
- The sediment produced on storage must be easily re-suspended by the use of moderate agitation/shaking.
- The suspension may be required to thicken in order to reduce the rate of settling of particles but the viscosity must not be too high that is not suitable for removing the dose from container.
- The suspended particles should be small and uniformly sized in order to give a smooth, elegant product, free from a gritty texture.
- The suspension should resist microbial attack during storage and also maintain during the shelf-life all organoleptic properties as initially.
- Topical suspension should spread easily when applied.

Advantages

- It is easy to dispense unstable or degradable drugs in solution form.
- Suspension is the only choice if the drug is not soluble in water and non-aqueous solvent is not acceptable, e.g. corticosteroids suspension.

- Suspension is most suitable for drugs having unpleasant taste and odor e.g. Chloramphenical palmitate (bitter taste).
- The insoluble solids act as a reservoir and continuously supply the drug into solution, which is absorbed over a long period e.g. Protamine zinc-Insulin.
- Drug in suspension exhibits a higher rate of bioavailability compared to the same drug of equivalent dose formulated in tablets or capsules. This is due to larger surface area and high dissolution. e.g. antacid suspension.

Disadvantages

- Sedimentation of solids occasionally gives poor form of product. It may lead to caking (formation of compact mass), which is difficult to dispense.
- Dose precision cannot be achieved unless suspensions are packed in unit dosage forms.
- Sometimes microbial contamination takes place if preservation not added in accurate proportion.
- A suspension being a bulky product, transportation cost is high.

Purpose of suspension

- Many people have difficulty in swallowing solid dosage forms and therefore require the drug to be dispensed in a liquid. If the drug is insoluble or poorly soluble in a suitable solvent their formulation as a suspension is usually required.
- The degradation of a drug in the presence of water may also preclude its use as an aqueous solution in which case it may be possible to synthesize an insoluble derivative which can be then be formulated as suspension. eg. oxytetracyline hydrochloride is hydrolyzed rapidly in aqueous solution.
- The prolonged contact between the solid drug particles and dispersion medium can reduce the efficiency of some drugs e.g. Ampicillin. The pharmacist makes the product up to volume with water immediately before issue to the patient. Shelf-life of product is 7 days at room temperature and 14 days at refrigerator.
- Some materials are required to be present in the gastrointestinal tract in a finely divided form, their formulation as suspensions will provide the desired high surface area e.g. kaolin, magnesium carbonate, magnesium trisilicate etc. used for the adsorption of toxins or to neutralize excess acidity.
- The adsorption properties of fine powders are also used in the formulation of some inhalations. The volatile components of menthol and eucalyptus oil would be lost from solution very rapidly during use. Prolonged release suspension would contain volatile ingredients adsorbed on light magnesium carbonate.
- Tastes and odors of drugs are more noticeable if in solution than in an insoluble form e.g. paracetamol suspensions are particularly more suitable for children as compared to paracetamol elixir. Insoluble chloramphenicol palmitate is successfully formulated in the form of suspension.

- Suspension of drugs can also be formulated for topical application e.g. Calamine lotion
- Suspension can also be formulated for parenteral administration to control the rate of absorption of the drug e.g. depot, implants.
- Vaccines are often formulated as suspension for induction of immunity. They may consist of dispersions of killed micro-organisms as in Cholera vaccine, Diphtheria and Tetanus vaccines
- X-ray contrast media are also formulated in the form of suspension e.g. barium sulphate suspension for alimentary tract examination.

Classification of Suspensions

A. On the basis of Preparation

a. Flocculated suspensions b. Deflocculated suspensions

B. On the basis of route of administration

a. Orally administered suspensions b. Topical suspensions
c. Sterilized (injectable and ophthalmic) suspensions

C. On the basis of preparation

a. Dispersed suspensions b. Open network suspension aggregates
c. Closed suspensions

Table 11.1: Comparison of Flocculated and Deflocculated Suspension

S.No.	Deflocculated suspension	Flocculated suspension
1	Particles exist in suspension form as separate entities	Particles form loose aggregates and settle down in the container
2.	Rate of sedimentation is slow, since each particles settles separately and particle size is minimal	Rate of sedimentation is high, since particles settle as a floc, which is a collection of particles
3.	A sediment is formed slowly, may take months	A sediment is formed rapidly, within minutes
4.	The sediment eventually becomes very closely packed, due to weight of upper layers of sedimenting material. Repulsive forces between particles are overcome and a hard cake is formed which is difficult to re-disperse.	The sediment is loosely packed and possesses a scaffold-like structure. Particles do not bind tightly to each other and a hard dense cake does not form. The sediment is easy to re-disperse so as to reform the original suspension
5.	The suspension has a pleasing appearance because the suspended particles remain suspended uniformly for long time. The supernatant also remains cloudy, even when settling is apparent.	The suspension is somewhat unsightly, due to rapid administration and the presence of an obvious, clear supernatant region. This can be minimized if the volume of sediment is made large.

Dispensing of Suspensions

Mainly four types of materials are used in dispensing of the suspension –

a. Suspensions containing diffusible solids

Insoluble lightweight powdered substances are readily mixed with water and remain suspended throughout the continuous phase after long time shaking and mixing. The uniform dispersion is based on the size distribution of the particles in continuous phase.

Examples of diffusible substances are Calcium carbonate, Magnesium trisilicate, Bismuth carbonate, Light magnesium carbonate, Kaolin, Rhubarb Powder.

Dispensing method

Solid powder is finely divided by triturating in pestle and mortar. Make a cream of fine power with small part of vehicle and add more vehicle with stirring or slow trituration. Remove foreign particles, if visible in suspension, by muslin cloth. Mix rinsing in the mortar and pestle and add other liquid ingredients, make up the volume by adding vehicle and mix properly by shaking the final product. Store in suitable container with label having 'shake well before use' instruction and dose.

Example 01 : Dispense the suspension.

Rx

Bismuth carbonate	2.00 g
Sodium bicarbonate	1.40 g
Belladona Tincture	1.00 ml
Purified water q.s. to	60.0 ml

Example 02 : Dispense the suspension.

Rx

Light Kaolin	6.00 g
Light magnesium carbonate	1.50 g
Sodium bicarbonate	1.50 g
Peppermint water q.s. to	50.00 ml

b. Suspensions containing indiffusible solids

Indiffusible solid substances will not remain distributed throughout the vehicle for enough time to ensure uniformity of dose. The stability of suspension and uniformity of dispersed substance are enhanced by increasing the viscosity of continuous phase by adding thickening/suspending agent.

Examples of indiffusible substances include Aspirin, Chalk, Phenobarbitone, Succinylsulphathiazole, Sulphadimidine (for oral use); and Calamine, Zinc oxide, Precipitated sulphur, Hydrocortisone, Triamcinolone acetonide (for external use).

Dispensing method

Solid powders are finely divided by triturating in pestle and mortar with thickening agent. Make a cream of fine power with 50% of vehicle and add more vehicle with stirring or triturating slowly. Remove foreign particles if visible in suspension by muslin cloth. Mix rinsing of mortar and pestle and add other liquid ingredient make up the volume by adding vehicle and mix properly by shaking the final product. Store in suitable container with label having 'shake well before use' instruction and dose.

Table 11.2 Common Suspending Agents in Dispensing Practice

Type and name	Form in which used	Concentration	Uses	Characteristics
1. Organic Natural: Gum Tragacanth	a. Powder b. Mucilage 12.5% v/v c. Compound powder 15% w/w	0.2% *w/v* 25% *v/v* 2-4% *w/v*	To suspend heavy indiffusible solids and resinous tinctures	Forms viscous gel in water. Mucilage is used when the vehicle is water or chloroform water. It is desirable to add a preservative.
Gum acacia	(a) Mucilage 40% w/v (b) Compound powder 20% w/w	6-12% *v/v* 2-4% *w/v*	To suspend light powders and resinous tinctures	Storage of the mucilage results in fall of pH below 4. It is rarely used for external purposes. Compound powder is used when the vehicle is other than water.
Starch (Wheat, corn, rice or potato)	a. Mucilage 2.5% w/w b. Compound powder 20% w/w	2-4% *w/w* 2-4% *w/w*	Not used orally. Makes good jellies for external use.	Good suspending agent for barium meal. Possesses good gelatinizing properties.
Sodium alginate	Mucilage 1% w/v		Used for suspending anionic substances	Viscosity is maximum after 1 hour of preparation and falls to a constant value after 24 hours.

Table 11.2 *Contd....*

Agar	Powder	1% *w/v*	Bulk laxative	In 1% concentration it produces a jelly like mass.
Gelatin	Powder	2-4% *w/v*	Used in pastes and external preparations.	There are two types, Pharmagel A and B. Isoletectric point of A is 7-9 and is compatible with cations. Isoelectric point of B is 5-7 and is compatible with anions.
Semisynthetic: Methyl cellulose	Mucilage 2% w/v in hot water	0.5-2% *w/v*	Used both for internal and external preparations.	Mucilage is clear to opalascent, It is susceptible to microbial attack; 0.001% phenyl mercuric nitrate is used to preserve it. On heating to 50^0C the mucilage gels and on cooling it becomes a sol. It is incompatible with phenol, tannic acid, chlorocresol, resorcinol and silver nitrate.
Sodium carboxymeth-yl cellulose	Mucilage 2% *w/v* in cold water	0.25-1% w/v	Used for oral, external and parenteral preparations.	Susceptible to pH less than 5 and more than 10 when viscosity is affected. It gets precipitated below pH 3. It is sterilizable by dry heat
II. Inorganic Bentonite	Suspension 5% *w/v* as stock suspension	1% *w/v*	Used for external preparations.	It should be sterilized before use. Bentonite is incompatible with electrolytes and positively charged particles.
III. Synthetic Carboxyvinyl polymer	Gel	0.1-0.4% *w/v*	Used for internal and external preparations, also used for gelling alcohol, glycols etc.	It possesses high viscosity between pH 6-11. The viscosity gets markedly reduced below pH 3.

Example 03 : Dispense the following suspension.

Rx

Bismuth carbonate	2.0 g
Chalk	2.0 g
Kaolin	8.0 g
Tincture catechu	4.0 ml
Purified water q.s. to	60.0 ml

Method of dispensing: Kaolin, chalk and bismuth carbonate are finely divided by triturating in pestle and mortar with tincture of catechu. Make a cream of fine power with 50% of purified water and add more purified water with stirring or triturating slowly. Remove foreign particles if visible in suspension by muslin cloth. Mix rinsing of mortar and pestle and add other liquid ingredient make up the volume by adding vehicle and mix properly by shaking the final product. Store in suitable container with label having 'shake well before use' instruction and dose.

c. Suspensions containing Precipitate forming liquids

Some liquid preparations containing resinous constituents, gums and small amounts of volatile components are precipitated on addition to water. Gum resins are oil soluble purified exudates of Myrrh, Benzoin, Galbanum, oppoponax, Tolu, Lobelia etc. The precipitated resin adheres to the side of the container and converted to non-dispersible form. To prevent this problem the pharmacist should adopt special precaution during dispensing. Two methods are commonly used for the prevention of precipitation of suspension.

A. Using Compound Tragacanth Powder

Mix finely powered substance, insoluble solid and gum intimately. Form a smooth cream with vehicle and dilute up to 50% of the final volume. Measure the precipitate forming liquid and pour in a slow stream into the center of the suspension with stirring. Avoid sticky liquid on the pestle and on the sides of the mortar. Precipitated resin particles are adsorbed by hydrocolloids over their surface conferring hydrophilic properties and preventing aggregation into clots. (Note – If electrolytes are present in the preparation, it should not be added until the resin has been protected by hydrocolloids)

B. Using Tragacanth mucilage

This method is quite easy to dispense resin-containing substances. Mix mucilage with an equal volume of vehicle in beaker and add precipitate forming liquid into the center of the mucilage with constant stirring. If any electrolyte is present, add and dilute well with vehicle.

Example 01 : Prepare and dispense Mixture of Lobelia and Stramonium.

Rx

Lobelia ethereal Tincture	8.0 ml
Tragacanth mucilage	10.0 ml
Potassium iodide	2.0 g
Stramonium Tincture	16.0 ml
Double strength Chloroform water	10.0 ml
Purified Water q.s. to	100 ml

Method of dispensing: Mix tragacanth with purified water and add Lobelia ethereal tincture and stramonium tincture with constant stirring. Add and mix potassium iodide and double strength chloroform water. Add sufficient purified water to make up the volume.

Practice Exercise

Example 01

Rx

Ammonium chloride		120 gr
Syrup of wild cherry	ad	3 fluid ounces

Label : 1 tablespoonful 3 times a day

Example 02

Rx

Ephedrine hydrochloride		60 mg
Syrup of tolu	ad	100 ml

One tablespoonful when the cough is severe.

Example 03

Rx

Pot citrate		5 g
Spt. ammon, aromat		15 ml
Spt. aeth, nitrosi		10 ml
Ext. glycyrrhiza liq.		30 ml
Aq. dest.	ad	200 ml

One dessertspoonful 6 times a day

Example 04

Rx

Sod. Salicylate		20 gm
Sod. citrate		10 gm
Syr. crange		15 ml
Water	ad	200 ml

M. ft. mist. Put 10 dose marks. One dose 3 times a day

Example 05

Rx

Codeine phos.	250 mg	
Syr. Lemon	50 ml	
Syr. Tolu	20 ml	
Chloform water	ad	150 ml

15 ml to be taken 3 times a day

Example 06

Rx

Aluminium hydroxide	20%
Magnesium oxide	10%
Water of peppermint	q.s.

M. ft. mist Mitte 4 ft. oz. One tablespoonful before meals.

Example 07

Rx

Bismuth subnitrate		8 gm
Nitric acid		18 ml
Ammonium carbonate		10 gm
Strong ammonia solution		
Purified water	aa q.s.	100 ml

M.ft. mist. 5 ml three times a day

(Refer to NF XII monograph Bismuth Magma)

Example 08

Rx

Sulphathiazole	5 gm
Syrup	20 ml
Water	50 ml

M. ft. mist. Mode dicto utenda.

Example 09

Rx

Mag. Carb.	15 gm
Citric acid	27.4 gm
Syrup	60 ml
Talc	5 gm
Lemon oil	0.1 ml
Pot. Bicarb.	2.5 gm
Purified water q.s.	350 ml

M.ft. mist. To be taken as directed

Table 11.3 Marketed Products

Generic Name	Company	Active Ingredients	Indications
Acigon	Nicholas Piramal	Each 10 ml contains Sodium alginate 440 mg, Dried aluminium hydroxide gel 160 mg, Magnesium Trisil 80 mg, Sodium bicarbonate 140 mg	Antacid
Adocid	Adoc Pharma	Each 5 ml contains Megaldrate 400 mg, semithicone 20 mg	Antacid
Diovol Forte	Wallace	Each 5 ml contains Dried aluminium hydroxide gel 300 mg, Magnesium hydroxide 250 mg, Activated dimethicone 40 mg, Deglycyrrhizinized Liquorice 400 mg	Antacid
Rcin	Lupin	Rifampicin 100 mg /5 ml	Antibiotic, Treatment of tuberculosis

Table 11.3 *Contd....*

Taurmox	Taurus Lab	Amoxycillin	Antibiotic, used in respiratory, genitor-urinary, skin and soft tissue infection.
Clamp	Dr. Reddy's Lab	Amoxycillin 200 mg and clavulanic acid 28.5 mg per 5 ml	Used in the treatment of respiratory and urinary tract infection
Cefspan	Glaxo-Smithkline	Cefixime 100 mg/5 ml	Infections of respiratory, urinary & biliary tract
Jucef-LB	Jollen Midicare	Cefixime 50 mg, Lactic acid bacillus 60 million spores	Infections of respiratory, urinary & biliary tract
Cefadic	Andic Lifesciences	Cefadroxil 125 mg	In the treatment of urinary tract infection caused by *E.coli*
Zedro	FDC	Cefadroxil 125 mg	In the treatment of urinary tract infection caused by *E.coli*
Zefdinir	German Remedies	Cefdinir 125 mg/5ml	Pharyngitis, tonsillitis
Roxeptin	IPCA	Roxithromycin 50 mg/5ml	Acute bronchitis, tonsillitis and genital infections

CHAPTER 12

OINTMENTS

I. SEMISOLID PREPARATIONS

Semisolid dosage forms include ointments, creams, pastes, suppositories and other forms of similar viscous consistency intended for external application. Semisolids may perform any one or more of the following functions

- vehicles for drugs
- emollients
- protective
- occlusive dressings on the skin.

OINTMENTS

Ointments are semisolid preparations for application to the skin and usually contain a medicament. Ointments are used topically for several purposes, e.g., as protectants, antiseptics, emollients, antipruritics, kerotolytics, and astringents. The vehicle or base of an ointment is of prime importance if the finished product is expected to function as any one of the above categories. The consistency of ointments should be such that they may be readily applied to the skin by inunction. The medicament may be in solution, suspension or emulsified in the base. Ointment vehicles serve as protective and emolliebnts for the skin. They usually exhibit plastic flow characteristics and hence when ointment is applied there is a definite yield value, the resistance to flow however drops as the application to the skin is continued. The present day concept of ointments is slightly different than earlier one in the sense that earlier ointments implied a semisolid preparation containing medicinal agents uniformly dispersed in a fatty base but presently ointments may be entirely free of oleaginous substances per se.

Ointments in the form of semisolid emulsions are also referred to as creams; and ointments and creams containing large proportions of insoluble powders are referred to as pastes.

In addition to topical ointments there are ophthalmic ointments, rectal ointments and vaginal creams depending upon the intended site of application. Thus the ointments are also applied to mucous membrane in addition to the skin.

In the case of a protective ointment, it serves to protect the skin against moisture, air, sun rays and other external factors. It is necessary that the ointment neither penetrates the human skin barriers nor facilitates the absorption of substances through this barrier.

An antiseptic ointment is used to destroy or inhibit the growth of bacteria. Frequently bacterial infections are deeply seated; a base which has the capacity to either penetrate or dissolve and release the medication effectively is therefore desired.

Ointments used for their emollient effect should be easy to apply, non-greasy and should effectively penetrate the skin.

Ideal ointment base

An ideal ointment base –

- should not retard wound healing,
- have a low sensiization index,
- pharmaceutically elegant,
- release the medicament efficiently at the site of application,
- have a low index of irritation,
- non-de-dehydrating, non-greasy and neutral in reaction,
- possess good keeping qualities,
- compatible with common medicaments,
- easily washable with water,
- have minimum number of ingredients,
- easy to compound and remain stable on storage, and
- economic and easy to transport

OINTMENT BASES

The earliest bases consisted of fats of animals or man and their mixtures with other substances but the modern day bases are mostly non-greasy, water-miscible and water-washable.

Classification

Although ointment bases can be classified in many ways, the simplest one based on composition is as follows.

A. Oleaginous bases.
B. Absorption bases.

C. Emulsion bases.
D. Water-soluble (hydrophilic) bases.

A. Oleaginous bases

Salient characteristics of these bases are -

- they are anhydrous,
- they are hydrophobic (do not absorb water readily),
- they are insoluble in water, and
- they are not removable by water.

These are the earliest ointment bases which consisted of vegetable and animal fats as well as petroleum hydrocarbons. A list of commonly used materials has been given here although in practice still a larger number of materials are used.

S. No.	Category	Substances
I.	Hydrocarbons	Petrolatum (white and yellow), Microcrystalline wax, Liquid paraffin, Paraffin, Ceresin, Plastibase (Jelene)
II.	Vegetable oils and animal fats	Coconut oil, Olive oil, Peanut oil, Sesame oil, Almond oil, Beeswax, Lanolin, Spermaceti wax
III.	Hydrogenated and sulphated oils	Hydrogenated castor, cottonseed, soyabean and corn oils. Hydrogenated sulphated castor oils
IV.	Alcohols, acids and esters	Cetyl alcohol, Stearyl alcohol, Oleyl alcohol, Lauryl alcohol, Myristyl alcohol, Oleic acid, Stearic acid, Palmitic acid, Myristic acid, Lauric acid, Glyceryl tristearate, Ethyl oleate, Isopropyl myristicate,Ethylene glycol, dilaurate/distearate/ dioleate
V.	Sillicones	Dimethylpolysiloxanes,Methylphenylpolysiloxanes, Stearyl esters of dimethylpolysiloxanes

Oleaginous bases are expected to provide a film, which resists soap and water yet readily removable by solutions of surfactants. This can possibly be achieved by emulsifying the silicones or other hydrophobic film formers so that when the protective ointment is properly applied, an invisible protective film is left on the skin. Film forming agents are exemplified by polyvinylpyrollidone, polyvinyl alcohol and the cellulose derivatives.

B. Absorption bases

The term absorption as applied here implies the hydrophilic or water absorbing properties of the base and not the absorption of medicaments from the bases. These bases are generally anhydrous but capable of absorbing several times their own weight of water ultimately forming *w/o* type of emulsions.

Absorption bases vary in their composition and are usually mixtures of animal sterols with petrolatum. Eucerin and Aquaphor are the commercial bases consisting of combination of cholesterol and/or other suitable lanolin fraction with white petrolatum. Anhydrous absorption bases can also be formulated by the addition of lipophilic surfactants to petrolatum and anhydrous water-removable bases can be formed by the addition of hydrophilic surfactants to petrolatum. Some important formulae of absorption ointment bases are given below.

Example 01

Cholesterol	3.0
Stearyl alcohol	3.0
White wax	8.0
White petrolatum	86.0

Example 02

Wool alcohols	6.0
Hard paraffin	24.0
Yellow or white soft Paraffin	10.0
Liquid paraffin	60.0

Example 03

Cholesterol	30
Cottonseed oil	30
White petrolatum	40

Example 03

White petrolatum	41.0
Microcrystalline wax	3.0
Fluid lanolin	10.
Span 80	4.75
Tween 80	0.25
Purified water	41.0

Absorption bases were primarily developed so as to have a product to which water or an aqueous solution of medicinal substances could be easily added. These bases are usually highly compatible with the majority of drugs used topically. The limited popularity of absorption bases however is attributed to their greasiness.

C. Emulsion bases

These may be either *o/w* or *w/o* type emulsions.

(a) Water-in-oil type emulsion (Hydrophobic ointment)

The *w/o* type emulsion bases such as lanolin and cold cream are used as emollients. The aqueous phase hydrates the skin and the oily phase forms an occlusive covering which prevents loss of water by evaporation. Emulsion bases also serve as vehicle for medicaments such as sulphur, ammoniated mercury, balsam of peru, zinc oxide etc. The main drawback of *w/o* emulsion bases is their greasy and sticky nature and therefore they are less popular than *o/w* type of bases.

Earlier cold creams consisted of oil (40 to 70%), wax or spermaceti (5 to 15%), and water (20 to 35%). Thus a large proportion of water was loosely held in the water-in-oil mixture. More stable creams were later formulated employing borax which formed the sodium soap by reacting with the fatty acids present in the beeswax. Presently cold creams are also formulated by employing non-ionic surfactants alone or in combination with beeswax. When cold creams are applied, slow evaporation of the water causes a pleasant cooling sensation and hence these creams are given the name `cold creams'. A simple formula for borax-beeswax cold cream is as follows.

Mineral oil	50.0
Beeswax	14.0
Borax	0.7
Purified water	35.3

(b) Oil-in-water ointment (Hydrophilic Ointment)

Oil in water type emulsion bases are used as vehicles for medicinal agents. Water being in the external phase they are easily removed with water alone from skin and linen. They are non-grasy and non-sticky. Vanishing creams are often used as cosmetics.

The vanishing type of cream bases contain a large proportion of water which may be as high as 80% and this seems to account for the high release of medicaments from such bases. Vanishing creams essentially contain about 20% stearic acid (triple pressed) and a part of it is reacted with alkali to form soap *in-situ.* About 5 to 10% glycerin is also included in the formulation as humectant which can be substituted either partially or wholly by propylene glycol. The typical sheen of vanishing cream is due to stearic acid. Truly speaking, vanishing cream should be regarded as dispersion and not an emulsion. Two simple formulae for vanishing cream are given below.

Example 01

Stearic acid	20.0
Potassium hydroxide	1.4
Glycerin	10.0
Purified water	70.0

Example 02

Stearic acid	15.0
White wax	2.0
White soft paraffin	8.0
Triethanolamine	1.5
Propylene glycol	8.0
Purified water	65.5

D. Water-soluble bases

These bases are prepared from mixture of low and high molecular weight polyethylene glycols which range in their consistency from liquids to solids. Their water solubility is due to the presence of many polar groups and other linkages. They are non-volatile, unctuous, inert and possess the ability to form an emollient surface. They neither hydrolyse and deteriorate nor support mould growth.

Medicaments like benzoic and salicylic acids, phenol, tannic acid, bacitracin etc. have a solubilizing effect on bases consisting of high molecular weight polyethylene glycols. Although the diffusion of medicaments through such bases occurs readily yet the percutaneous absorption is very little. Some formulae for water-washable ointments containing polyethylene glycols are given below.

Example 01

PEG 400 monostearate	26.0
PEG 400	37.0
PEG 4000	37.0

Example 02

PEG 4000	42.5
PEG 400	37.5
1, 2, 5-Hexanetriol	20.0

Example 03

PEG 400	60
PEG 4000	40

Example 04

PEG 4000	11.2
Stearyl alcohol	20.8
Glycerin	17.0
Sodium lauryl sulphate	0.6
Purified water	50.4

Some of the water-soluble bases are also prepared by employing glyceryl monostearate (GMS), cellulose derivative, sodium alginate, bentonite, colloidal magnesium aluminium silicate, and Carbopol 934. Carbopol 934, and acid polymer disperses readily in water to yield an acid solution of low viscosity. It is physiologically inert, non-irritating and non-sensitizer. It exhibits excellent compatibility with materials frequently incorporated in ointment formulations. Some examples of ointment bases employing materials like GMS, hydrocolloids and Carbopol 934 etc. are given below.

Example 01

Calcium citrate	0.05 g
Sodium alginate	3.0 g
Methyl paraben	0.20g
Glycerin	45.0 g
Purified water to make	100 g

Example 02

Petrolatum	32.0 g
Bentonite	13.0 g
Sodium lauryl sulphate	0.5 g
Purified water	54 g
Methyl paraben	0.1 g

Example 03

Mineral oil	10
White petrolatum	30
GMS	10
Cetyl alcohol	05
Glycerin	05
Purified water	40

Example 04

Methocel 90 HC 4000	1.0 g
Carbopol 934	0.3 g
Propylene glycol	20.0 ml
Methyl paraben	0.15 g
Purified water q.s	100 ml
Sodium hydroxide q.s pH 7.0	

Each ointment base type has different physical characteristics and therapeutic uses based upon the nature of its components. The following table summarizes the composition, properties, and common uses of each of the five types of bases.

Table 12.1: Properties of ointment bases

Properties	**oleaginous bases**	**absorption bases**	**w/o emulsion bases**	**o/w emulsion bases**	**water miscible bases**
Composition	oleaginous compounds	oleaginous base & *w/o* surfactant	oleaginous base & water (< 45% *w/w*) & *w/o* surfactant (HLB ≤8)	oleaginous base & water (> 45% *w/w*) + *o/w* surfactant (HLB ≥9)	Polyethylene Glycols (PEGs)
Water Content	anhydrous	anhydrous	hydrous	hydrous	anhydrous, hydrous
Affinity for Water	hydrophobic	hydrophilic	hydrophobic	hydrophilic	hydrophilic
Spreadability	Difficult	difficult	moderate to easy	easy	moderate to easy
Washability	Non-washable	poorly washable	poorly washable	washable	washable
Stability	oils poor; hydrocarbons better	oils poor; hydrocarbons better	unstable, especially alkali soaps and natural colloids	unstable, especially alkali soaps and natural colloids; nonionics better	stable
Drug Incorporation Potential	solids or oils (oil solubles only)	solids, oils, and aqueous solutions (small amounts)	solids, oils, and aqueous solutions (small amounts)	solid and aqueous solutions (small amounts)	solid and aqueous solutions

Table 12.1 *Contd....*

Drug Release Potential*	Poor	poor, but > oleaginous	fair to good	fair to good	good
Occlusiveness	Yes	yes	sometimes	no	no
Uses	protectants, emollients (+/-), vehicles for hydrolyzable drugs	protectants, emollients (+/-), vehicles for aqueous solutions, solids, and non-hydrolyzable drugs	emollients, cleansing creams, vehicles for solid, liquid, or non-hydrolyzable drugs	emollients, vehicles for solid, liquid, or non-hydrolyzable drugs	drug vehicles
Examples	White Petrolatum, White Ointment	Hydrophilic Petrolatum, Anhydrous Lanolin, Aquabase, Aquaphor, Polysorb	Cold Cream type, Hydrous Lanolin, Rose Water Ointment, Hydrocream, Eucerin	Hydrophilic Ointment, Dermabase, Velvachol, Unibase	PEG Ointment, Polybase

Preparation of ointments

Ointments can be prepared either by mechanical incorporation or by fusion methods. Irrespective of the method employed for the preparation, ointments should be smooth and free from granular or gritty particles. In compounding of ointments, the following general considerations are observed.

(i) If insoluble substances are to be incorporated in the ointment base then they should be in impalpable powder form.

(ii) For efficient incorporation of insoluble substances they should first be levigated with a little quantity of base to form a smooth cream and then incorporated into the remainder of the base.

(iii) Water-soluble salts are best incorporated by dissolving them in a small quantity of water and then incorporating in the base.

(iv) Drugs soluble in ointment bases may also be incorporated by fusion (melting the highest melting point ingredient of the base and mixing the medicament into it). Remaining ingredients are then added and mixed by stirring.

A. PREPARATION BY MECHANICAL INCORPORATION

This can be achieved by the use of i) mortar and pestle, ii) ointment slab and spatula, and iii).an ointment mill. Mechanical method of incorporation is particularly advantageous when the substance to be incorporated into ointment base must be in a fine state of subdivision.

a. Mortar and pestle

This method is used to a limited extent in compounding practice particularly when large quantities of liquids are to be incorporated in a base or when exceptionally large quantities of the ointments are to be prepared. Compounding a homogeneous ointment in a mortar and pestle is not as simple as compounding of a powder.

b. Ointment slab

In this case both mixing and size reduction of insoluble medicaments are better than the previous method. The powder is first rubbed with a small quantity of the base to form a concentrated ointment base containing a finely divided powder uniformly distributed in it. The concentrated ointment is then gradually diluted with remaining quantity of the base by rubbing with a spatula. A small quantity (approximately 5%) of oil or oil-soluble substances can be used as a levigating agent. Large amounts of levigating agents may cause undue softening of the finished preparation. The spatula should be of stainless steel with a long, broad flexible blade. When steel spatula cannot be used for reasons of reacting with certain drugs like iodine, salicylic acid, and mercury salts etc., a hard rubber spatula or a wooden tongue depressor may be used.

c. Ointment mill

Ointment mills are particularly suitable for large scale manufacture of ointments although small mills are available for laboratory scale ointment preparation. Ointments containing gritty particles are also passed through the ointment mill to ensure further uniformity and smoothness. Usually the powdered medicaments are sifted into the softened or melted base in a change can mixer, stirred into the softened or melted base in a change can mixer, stirred until congealed and then run through any ointment mill. Most popular ointment mill is the triple roller mill in which the ointment is made to pass through the narrow clearance between the rolls. This mill can be sterilized by wiping with 5% aqueous phenol solution and storage under UV light before use. There is a provision for cooling the rolls so that melted materials introduced as a liquid will emerge as an ointment.

B. PREPARATION BY FUSION

When waxy material and hard bodies are to be incorporated in soft oleaginous materials, fusion is the best technique. It consists of subdividing the waxy components and melting together all components over a water bath starting from one having a highest melting point. Remaining components are then added in order of their decreasing melting points till all the components are added up. Thus all the components are not unduly exposed to higher temperatures. The mixture should be continuously stirred until congealed to ensure a homogeneous preparation. Powdered ingredients, if any, are then added using a small quantity of the base as a levigating agent.

PACKAGING AND LABELLING

1. Ointment jars

a. Straight-sided screw cap jars of glass or plastic.
b. Clear, amber or opaque glass containers
c. White, opaque, plastic usually high-density polyethylene jar.
d. Metal or composition plastic tops

2. Ointment tubes

a. Made of tin or aluminium or plastic materials e.g. polyethylene, polypropylene.
b. Ointment tube should be packed in a winged plastic board box.
c. The box serves to hold and protect the ointment tube and to carry the label.
d. The ointment tube is identified with an inked-on prescription number so that both tube and box are identified.

On large scale tubes are labeled in a variety of ways. Paper labels may be used. Label may be silk-screened onto plastic surfaces. Expiry dates and code lot numbers may be stamped on as a part of the tube crimping procedure.

Stability

The ointments can be dispensed in wide-mouth jars or tubes of adequate size or in collapsible tubes. While dispensing in jars, care should be exercised not to allow the contact of the ointment with the cap liner. The cap should be tightly fitted after use so as to avoid evaporation of water.

The problems of stability of ointments are mostly concerned with the initial and `in-use' microbial contamination and its increase. Many ophthalmic ointments are found to be heavily contaminated with pathogenic micro-organisms. The main source of microbial contamination in ointments is water which supports the growth of micro-organisms.

To safeguard the stability of the packaged product the following points are borne in mind.

(i) In general, the pharmacist or the manufacturer should follow Good Manufacturing Practice (GMP).
(ii) Use of preservatives to protect against the contamination, deterioration or spoilage of ointment bases by bacteria and fungi.
(iii) Use of antioxidants when there is possibility of oxidative degradation of the base.
(iv) Use of chelating agents where the presence of traces of metallic ions is anticipated. The traces of metallic ions, if present, may catalyse oxidative degradation.
(v) If the metallic ions are chelated their catalytic effect is nullified.

(vi) The immediate container should not permit evaporation of water from the packaged ointments otherwise an emulsion base may lose aqueous phase and others may become dry and hard.

(vii) The containers should ensure not only the sterility of ophthalmic ointments initially but also up to a time till whole of the preparation is consumed.

(viii) Due to wide variations in the climatic conditions in different regions in tropical countries, maintenance of desirable consistency of an ointment is also an important consideration.

(ix) Most of the problems related to the stability of packaged ointments can be solved by dispensing them as single application capsules although it works out to be more expensive. This is particularly recommended in case of ophthalmic ointments where sterility and absence of particles are the prime considerations.

Ophthalmic ointments

Eye ointments should be sterile and supplied in small sterile tubes with a fine nozzle for convenience in application. The tubes should be thoroughly cleaned and free from metallic and dust particles. These ointments are intended for application into the eye for the effect of a variety of medicaments on the outside and edges of the eyelids, the conjunctiva, the cornea and the iris. Most of these ointments contain petrolatum, petrolatum-mineral oil and petrolatum-anhydrous lanolin bases. Absorption and emulsion bases may irritate the eye due to the emulsifier/surfactant present in the base.

Sterility of ophthalmic ointments is a legal requirement and hence tests for sterility should always be performed on packaged products. Immediate container for ophthalmic ointment should be sealed and tamper-proof so as to ensure sterility at time of first usage.

The active ingredients should be finely divided and sterile. Petrolatum bases can be sterilized in a hot air oven at 175^0C for 2 hours. The processing should be carried out under aseptic conditions employing sterile apparatus and equipment. For small scale preparations either an aseptic hood or a laminar flow unit is satisfactory. An easy method for sterilizing ointment tubes consists of keeping them immersed in 70% alcohol for 24 hours prior to use. Current trend in ophthalmic ointments is to pack them in single application capsules so as to preclude contamination during use products. Such single application ointment capsules contain a quantity sufficient for single use and have to be punctured with a sterile needle just before use and discarded afterwards.

Rectal ointments

The usual ointment bases need modification if they are to be applied rectally. Rectal ointment should be very soft in consistency and sufficient thin so that they can pass easily through a rectal nozzle without bursting the tube. Replacement of the 25% base with liquid paraffin usually provides desired thin and soft consistency in ointments containing soft paraffin, olive oil or arachis oil for replacing Simple Ointment, to render it suitable for rectal application. The present trend is towards the formulation of water-soluble rectal ointment bases.

GENERAL COMMENTS ON COMPOUNDING OINTMENT BASES

a. Some quantity of an ointment may be lost in the compounding process between 2 and 4 grams. The ointment is lost as it adheres to ointment tiles, beakers, or ointment pads, spatula etc. To compensate for this loss, make an excess of the ointment. A general rule might be to add all ingredients in 10% excess of the prescribed amount.

b. Melt ingredients on a water bath (not more than 100°C) or special low temperature hotplate (full range is 25°C to 120°C). Most ingredients used in ointment bases will liquefy at around 70°C. These two heating devices provide adequate control over the heating and will ensure that the ingredients are not over heated.

c. If oil and aqueous phase are being mixed together to make an ointment, it is helpful to heat the aqueous phase a few degrees higher than the oil phase prior to mixing because aqueous phase tends to cool faster than the oil phase and may cause premature solidification of some ingredients. However, use the lowest temperature possible and keep the time of heating as short as possible. This will minimize the quantity of water lost through evaporation.

d. If a number of ingredients required melting melting, the ingredient with the highest melting point should be melted first. Then gradually reduce the heat to melt the ingredient with the next lowest melting point. Continue this process until all ingredients have been added.

e. The cooling step in an ointment's preparation is an important part of the compounding process.

   - Do not cool by putting the melt in water or ice. It will change the consistency or homogeneity of the final product, making it more stiff than desired.
   - If volatile ingredients such as oils, flavors, or drugs are required, add them when the product is cool to the back of the hand and apply just enough heat to evaporate the volatile substance.
   - Ointments should be cooled until just a few degrees above solidification before they are poured into tubes or jars. They should be thick, viscous fluids. This will minimize layering of the ointment in the packaging container.

Example 01 : Oleagineous base

White Wax	5 %
White Petrolatum	95%

Method of Preparation : Melt the white wax on a hot plate (at 70 - 75°C). When the wax has completely melted, add the petrolatum and allow the entire mixture to remain on the hot plate until liquefied. Following liquefication, remove from heat and allow the mixture to congeal. Stir the mixture until it begins to congeal.

Example 02: Absorption Base

Cholesterol	3%
Stearyl Alcohol	3%
White Wax	8%
White Petrolatum	86%

Method of Preparation : Melt the stearyl alcohol, white wax, and petrolatum together on a hot plate and add the cholesterol to the mixture; stir until completely dissolved. Remove the mixture from the hot plate and stir until congealed.

Example 03 : Water-in-oil emulsion base

White wax	12.0%
Cetyl Esters Wax (or Spermaceti)	12.5%
Mineral Oil	56.0%
Sodium Borate	0.5%
Water	19.0%

Method of Preparation : Melt the white wax and spermaceti on a hot plate and add the mineral oil to this mixture and bring the temperature to 70°C. Dissolve the sodium borate in water. Heat the sodium borate solution to 70°C. When both phases have reached the desired temperature, remove both phases from the hot plate and add the aqueous phase slowly and with constant stirring to the oil phase. Stir briskly and continuously until congealed.

Example 04 : Oil in water emulsion base

Sodium Lauryl Sulfate	1.0%
Propylene Glycol	12.0%
Stearyl Alcohol	25.0%
White Petrolatum	25.0%
Purified Water	37.0%

Method of Preparation : Melt the stearyl alcohol and white petrolatum on a hot plate at 70°C. Dissolve remaining ingredients in water and heat the solution to 70° C. Add the oleaginous phase slowly to the aqueous phase, stirring constantly. Remove from heat and stir the mixture until it congeals.

Example 05 : Water Soluble Base

Polyethylene Glycol 400	60%
Polyethylene Glycol 4000	40%

Method of Preparation : Melt the PEG 400 and PEG 4000 on a hot plate and heat the mixture to about 65°C. Remove from the hot plate and stir until congealed.

Practice Exercises

Example 01 : To prepare Emulsifying Ointment

Liquid paraffin, Emulsifying wax	2.00 g
White soft paraffin	3.00 g
	5.00 g

Method of Preparation : Melt together liquid paraffin, emulsifying wax, and white soft paraffin. Stir until cool.

Uses : Pharmaceutical aid.

Example 02 : To prepare Simple Ointment

Wool fat	0.50 g
Cetostearyl alcohol	0.50 g
Hard paraffin	0.50 g
White soft paraffin or yellow soft paraffin	8.50 g

Method of Preparation : Mix wool fat, cetostearyl alcohol, hard paraffin, and white soft paraffin or yellow soft paraffin in a container. Heat the mixture gently with stirring until homogeneous. Stir continually until cold.

Uses : Pharmaceutical aid.

Example 03 : To prepare Paraffin Ointment

White beeswax	0.20 g
Hard paraffin	0.30 g
Cetostearyl alcohol	0.50 g
White soft paraffin	9.00 g

Method of Preparation : Mix white beeswax, hard paraffin, cetostearyl alcohol, and white soft paraffin. Heat gently with stirring until homogeneous, and stir until cold.

Uses : Pharmaceutical aid and protective.

Example 04: To prepare Wool Alcohol Ointment

Wool alcohol	0.60 g
White soft paraffin or yellow soft paraffin	1.00 g
Hard paraffin	2.40 g
Liquid paraffin	6.00 g

Method of Preparation : Melt together wool alcohol, white soft paraffin or yellow soft paraffin, hard paraffin, and liquid paraffin. Heat gentle and stir until cold.

Uses : Pharmaceutical aid, protective

Example 05 : To prepare Salicylic Acid Ointment

Salicylic acid, finely sifted	0.20 g
Wool alcohol ointment	9.80 g

Method of Preparation : Melt the wool alcohol ointment. Add gradually the salicylic acid and stir until cold.

Uses : Local anti-infective

Example 06 : To prepare Zinc Ointment

Zinc oxide, finely sifted	1.50 g
Simple ointment	8.50 g

Method of Preparation : Triturate the zinc oxide with a portion of the simple ointment until smooth. Gradually add simple ointment sufficient to produce 10 g.

Uses : Astringent, protective and antiseptic

CHAPTER 13

MISCELLANEOUS PREPARATIONS

1. TABLETS	6. CAPSULES	11. OPHTHALMICS
2. TABLET TRITURATES	7. CREAMS	12. PAINTS
3. LOZENGES	8. JELLIES	13. INHALATION
4. PILLS	9. SUPPOSITORIES	14. SPRAYS
5. PASTILLES	10. PASTES	

1. TABLETS

Tablets are a solid, unit dosage form prepared by compression using tablet compression machine. Tablet can be defined as solid, flat or biconcave disc (also available in various shapes) prepared by compressing a drug or a mixture of drugs with or without suitable diluents. About 90% of drugs are available in the form of tablets to produce a therapeutic effect when administered by the oral route. They vary in shape and differ greatly in size and weight, depending on the amount of medicinal substances and the intended mode of administration.

Tablet fabrication by compression was initiated in 1843 by Brockedon. Since then the popularity of this dosage form has been increasing and today tablets remain the most popular of all the dosage forms, intended for oral use. This may be attributed in part to the availability of variety of compression machines and advances in tablet technology.

Common Abbreviations of Tablets

- Sugar Coated Tablets [SCT]
- Multiple Compressed Tablets [MCT]
- Film Coated Tablets [FCT]
- Enteric Coated Tablets [ECT]
- Chocolate Coated Tablets [CCT]

- Multiple Compressed Tablets [MCT]
- Buccal Tablets [BT]
- Sublingual Tablets [ST]
- Effervescent Tablets [ET]
- Dispensing Tablets [DT]
- Hypodermic Tablets [HT]

Advantages

Tablet dosage form has number of potential advantages over the other solid dosage forms as well as liquid dosage forms such as :

1. Unit dosage form (dosage accuracy). 2. Compactness of dosage. 3. Easy to swallow. Highly soluble. 4. Flexibility of dosage form. 5. Easy to prepare. 6. Economic for packaging, shipping and storage.

Disadvantages

1. Highly amorphous substances are very difficult to compress.
2. Poor wetting and slow dissolution drugs can not be placed in the form of tablets.
3. Objectionable odor, bitter tasting and humectant substances need special treatment for compression.

CLASSIFICATION OF TABLETS

Tablets are classified on the basis of shape and size, process involved in its preparation and route and other characteristics.

I. Shape and size	II. Process
1. Round tablets : a) flat surface, b) concave surface, c) convex surface 2. Oval tablet : a) oral route, b) other than oral route tablets 3. Oblong tablet : suppositories 4. Cylindrical tablet : suppositories 5. Triangular tablets a) Lozenges, b). chewable tablets	1. Compressed Uncoated tablets 2. Compressed Coated tablets a). sugar coated, b). film coated, c). enteric coated

III. Route and other special characteristics

1. Oral tablets for ingestion	2. Tablets used in oral cavity
a. Compressed tablets (CT) b. Multiple compressed tablets (MCT) c. Prolonged action tablets d. Sustained release tablets e. Delayed action tablets f. Chewable tablets g. Coated tablets	a. Buccal tablets b. Sublingual tablets c. Troches and Lozenges d. Dental cones
3. Tablets administered by other than oral route	**4. Special tablets**
a. Suppositories b. Implant	a. Effervescent tablets b. Dispersible tablets c. Dispensing tablets d. Hypodermic tablets e. Tablet triturates (TT) f. Soluble tablets

COMPOUNDING

Compounding of tablets requires following additives, in addition to the drug substance.

Diluents : Diluents are substances to increase bulk and convert in the compressible form, when drug material is potent or inadequate to provide a suitable shape and size to tablet. A tablet diluent must be compatible, inert, economic, easily available and organoleptically acceptable. It should not affect the bioavailability of a drug adversely.

Examples of tablet diluents include dibasic calcium phosphate, calcium sulphate, lactose, lactose anhydrous, lactose spray dried, mannitol, sorbitol, sucrose, dextrose etc. Examples of directly compressible diluents include Sta-Rx-1500, Emdex (contains dextrose 90 to 92% and maltose 3 to 5%), Celutab (dextrose & maltose), Avicel (Microcrystalline cellulose), Di-Cal (Dicalcium phosphate dihydrate), Cab-O-Sil (Colloidal silica).

Binders and Adhesive : These materials are used in dry or liquid form to reduce the amorphous nature of substance and convert into compressible form (wet granulation).

Example include acacia, tragacanth, gelatin, alginates, methylcellulose, hydroxypropyl-methylcellulose, hydroxypropylcellulose, PVP, Starch, sorbiol, ethylcellulose, pregelatinized starch, glucose, iris moss, ghatti gum, arabogalactan, waxes, etc.

Disintegrants : Most of the tablets contain disintegrating agent. Disintegrating agents facilitate the disintegration of the tablet in small particles in the gastrointestinal tract. Breaking of tablet is based on the swellability, adsorption of water or chemical reaction. Examples include soluble starch, pre-gelatinized starch (PGS), veegum HV, bentonite, microcrystalline cellulose, sodium carboxy methylcellulose, PVP, guar gum, Ispaghula, primogel, explotab, aerosil, natural sponge citrus pulp, Alginic acid and alginates, Ion exchange resin, magnesium aluminium silicate, modified corn starch, sodium dodecyl sulphate, sodium starch glycollate, etc.

Glidants : Glidants act as a flow promoter and reduce the friction between particles. It improves the flow properties of granules or powder through hopper to die. It is not deformed by compression pressure of the tablet machine. Examples include talc, starch, magnesium stearate, calcium stearate, boric acid, sugar, lycopodium and sodium chloride.

Lubricants :

Lubricants reduce inter-particular friction. It improves the ejection of tablet from die wall and reduces the sticking problems and smooth tablets are produced. Examples include Talc, magnesium stearate, calcium stearate, stearic acid, polyethyleneglycols, starch derivatives.

Antiadhesives or Antisticking agents : These materials are used to reduce the adhesion of the tablet surface to dies and punches during the compression of tablets. The pressure of the machine deforms these materials. It reduces sticking, picking and chipping problems. Examples include paraffin, stearic acid, cocoa butter, soaps, starch derivatives.

Coloring agent : Colours are selected from 'permitted' list and are added to promote elegance and also to mask differences in colour or speckling when either the drug or an additive is off white. Pastel shades are commonly used as these shades help in achieving uniform colour distribution. Coloring materials or dyes are used in tablet formulation mainly for three purposes; disguising of off color drugs, product identification and production of more elegant products. Colours may be added either to the vehicle used for granulation or to the mixture of powders prior to granulation. The first approach is known to give better results provided migration of dye to the top of granules along with solvent during drying does not occur. When wet granulation is not to be employed, lake dyes (dyes adsorbed on alumina or aluminium hydroxide) are recommended. Fading of the colour on standing and exposure to light leading to mottling of tablets is the common problem with dyes. Examples include water soluble dyes and many other FD&C approved colors or dyes.

Flavoring agent : These substances are not necessary for the formulation of compressed tablets. The proportion of flavours should generally be limited to 0.5% because excessive amounts may interfere with the free flow or cohesion of the granules. Special tablets require flavoring agents such as chewable tablet, lozenges, etc. Examples include flavoring oils like cinnamon, coriander, and caraway etc.

Sweeteners : Chewable tablets have sweetening agents because such tablets remain in the mouth and are not swallowed. Examples include saccharin sodium, aspartame, sugar, etc.

COMPRESSED TABLETS

For making compressed tablets, it is necessary to prepare the material in a dry, granular form to render it suitable for passing through a compression machine. Following general processes are employed for this purpose.

I. Wet granulation

1. The drug or a mixture of drugs in powder form is mixed; diluent and half quantity of disintegrating agent are added. The material in the desired degree of fineness is mixed and damped with a suitable moistening agent selected with regard to its effect on the chemical and physical nature of the material.
2. The moistened material is made into granules by passing it through a sieve # 12, 16, 22 etc.
3. The granules are dried in a current of air, at a suitable temperature generally not exceeding 60°C.
4. The dry granules are passed through suitable sieve to get uniform granules and added half quantity of disintegrant, lubricant, antiadhesive, and glidant.
5. These granules are mixed well and are suitable for compression to get the desired type of tablets.

II. Dry granulation

1. The drug or a mixture of drugs in powder form is mixed. If necessary, add a suitable inert substance to act as diluent along with half quantity of disintegrating agent and lubricant.
2. Compress the powder materials in the form of large tablets.
3. These large tablets are broken up into granules of a suitable size.
4. These granules are passed through set of sieves to get granules of uniform size.
5. The remaining quantities of disintegrant, lubricant and glidant are added and mixed well. The granules can be compressed using tablet machine.

III. Direct compression

1. The drug or a mixture of drugs in powder form is mixed. If necessary, add a suitable inert substance to act as diluent direct compressible disintegrating agent, glidant and lubricant.
2. Pass the powder material through a suitable sieve.
3. Compress the powder materials in the form of tablets.

Table 13.1 : Stages involved in various granulation methods

Wet granulation	Dry granulation	Direct compression
Raw material (drug)	Raw material (drug)	Raw material (drug)
Weighing and measuring	Weighing and measuring	Weighing and measuring
Screening	Screening	Screening
Manual feeding	Blending (slow-speed planetary mixer)	Manual feeding
		-
Blending (slow-speed planetary mixer)	Compress slug	-
		-
Wetting (hand addition)	-	-
Subdivision (comminutor)	Subdivision (comminutor)	-
Drying (fluid bed dryer)	-	-
Subdivision (comminutor)	-	-
Premixing (barrel roller)	Premixing (barrel roller)	-
Lubrication (ribbon blinder)	Lubrication (ribbon blinder)	-
Manual feeding	Manual feeding	-
Compression	Compression	Compression

EVALUATION PARAMETERS

Shape and size : Thickness of the tablets should be controlled within ± 5% variation with a standard value. It may change with die-wall, particle size, distribution, packing of particles and compressive load. The crown thickness of tablets may be measured by micrometer (sliding caliper scale). This test is necessary for packaging of tablets as well as drug content uniformly.

1. **Organoleptic properties** : Some tablets may contain organoleptic substances such as flavoring agent, coloring agent and sweetener. Color uniformity of the tablet can be evaluated by reflectance spectrophotometry, tristimulus colorimetry or microreflectance photometery.

2. **Hardness :** Suitable hardness is necessary for handling in manufacturing, packaging and shipping. Hardness of the tablets can be measured by Monsanto tester, Strong-cobb-tester, Pfizer tester and Erweka tester.

3. **Friability :** Friability is another measurement of tablet strength as tablet hardness is not an absolute indicator of strength. Roche friabilator is used as laboratory equipment for the determination of friability. It has a plastic chamber that revolves at 25 rpm, tablet drops a distance of six inches with each revolution and operated for 100 revolutions. Compressed should not lose more than 1.0% of their weight.

4. **Weight variations** : It is measured to ensure that tablet contains the proper amount of drug and is a satisfactory test for determination of content uniformity of tablets.

Usually ten tablets are taken for this test. In USP, 20 tablets are weighed individually and average weight of tablets is calculated.

USP limit		IP limit	
Average weight of tablets (mg)	Maximum variation	Average weight of tablets (mg)	Maximum variation
130 or less	± 10.0%	80 or less	± 10.0%
130 to 324	± 7.5%	80 to 300	± 7.5%
More than 324	± 5.0%	More than	± 5.0%

6. **Disintegration :** Breaking of tablets into smaller particles or granules is known as disintegration and time taken for breaking of tablets in a suitable medium is called disintegration time (DT). IP apparatus consists of 6 glass tubes each 3 inches long, open at top and has 10 mesh screen at the bottom end of basket rack. One tablet is placed in each tube and placed in a one liter beaker of water, simulated gastric fluid or simulated intestinal fluid at 37 ± 2°C. It moves up and down through a distance of 5 to 6 cm at 28 to 32 cpm. Uncoated tablets have disintegration times as low as 5 minutes. Majority of tablets have DT of 30 minutes. Disintegration time of enteric coated tablet is one hour in simulated gastric fluid and two hours in simulated intestinal fluid.

7. **Dissolution** : The rate of absorption depends on the dissolution of the product. It is directly proportional to the bioavailability of the products. For dissolution study two types of apparatus are used, basket assembly and paddle assembly. It consists of a hemispherical flask of 1000 ml capacity, temperature is maintained at 37 ± 0.5°C, $t_{90\%}$ obtained within 30 min. is satisfactory.

8. **Drug content** : Drug uniformity in tablet is determined by assay. It is calculated on batch to batch or lot to lot basis. It is estimated by the titration, spectrophotometer and HPLC.

Table 13.2 : Tablet Defects

Defect	Description	Causes	Remedy
Capping	Partial or complete separation of top or bottom surface of the tablet from the main body is called capping. This type of problem is generally found after compression.	a. Entrapment of air, b. deformational problems c. incorrect set up of tablet press	a. Reduce the speed of press b. increase percentage of moisture

Table 13.2 *Contd....*

Lamination	Separation of a tablet into two or three layers is called as lamination	a. entrapment of air b.deformational properties of formulations c. direct compression d. low moisture content (less than 5%).	a. Reduce the speed of press b.Increase percentage of moisture.
Picking	Removal of surface material from the punch surface is called picking	a. Embossing or engraving of punch tips b. Convex type of punch c. insufficient anti-adhesive	a. Reduce convex curve of punch b. uniform distribution of anti-adhesive c. Reduce letters like A, O, Welcome, etc. on punch.
Sticking	Some material of tablet adhering inside the die wall, is called sticking	a. insufficient lubricant b. Excessive moisture content	a. mix sufficient lubricant b. Reduce moisture content
Chipping	Serious problem of sticking is called chipping. The tablet produced has rough surface due to this problem. It creates difficulty in free movement of punches	Low melting point substances	Add higher melting point substances e.g. stearic acid.
Mottling	Unequal distribution of color in tablet is called mottling.	a. Migration of dye b. Unequal distribution of color c. large particle size	Add anti-leaching dye substances in the product such as acacia, tragacanth etc.
Poor flow	Incomplete filling of dies by the powder material due to poor flow of material from hopper to die wall.	a. speed of tablet machine b. Different density of powder material as well as additives.	Addition of glidant e.g. talcum, colloidal silica.
Double Impression	One dark and one lighter impression on tablet surface are called double impression.	Uncontrolled movement of lower punch.	Regulation of the punch movement as well as speed of the machine.

2. TABLET TRITURATES

Tablet triturate (Molded tablets) are generally prepared by mixing the active drug with lactose, dextrose, sucrose, mannitol, or some other appropriate diluent that can serve as the base. This base must be readily water soluble and should not degrade during the tablet's preparation. Lactose is the preferred base but mannitol adds a pleasant, cooling sensation and additional sweetness in the mouth. The base ordinarily used for molded tablet triturates is lactose containing 10% - 20% sucrose, the latter being added to make a firmer tablet. Drugs that react chemically with sugars require special bases such as precipitate calcium carbonate, precipitated calcium phosphate, kaolin, or bentonite. A liquid is added to moisten the powder mixture so it will adhere while being pressed into the mold cavities. Mixtures of alcohol and water in varying proportions (typically about 50 - 80% alcohol) are employed; the alcohol will speed up the drying of the liquid and the water will cause the sugars to dissolve and bind the tablet. If the tablet contains ingredients that are very soluble in water, water can be omitted altogether and alcohol alone can be used.

One of the advantages of Tablet triturate is that they quickly disintegrate in the presence of moisture. And since the tablets are actually compressed powder mixtures, the pharmacist can easily adjust the composition for any number of dosages. Their chief disadvantage is their small size which will limit their use to substances effective in small doses.

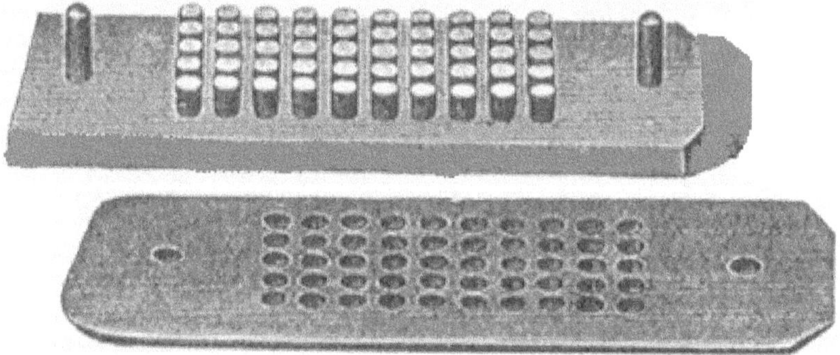

Fig. 13.1 Tablet Triturate Mould

Tablet triturate molds are made of metal. There are two plates, the cavity plate is the plate that has only holes and the peg plate that has pegs. The mold will indicate the capacity of one cavity in the cavity plate but that indication is only an approximation. Typical die plate cavity sizes are 60 mg and 100 mg.

Properties of an ideal tablet

The objective of formulation and fabrication of tablet is to deliver the correct amount of drug in proper form at or over proper time.

1. Tablet should be elegant, free from defects such as cracks, chips, contamination and discoloration.
2. Tablets are stable dosage form and maintain its physical integrity over time.
3. No alteration in the chemical and physical properties of medicinal agent during the storage of dosage form.
4. It should be capable to maintain the uniformity its production, packaging, shipping and dispensing.
5. An ideal tablet should be able to release the medicament(s) in body in predictable and reproducible manner.

3. LOZENGES

Lozenges resemble tablets and provide a prolonged effect of the drug. They are sucked in the mouth to disintegrate slowly releasing the medication for local action. The base however is different than that for the pastilles and consists of gum, starch and sugar along with a suitable liquid excipient which dries. In industry, the lozenges are formulated like tablets using higher proportion of gum and compressing them harder. The traditional method of compounding is by moulding the lozenge mass in suitable shape and size. A hard dough is prepared using appropriate quantity of the drugs and excipients providing for losses, water or alcohol are used for moistening which provides rapid drying. The mass is rolled flat on a tile using a dusting power, if necessary. The lozenges are then cut from the flat mass with the help of a lozenge cutter. Lozenge cutters are available that provide different shapes and sizes. They are allowed to dry and packed in containers similar to those employed for pastilles.

For making pastilles, the moulds are calibrated for the weight of the base they can hold when filled to the brim. The quantities of the medicaments and the excipients are accordingly weighed, providing for losses. Similarly for moulded lozenges, the mass should be spread over an area from which lozenges in required number may be cut to provide correct quantity of medication in each lozenge.

Rx	
Sulphadiazine	200 mg
Ol. menth. pip.	0.01 ml
Gum Tragacanth	
Sucrose	
Water	aa q.s.
Mitte tales 20 lozenges. Label: Suck occasionally.	

4. PILLS

Pill is an old dosage form of presenting solid medication. Inconvenience associated with the administration of powders led to the use of pills by converting the powder into a spherical shape with the help of a liquid and excipients. Historically, the pills have been into use for the last 200 years and till the advent of compressed tablets pills were a very popular dosage form. Almost 60% of the prescriptions at one time comprised of pills. The word 'pill' has become so deep-rooted in medical practice that today when pills are seldom used and prepared in dispensing practice or by the industry, the term 'pill' is at times used for a tablet. However pills continue to be popular is homeopathic and ayurvedic medicine A century ago, making good pills was considered to be a great pharmaceutical art and only experienced pharmacists were known to be able to roll attractive looking pills. At one stage the pharmacist was considered to be a pill maker. The pills were provided with coatings of a variety of substances e.g. sugar, salol, talc, silver and gold leaf, and varnish. From the dispensing counter, the pill reached the pharmaceutical industry and machinery was designed to manufacture pills on large scale prior to the introduction of compressed tablets.

Pills are generally spherical in shape, sometimes oval. The only positive aspect of this dosage form was its shape that facilitated swallowing. A large pill meant for veterinary use is called a **bolus**. Freshly made pills provided rapid disintegration in the gastro-intestinal (GI) tract but manufactured, particularly coated pills were most unpredictable as regards their disintegration time. Further, variation in the weight of individual pills is more than that in the tablets and capsules. The pills were kneaded to make a mass with hand which from modern standards is considered an unhygienic practice.

It is interesting that the basic principles of pill making and coating are presently being applied to tablet making and coating and fabrication of sustained release dosage forms. In the process of evolution of unit dosage forms of medicaments, pills may be considered as predecessors of tablets.

In compounding pills the drug(s) and excipients are taken for two additional pills than the number of pills that are to be supplied. The excipients used in pills are many and include diluents e.g. glycyrrhiza, lactose and gums or their combinations. The quantity of the diluent to be used is a matter of experience, the object being to produce a pill of reasonable size. Although no norms are prescribed, yet the average weight of a pill is expected to be within 120 to 150 mg. The drug, the diluent and other excipients are made into a suitable mass which should be plastic, firm and adhesive. These properties are essential to keep the mass cohesive to enable the pill to retain its shape. Liquid excipients also called moistening agents include mucilages, honey, syrup, syrup of liquid glucose, water, alcohol and glycerin. Water alone is not used as it does not assist coherence on drying. This is also true with alcohol and the pills tend to be hard on drying. Sometimes solid excipients that are absorbents are used e.g. glycurrhiza, calcium phosphate, acacia and oxides and carbonates of magnesium. Oleaginous substances like waxes and oils are used as excipients in some preparations. After a mass of proper consistency is obtained, it is rolled on a pill tile to yield a pill pipe in the shape of a pencil. Dusting Powders e.g. lycopodium, magnesium carbonate or starch may be used to prevent sticking of the tile or the roller. The choice of the dusting material depends upon the colour of the pill. The dusting powders are expected not to show themselves conspicuously over the surface of the pill. The pipe is rolled in uniform diameter to a length of two more cutters than the number of pills to be prepared. It may be remembered that the ingredients were also taken for two extra pills. The pipe so rolled is placed next to the edge of the pill cutter and pressed with the roller to cut it in small pieces. The cut mass at the two ends will be lesser in weight as compared to others and hence it is rejected. The rest of them are removed one by one from the cutter and rolled round in the palm of one hand with the help of the index finger of the other hand. Appropriate quantity of the dusting powder may be applied to the palm and the finger to prevent sticking. Sometime, pill rounders are also used for the purpose to provide a perfectly round shape. Pearl, silver or gold coating may be provided to the pills by adding a small quantity of talcum powder or a silver or a gold leaf, respectively, keeping the pills in the rounder. A drop or two of water may be sprinkled, if necessary. The lid is placed in position and the rounder gently rotated to provide a uniform coating. Two to three of such coats yield a good finish to the product. At the dispensing counter varnish, sugar or enteric coating can be provided by dipping individual pills attached to a pin in the solution of these materials, the pills and sealing the pin hole with the solution applied with a thin brush. Pills are supplied in cylindrical paper board boxes or wide-mouthed plastic or glass containers of a proper size and a tight-fitting lid.

PRACTICE EXERCISES

Rx

Aloe	3 gr
Excipient	q.s.

Mitte tales pilula numero xii.

Rx

Calomel	1 gm
Pulv. Ipecac.	100 gm

Make a pill mass and divide in 10 pills

Rx

Belladona extract	½ grain
Opium	½ grain

Supply 8 pills. To be used as directed.

5. PASTILLES

Pastilles are preparations which are kept in the mouth and slowly allowed to dissolve thus gradually releasing the medication for local action generally in the throat. The base is composed of glycerin and gelatin. The drug may be either in solution or in suspension form in the base. In extemporaneous dispensing the pastilles are prepared by pouring hot molten mass in moulds and allowing to cool when it sets in a soft mass. They can be scooped out of the mould easily because the mould is previously wiped with a cloth moistened with liquid paraffin, which prevents sticking to the mould surface. They are then wrapped in a waxed or cellophane paper. Pastilles manufactured by the pharmaceutical industry are relatively harder as they contain a greater proportion of gelatin. As they are harder, a longer time is required for dissolution in the mouth. Since the pastilles are designed to remain in the mouth for a long time, they are sweetened and flavoured to make them agreeable in taste and partially mask the taste of the medicament(s). The pastilles are packed in air-tight containers and stored in cool, dry place since they are liable to absorb moisture and become damp which, in absence of a preservative, may encourage mould growth.

Rx

Penicillin	100,000 I.U.
Menthol	0.001 gm
Glycerin	
Gelatin	
Water	aa q. s.

Send 12 such pastilles. Keep in mouth and let dissolve slowly.

6. CAPSULES

The word capsule is derived from the Latin capsula meaning a small box. The word is used to describe an edible package made from gelatin that is filled with medicines to produce a unit dose mainly for oral use. Capsules are defined as solid dosage form in which one or more medicament with or without inert substances are enclosed within a small gelatin shell.

The capsule shells are composed of gelatin or other materials, the consistency of which may be adjusted by the addition of substances such as glycerol and sorbitol or a mixture of both. It contains excipients such as surface-active agents, opaque fillers, anti-microbial preservatives, sweetening agents, flavoring agents and coloring agents. The contents of capsules may be of solid, liquid or paste-like consistency. Capsules consist of one or more medicaments, with or without excipients such as solvents, diluents, lubricants or disintegration of the shell.

There are two types of capsules

I. HARD GELATIN CAPSULES

It consists of mainly two pieces, a cap and a body that fit inside the other. It is manufactured from a mixture of gelatin, colorants and sometimes may contain opacifying agents and is filled in separate operation. Empty capsules are sold by sizes from 000 the largest, to size 5, the smallest. The most popular sizes in practice are size 0 to 5 for human use.

Table 13.3 : Different Size of capsules and volume filled in ml

S.No.	Capsule No.	Volume in ml
1.	000 Largest size	1.36
2.	00	0.95
3.	0	0.67
4.	1	0.48
5.	2	0.37
6.	3	0.27
7.	4	0.20
8.	5 Smallest size	0.13

In dispensing practice it is advised that the pharmacist should note down the size of the capsule on the prescription so that he would use the same size in case the prescription is refilled.

Number 10,11 and 12 capsules are also manufactured for veterinary use only

Hard gelatin capsules contain about 12 to 16% water and require storage under controlled conditions of temperature and humidity. Capsules become flaccid and lose their shape if stored under high humidity whereas under low humidity they become brittle.

Capsule shells are prepared by two methods:

1. Plate Process, and 2. Rotary Die Process

Following materials are filled in hard gelatin capsules:

1. Dry solids : Powder, granules, pellets, tablets
2. Semisolid : Thixotropic mixture, thermo-softening mixtures, pastes, etc.

Advantages of Capsules

1. Ease of use due to the fact that it is smooth, slippery and easy to swallow and tasteless for drugs.
2. Suitable for substances having bitter taste and unpleasant odor.
3. As produced in large quantities it is economic, attractive and available in wide range of colors.
4. Minimum excipients required.
5. Little pressure required to compact the material.
6. Unit dosage form.
7. Easy to store and transport.

Disadvantages of Capsules

1. Not suitable for highly soluble substances like potassium chloride, potassium bromide, ammonium chloride, etc.
2. Not suitable for highly efflorescent or deliquescent materials.
3. Special conditions are required for storage.

Determination of Capsule Fill Weight

Capsule fill weight is determined applying following formula

Capsule fill weight = Tapped bulk density of substance × capsule volume

Example- I

A formulation has a theoretical fill weight of 325 mg and tapped bulk density of the substance is 0.75 g/ml while bulk density of inert substance is 0.80 g/ml.

Given

1. Weight of substance in each capsule = 325.0 mg
2. Bulk density of substance = 0.75 g/ml
3. Bulk density of inert substance = 0.80 g/ml

$$\text{Volume occupied by fill weight} = \frac{\text{Weight of substance in each capsule}}{\text{Bulk density of substance}}$$

$$\text{Volume occupied by fill weight} = \frac{0.325}{0.325} = 0.43 \text{ ml}$$

Volume of size '1' capsule = 0.48 ml (from Table 1.)

Volume occupied by drug = 0.43 ml (by calculation)

Volume unoccupied = 0.48 – 0.43 = 0.05 ml

Weight of diluent or inert substances = volume × bulk density

= 0.05 × 0.80 = 0.040 g = 40.0 mg

Send ten capsules of the given materials (Always weigh substance for one extra capsule as material is lost during powdering, mixing, and handling of the substance)

Weight for 11 capsule of substance = 325 × 11 = 3.575 g

Weight of diluent or inert substance = 40 × 11 = 0.440 g

Total weight of filling substance in the hard empty shell = 4.015 g

Example II

Fill the substance containing drug in each capsule, of size '1' capsule 280 mg of bulk density 0.70 g/ml. Determine how much amount of inert substance is required to fill 10 capsules while bulk density of inert substance is 0.85.

Solution : similar problem as in example I.

Example III

Which number of capsule is to be used for 375 mg material having bulk density 0.75 g/ml. Bulk density of inert substance is 0.68. Calculate the total g/ml required for 10 capsules.

Given

Weight of substance in each capsule = 375.0 mg

Bulk density of substance = 0.75 g/ml

Bulk density of inert substance = 0.68 g/ml

$$\text{Volume occupied by fill weight} = \frac{\text{Weight of substance in each capsule}}{\text{Bulk density of substance}}$$

$$\text{Volume occupied by fill weight} = \frac{0.325}{0.75} = 0.466 \text{ ml}$$

For filling this volume of substance '1' number capsule is most appropriate because

Volume of size '1' capsule = 0.48 ml (from Table 1.)

Volume occupied by drug = 0.466 ml (by calculation)

Volume unoccupied = 0.48 – 0.466 = 0.014 ml

Weight of diluent or inert substances = volume × bulk density

= 0.014 × 0.68 = 0.040 g = 0.00952 g = 9.52 mg

Send ten capsules of the given materials

Weight for 11 capsule of substance $= 375 \times 11 = 4.125$ g

Weight of diluent or inert substance $= 9.52 \times 11 = 0.105$ g

Total weight of filling substance in the hard empty shell $= 4.230$ g

Evaluation of Capsules

1. Drug content : Determine by assay process for the drug.
2. Weight variations : Determine by simple weighing of 20 capsules using digital balance, should be within the limit of 90% to 110% in weight.
3. Disintegration : Disintegration test is usually not required for capsules unless it is treated to resist solution in gastric fluid. In such cases it must meet the requirements for disintegration of enteric-coated tablets.
4. Dissolution test : Use dissolution apparatus basket assembly for determination of dissolution test.

Storage

Capsules should be kept in well-closed containers at a temperature not exceeding 30°C.

Filing Equipments

1. Eli Lilly Co., Indianapolis, IN.
2. Farmatic SNC, Bologna, Itlay
3. Hoflinger and Karg, Waiblingen, Germany
4. mG_2 S.P.A., Bologna, Itlay
5. Osaka, Osaka, Japan
6. Macofar SAS, Bologna, Itlay
7. Perry Industries, Green Bay, WI
8. Zanasi Nigris, S.P.A., Bologna, Itlay
9. Parke-Davis and Company, Detroit, MI

Other Machines

1. Rotoweigh : Capsule weighing machine
2. Rotosort : Filled capsule sorting machine
3. Seidenader Model PM 60 : Unfilled capsules cleansing and polishing machine
4. Erweka KEA : Capsule deducting and polishing machine

5. Hartnett Model B : Capsule imprinting machine
6. Markem Model 280 A : Capsule imprinting machine

Most of these machines are suitable for large scale manufacturing of capsules. For dispensing, hand operated capsule filling machines are available in various sizes.

II. SOFT GELATIN CAPSULES

The shells of soft capsules are thicker than those of hard capsules. It consists of a single part and may be of various shapes. The shells are usually formed, filled and sealed in a combined operation but in some cases, shells for extemporaneous use may be performed. The shell material may contain medicament. It may be used for enclosing liquid material while solids are usually dissolved or dispersed in a suitable excipient to give a paste like consistency. Soft gelatin capsule are also known as **soluble elastic** or **soft elastic capsule**. Their composition differs from hard gelatin capsules in that the sugar is replaced by a plasticizer like glycerin, sorbitol or a similar polyol. Soft gelatin can be modified to impart enteric, chewable and with some drugs sustained release properties. They have also been employed as a suppository dosage form for rectal or vaginal administration. Single dose application of topical and ophthalmic preparations, rectal ointments and medications for ear and nose can be packaged in soft capsules. In cosmetic industry these capsules may be used for the packaging of perfumes, shampoos, various skin creams, suntan oils etc. Soft capsules provide an attractive, odourless and tasteless from for prescribing the medication.

Soft gelatin capsules are available in oblong, spherical, elliptical and other shapes. Spherical or oval capsules are also known as **pearls** or **globules**. They are also available in different sizes to contain from 0.1 to 30 ml volume.

Following types of liquids are encapsulated in soft gelatin capsules-

1. Water-immiscible, volatile and nonvolatile liquids e.g. vegetable and animal oils, aliphatic hydrocarbons, chlorinated hydrocarbons, ethers, esters, alcohols and organic acids.
2. Water-miscible, nonvolatile liquids e.g. polyethylene glycols and non-ionic surfactants such as tween-80.
3. Water–miscible and relatively nonvolatile compounds e.g. propylene glycol, isopropyl alcohol.

Example No. 01: Amoxycillin capsule

Rx	
Amoxycillin trihydrate	250 mg
Diluent	q.s.

Dose : 2 to 3 capsule daily

Example No. 02: Ibuprofen capsule

Rx	
Ibuprofen	300 mg
Diluent	q.s.

Dose : Ibuprofen 200-600 mg twice daily

Example No. 03: Chlortetracycline capsule

Rx	
Chlortetracycline	250 mg
Diluent	q.s.

Dose : 1 to 3 capsules daily in divided doses.

Example No. 04: Paracetamol capsule

Rx	
Paracetamol	250 mg
Diluent	q.s.

Dose : 1 to 3 tablets

7. CREAMS

The term cream is used in different senses. A concentrated layer separated from milk is called cream, milk of magnesia is often referred to as a cream and certain ointments are also known as creams. Many cosmetic preparations are also called creams e.g. vanishing cream, cold cream, hand cream etc. In pharmaceutical practice the term 'cream' is applied to viscous emulsions or semi-solid preparations consisting of solutions or dispersions of one or more medicaments in suitable base and intended for application to the skin or mucous membrane. They are applied to the skin for protective, beautifying, therapeutic or prophylactic purposes. Creams may contain suitable antimicrobial or preservatives unless the medicaments or basis have sufficient intrinsic bactericidal and fungicidal activity.

Creams are mainly two types

1. water-in-oil (w/o) 2. oil-in-water (o/w)

Dilution of creams

Sometimes dilutions of proprietary creams are required. Care should be taken in diluting creams particularly to prevent microbial contamination. For dilution of creams, appropriate diluent should be used and heating should be avoided during mixing of diluent in the creams. Sometimes use of diluent may affect the stability of creams. Diluted creams should be used within two weeks of their preparation.

The stability and activity of cream may be impaired by the dilution such as :

1. Diluent without antimicrobial agent reduces the overall concentration of the preservative in the preparation.
2. Sometimes creams change from o/w to w/o by the diluent property.
3. Change of pH by dilution may cause precipitation or degradation of medicaments.
4. Choice of wrong diluent may cause poor solubility of medicament.
5. The activity of medicament may be reduced due to complex formation with the diluent.
6. It may invert the activity of emulsifying agents.

CONTAINER

Cream should be supplied in suitable containers fitted with a closure which reduces contamination of micro-organisms and evaporation of water while the product is not in use. For commercial purpose creams should be supplied in suitable collapsible tubes.

LABELING : Comply with the general requirements for labeling and should also specify i)expiry date, and ii) storage conditions

STORAGE : Creams should be stored at temperature not exceeding 25°C. They should not be allowed to freeze.

Example 01 : To prepare Aqueous Cream

A.

Emulsifying ointment	30.0 g
Chlorocresol	0.1g
Purified water, freshly boiled and cooled	69.9 g

B. Emulsifying Cream

Emulsifying wax	30.0 g
White soft paraffin	50.0 g
Liquid paraffin	20.0 g

Method of Preparation : Emulsifying ointment is prepared by melting all ingredients together and stirring until cold. Dissolve chlorocresol in small amount of purified water with the aid of gentle heat. Melt the emulsifying ointment and add the solution of chlorocresol while still warm.

Uses : Pharmaceutical aid

Example 02 : To prepare Buffered cream

Emulsifying ointment	30.0 g
Sodium phosphate	2.5 g
Citric acid monohydrate	0.5 g
Chlorocresol	0.1g
Purified water, freshly boiled and cooled	66.9 g

Method of Preparation : Dissolve sodium phosphate, citric acid monohydrate and chlorocresol in purified water with gently heat. Melt the emulsifying ointment with heat. Heat both solution and emulsifying ointment at the same temperature and mix with stirring gently until cold.

Uses : Pharmaceutical aid

Example 03 : To prepare Aqueous Calamine Cream

Calamine	4.0 g
Zinc oxide	3.0 g
Arachis oil	30.0 g
Emulsifying wax	6.0 g
Purified water, freshly boiled and cooled	57.0 g

Method of Preparation : By gentle heat dissolve emulsifying wax in arachis oil and add 45.0 ml of purified water at the same temperature, Stir until cool. Triturate calamine and zinc oxide with remaining quantity of purified water. Add this mixture in the cream and mix uniformly.

Uses : Astringent and protective

Example 04 : To prepare Cetrimide cream

Cetrimide	0.5 g
Cetostearyl alcohol	5.0 g
Liquid paraffin	50.0 g
Purified water, freshly boiled and cooled	100.0 g

Method of Preparation : Dissolve the cetostearyl alcohol in the liquid paraffin with the aid of gentle heat (A). At the same temperature in another beaker dissolve cetrimide in purified water (B). Add warm oily phase (A) into aqueous phase (B) with stirring until cold.

Example 05 : To prepare Cold Cream

Cetyl esters wax	12.5 g
White wax	12.0 g
Mineral oil	56.0 g
Sodium borate	0.5 g
Purified water	19.0 g

Method of Preparation : Reduce size of cetyl esters wax and white wax in small pieces. Melt them on a steam bath with the mineral oil and continue heating until the temperature of the mixture reaches 70°C (A). Dissolve the sodium borate in purified water and heat at 70°C in separate flask (B). Gradually add aqueous solution (B) to the mixture of oily phase (A) with continuous and rapid stirring until it has congealed.

Uses : Emollient and cleansing cream.

Example 06 : To prepare Vanishing cream

Stearic acid	13.0 g
Stearyl alcohol	1.0g
Cetyl alcohol	1.0g
Methylparaben	0.10 g
Propylparaben	0.05 g
Potassium hydroxide	0.90 g
Purified water, sufficient to produce	100.0 g

Method of Preparation : Melt stearic acid, stearyl alcohol, and cetyl alcohol at 75°C in a conical flask. (A). Dissolve potassium hydroxide in purified water at 75°C in another conical flask and add preservative (B). Add (A) into (B) at 75°C slowly with continuous stirring. Slowly stir the mixture until a smooth cream is formed at room temperature.

Category : Protective

8. JELLIES

Jellies are transparent or translucent semisolids to thick viscous fluids that consist of sub microscopic particles in a somewhat plastic or rigid vehicle. They may be prepared from natural gums such as tragacanth, pectin, alginates or from synthetic derivatives of natural substances such as methylcellulose and sodium carboxymethylcellulose. Some of them are medicated or contain aromatics. Tragacanth is used in the preparation of Ephedrine Sulphate jelly. The jellies are mainly used as lubricants for surgical gloves, catheters and rectal thermometers and in haemorrhoids. They are now becoming popular for contraception purposes and contain surfactants to enhance the spermicidal properties of the jelly. Methyl salicylate and eucalyptol are commonly used aromatics which provide a desirable odour to the preparation.

Spermicidal agents commonly included in contraceptives are phenylmercuriec acetate, nonylphenoxypolyethoxyethanol, methoxyppoly-ethylene glycol 550 laurate and paraformaldehydde.

9. PASTES

Pastes differ from ointments and creams in showing essentially dilatant flow due to the high concentration of insoluble medicament present in them. They are characterized by definite yield value and increase in the resistance to flow with increased force of application. As compared to ointments they are usually stiffer, less greasy and more absorptive. As they absorb serum secretions, pastes are used for acute lesions having a tendency to ooze.

Historically the pastes were introduced in about 1900; Unna's and Lassar's pastes are still used in practice.

The usual concentration of insoluble powders in pastes may be 20% or more and may consist of starch, zinc oxide, calcium carbonate etc. Zinc Oxide Paste USP contains as high as 50% of powdered medicament. Pastes are chiefly used as vehicles for atringent and antiseptic agents. They are not suitable for application to hairy parts like scalp because they form a densely melted mass.

Example 01 : To prepare Compound Aluminium Paste

Aluminium powder	20.0 g
Zinc oxide	40.0 g
Liquid paraffin	40.0 g

Method of Preparation : Mix the aluminium powder and zinc oxide with liquid paraffin until smooth.

Uses : Mild astringent, protective and antiseptic

Example 02 : To prepare Resorcinol and Sulphur Paste

Resorcinol, finely sifted	5.0 g
Precipitated sulphur	5.0 g
Zinc oxide, finely sifted	40.0 g
Emulsifying ointment	50.0 g

Method of Preparation : Prepare emulsifying ointment and triturate the resorcinol, precipitated sulphur and zinc oxide with a portion of the emulsifying ointment until smooth. Gradually incorporate the remaining quantity of the emulsifying ointment.

Uses : Anti-fungal, antibacterial, protective

Example 03 : To prepare Compound Zinc Paste

Zinc oxide, finely sifted	25.0 g
Starch, finely sifted	25.0 g
White soft paraffin	50.0 g

Method of Preparation : Melt white soft paraffin in a glass container. Incorporate zinc oxide and starch and stir until cold.

Uses : Protective, astringent and antiseptic

Example 04 : To prepare Zinc and Salicylic Acid Paste (**Lassar's Paste)**

Zinc oxide, finely sifted	24.0 g
Salicylic acid, finely sifted	2.0 g
Starch, finely sifted	24.0 g
White soft paraffin	50.0 g

Method of Preparation : Melt white soft paraffin in a glass container. Incorporate the zinc oxide salicylic acid, and starch stir until cold.

Example 05 : To prepare Zinc and Coal Tar Paste

Emulsifying wax	5.0 g
Zinc oxide, finely sifted	6.0 g
Coal tar	6.0 g
Starch	38.0 g
Yellow soft paraffin	45.0 g

Method of Preparation : Melt the emulsifying wax at 70°C and add coal tar and 22.5 g of yellow soft paraffin and stir at 70 °C until completely melted. Add the remainder of the yellow soft paraffin and cool at 30 °C. Add zinc oxide and the starch with constant stirring and stir until cold.

10. SUPPOSITORIES

Suppositories are solid or semisolid dosage forms, usually medicated, for insertion into body cavities like rectum, vagina or urehral tract. They are designed to melt, disintegrate or dissolve at the body temperature. Suppositories intended for vagina, urethra or nasal cavity are also referred to as pessaries, urethral bougies and nasal bougies, respectively. Distribution of a drug from suppositories may be either local or systemic. Pessaries are also made as compressed tablets, which disintegrate in the body fluids. They are frequently used for local effects for relief of hemorrhoids or infection in the rectum, the vagina or the urethra.

Historically suppository dosage from dates back to 2600 B.C. and were reported in the works of Hippocrates and in Papyrus Ebers, Theobroma oil and glycerinated gelatin mixtures were recommended as suppository vehicles in 1852 and 1871, respectively. Suppositories account for about 1% of all medications dispensed today.

Advantages of suppository medication

- When oral administration of a drug is not suitable as in infants or patients suffering from nausea, vomiting and gastrointestinal disturbances; suppositories serve as an alternate for drug administration.
- They have been used for a variety of conditions like hemorrhoids and local infections in vagina and rectum.
- Drugs like hypnotics, tranquillizers, antispasmodics etc. are often given as suppositories. This provides the advantage that the biotransformation of drugs in liver, pH conditions and gastrointestinal enzymes are avoided as the portal circulation is bypassed.
- Oral administration of phenylbutazone and indomethacin may cause gastric irritation hence these drugs are sometimes administered rectally.
- Suppositories have also been used for prolongation of drug action.
- Absoprtion of drugs from rectal mucosa directly into the venous circulation may bring about a faster onset of action as compared to oral administration.
- Undissociated drugs are absorbed more rapidly from gastric mucosa than the ionised ones.
- Rate of diffusion of drugs from the dosage form to the site of absorption depends upon nature of the medicament, its lipid/water solubility, physical state of the colon and the amount and nature of the solids and lipids present in the colon.

- In general, presence of surfactants may increase the rate of diffusion unless complexation takes place. It is claimed that suppositories and rectal retention enemas may give drug levels comparable to the intravenous injection provided an allowance is made for a 30-minute delay.

CLASSIFICATION

Suppositories are classified as -

1. **Rectal suppositories** : Rectal suppositories for adults are tapered at one or both ends and usually weigh about 2.0 g each. Infant suppositories usually weigh about one-half that of adult suppositories. Sedatives, tranquilizers, and analgesics are administered by rectal suppositories. They are used as hemorrhoid remedies dispensed over-the-counter. An adult suppository of 2.0 g weight is based on use of cocoa butter as the base. If other bases are employed in place of cocoa butter, weight may be increased or decreased.
2. **Vaginal suppositories (Pessaries)** : These are usually globular, or oviform and weigh about 4.0 to 8.0 g each. Vaginal medications are available in various physical forms like cream, liquids, and gels for the management of vaginal disorders. These suppositories are also known as pessaries.
3. **Urethral suppositories (Bougies)** : These are cylindrical dosage form, diameter 5.0 mm, and length 50 mm for female and 125 mm for male. Weight for urethral male suppository is 4.0 g while for female weight is 2.0 g. It is not popular dosage form and is rarely encountered. These are also known as urethral bougies.
4. **Nasal bougies -** These are similar to urethral bougies slightly thinner, not more than 8 cm in size and weigh about 1.2 g. In dispensing practice nasal bougies are prepared from gelato-glycerin base.
5. **Ear cones -** These are rarely used and whenever required they are prepared from cocoa butter.

SUPPOSITORY BASES

Ideal suppository base

1. It should possess the following properties-
2. It should melt at body temperature or dissolve or disintegrate in body fluids.
3. Higher melting point bases may be necessary for eutectic mixtures. Addition of balsams to suppositories is intended for use in tropical climates.
4. It should be inert, non-irritating and non-sensitizing.
5. It should release the medicament readily.
6. It should be compatible with a broad variety of drugs.
7. It should be stable on storage and transportation
8. It should have wetting and emulsifying properties.

9. It should be able to incorporate a high percentage of water in it i.e. a high water number.
10. It should shrink sufficiently on cooling to release itself from mold and should be moldable by pouring or by cold compression.
11. Fatty bases should have acid value below 0.2, saponification value in between 200 to 245, iodine value less than 7 and a small range between the melting and solidification points.

Classification of Suppositories Bases

Suppository bases can be broadly divided into following categories-

A. Oleaginous bases. B. Aqueous bases. C. Emulsifying bases.

A. Oleaginous bases

Theobroam oil or cocoa butter was introduced as base in 1852 and has been one of the most widely used bases. It satisfies most of the criteria of an ideal suppository base but it melts at 32^{0}C i.e. below the body temperature. Overheating alters its physical characteristics and it has a tendency to adhere to the mold when solidified. it may exist in 4 crystalline states.

α Form : This form is obtained by suddenly cooling the melted mass to 0^{0}C. Its melting point is 24^{0}C.

β Form : This form is obtained when cocoa butter is melted at 35 to 36^{0}C and slowly cooled. It melts at 18 to 23^{0}C.

β'Form : It reverts back to β form and melts at 34 to 35^{0}C.

γ Form : It is obtained by pouring a cool (20^{0}C) cocoa butter into a container before it is solidified and cooled at deep freeze temperature. It melts at 18^{0}C.

All the four forms are unstable and are converted to stable form over a period of several days. Thus extreme care should be exercised while melting and cooling cocoa butter. As a general rule, the minimal use of heat during the melting process is recommended.

Cocoa butter can take up to 20 to 30g of water per 100 g. The incorporation of emulsifiers such as Tween 61 (5 to 10%) increases the water absorption capacity of cocoa butter.

Drugs like volatile oils, cresote, phenol and chloral hydrate lower the melting point of cocoa butter considerably and hence some wax and spermaceti can be used to correct such a problem.

To overcome drawbacks of cocoa butter, hydrogenated palm kernel and soyabean oils have been suggested. Palm kernel oil is particularly suggested for use in tropical countries. Completely or partially hydrogenated cottonseed oil such as `Cotoflakes' and `Cotomar' together with hexanediol has also been suggested.

Edible hydrogenated vegetable oil in combination with some waxes has been worked out in India. Pharmacopoeia of India recommends Kokum fat as a major constituent of the official suppository bases.

B. Aqueous bases

i. Glycero – gelatin : It is a mixture of glycerin and water made into a stiff jelly by the addition of gelatin. The proportion of gelatin can be varied according to the intended use of the preparation.

   Gelato-glycerin bases dissolve in the body fluids liberating contained medicaments. Gelato-glycerin Mass BP contains 14% gelatin, 70% glycerin and water. USP formula contains 20% gelatin together with 70% of glycerin. For dispensing purposes, good quality powdered gelatin should be used. In order to control the consistency, glycerin can be partially or wholly substituted by propylene glycol and polyethylene glycols. The incompatibility of some medicaments can be avoided by the use of either Pharmagel A (cationic) or Pharmagel B (anionic). Glycerin suppositories being liable to mould growth, preservatives should be added.

ii. Soap glycerin : In this case, soap is employed instead of glycerin for hardening. Sodium stearate can incorporate up to 95% of glycerin. Sodium stearate (soap) is produced in situ by interaction of sodium carbonate with stearic acid. Soap glycerin suppositories are however hygroscopic.

iii. PEG bases : Different mixtures of polyethylene glycols are marketed under the trade names of Postonals, Carbo waxes and Macrogols. Some important PEG bases used in the preparation of suppositories are as follows.

I		III	
PEG 1000	96	PEG 1540	70
PEG 4000	4	PEG 6000	30
II		IV	
PEG 1000	75	PEG 1540	30
PEG 4000	25	PEG 6000	50
		Purified water and medicament	20

Base I is a low melting, rapidly disintegrating base and requires refrigeration during summer. Base II is much more stable, harder and gives a slower release. Base III is particularly suitable for those drugs having a melting point lowering effect on the base.

Base IV contains water and facilitates incorporation of water-soluble and PEG insoluble substances.

Most of the drugs commonly administered in suppository form are compatible with these bases. Polyethylene glycols are however incompatible with phenols and reduce the antiseptic effects of quaternary ammonium compounds.

C. Emulsifying bases

Massa Esterinum, Witepsol and Massupol are the trade names under which the emulsifying bases are marketed. Massa Esterinum is a mixture of the mono-, di- and tri-glycerides of the fatty acids having the formula $C_{11}H_{23}COOH$ to $C_{17}H_{35}COOH$. Witepsol bases consist of hydrogenated triglycerides of lauric acid with added monoglycerides. These are available in 9 grades. Massupol consists of glyceryl esters namely of lauric acid and addition of very small quantity of glyceryl monostearate.

All these bases are free from the drawbacks of cocoa butter and don't require any mold lubricant.

Water-dispersible bases essentially consist of surfactants. They melt at body temperature. Some formulae of dispersible bases containing surfactants are outlined below.

I		II		III	
Glyceryl monostearate	10	Glyceryl monostearate	15	Twenn 60	40
Tween 61	90	Twenn 61	85	Tween 61	60

Preparation of Suppositories

1. **Hand Mould Suppositories :** This is the oldest and simplest method of preparing suppositories. A skilled person is required for the preparation of suppositories.

   General process for preparation of suppositories is as follows :

   a. Mix measured quantity of medicinal substances with sufficient quantity of theobroma oil.

   b. Triturate and, if required, soften with diluted alcohol and rub until a smooth paste is formed.

   c. Add remaining quantity of theobroma oil and add wool fat for consistency.

   d. When the mass becomes plastic by vigorous kneading of the pestle quickly remove from the mortar with a spatula.

   e. Transfer with spatula to a piece of filter paper and keep in hands during the kneading and rolling procedure.

   f. Roll the mass by quick rotating movements of the hands and immediately place on a pill tile.

g. Rolling the mass on the tile with a flat board forms a cylindrical suppository.
h. Cut in pieces by spatula.
i. Give the shape by rolling one end on the tile with a spatula.
j. Pack in butter paper or in proper container and store in cool place.

2. Compression mould suppositories (Cold compression)

a. Mix theobroma oil and drug.
b. Mixture is forced into a mould under pressure, using a wheel-operated press.
c. Mould is removed, opened and replaced.
d. On large-scale cold-compression machines are hydraulically operated by water-jacketed cooling and screw fed.

3. Fusion or melt mould suppositories

a. Drug is dispersed or dissolved in a melted suppository base.
b. Pour the mixture into suppository moulds and allow cooling in ice bath.
c. Finished suppositories are removed by opening the mould.
d. Various types and sizes of moulds are available for preparation of suppositories. Moulds are made of aluminum alloys, brass or plastic and are available with from six to several hundred cavities.

4. Automatic mould Machine

All filling, ejection, and mould cleaning operations are fully automatic. The output of a typical rotary machine ranges from 3500 to 6000 suppositories per hour. The suppository mould is lubricated by brushing or spraying and then filled to a slight excess. Excess material is removed after the mass gets solidified and collected for re-use. All heating and cooling systems are fully automatic.

Suppositories are usually formulated on weight basis. The medicament replaces the portion of base having same density as that of theobroma oil. If the drug substance is heavier, it will replace a proportionally smaller amount of theobroma oil.

Example 1

Prepare six suppositories containing 0.1 g tannic acid in each suppository.

Density of tannic acid is 1.6 as compared with cocoa butter.

Weight of blank suppositories = 2.0 g

Cocoa butter replaced by drug = 0.1/1.6 = 0.062 g

Cocoa butter required for one suppository = 2.000 – 0.062 = 1.938 g

Actual weight of one suppository = 1.938 + 0.10 = 2.038 g

Weight of cocoa butter for 8 suppositories (take excess weigh of 2 suppositories as required) = 1.938 × 8 = 15.504 g

Weight of tannic acid for 8 suppositories (take excess weigh of 2 suppositories as required) = 0.10 × 8 = 0.80 g

Total weight of all suppositories = 15.504 + 0.80 = 16.304 g

Example 2

Prepare 0.1 g tannic acid 6 suppositories using polyethylene glycol as base. Density factor of cocoa butter is 1.6 and density factor of polyethylene glycol is 1.25.

Weight of polyethylene glycol suppository = 1.75

Cocoa butter replaced by drug = (0.1/1.6) ×1.25 = 0.078 g

Polyethylene glycol required for one suppository = 1.750 – 0.078 = 1.672 g

Actual weight of one suppository = 1.672 + 0.10 = 1.772 g

Weight of polyethylene glycol for 8 suppositories (take excess weigh of 2 suppositories as required) = 1.672 × 8 = 13.376 g

Weight of tannic acid for 8 suppositories (take excess weigh of 2 suppositories as required) = 0.10 × 8 = 0.80 g

Total weight = 13.376 + 0.80 = 14.176 g

Displacement value of medicaments

The quantity of medicament that displaces one part of cocoa butter is called displacement value. The volume of particular suppository mould is uniform but fill weight will vary according to the density of medicaments as compared with cocoa butter with which the mould was calibrated.

Determination of Displacement value

Weight of six suppositories of theobroma oil or any other base = a g

Weight of six suppositories containing, say 40 percent of drug(s) = b g

Calculate weight of theobroma oil = 60 / 100 × b = c g
Calculate drug(s) = 40/100 × b = d g
(a – c) g = the weight of theobroma oil displaced by d g of drug substances
Displacement value of the medicament = d / (a – c)

Table 13.4: Displacement Values (DV) of Solid Medicaments

Medicament	DV	Medicament	DV	Medicament	DV
Alum	2.0	Hydrocortisone	1.5	Phenol	1.0
Aminophyllin	1.5	Ichthamol	1.0	Quinine HCl	1.0
Bismuth oxynitrate	5.0	Iodoform	4.0	Resorcinol	1.5
Bismuth subgallate	2.5	Lead acetate	3.0	Salol	1.5
Boric acid	1.5	Lead Iodide	5.0	Silver Proteinate	1.5
Chloral hydrate	1.5	Mercury ointment	1.5	Tannic acid	1.0
Cinchocaine	1.5	Morphine HCl	1.5	Zinc oxide	5.0
Cocaine HCl	1.5	Opium	1.5	Zinc sulphate	2.0
Hydrocortisone	1.5	Peptone	1.5		

PACKAGING AND STORAGE

Suppositories are packaged in partitioned boxes or in tightly closed screw-capped glass container or wrapped individually in aluminium foil. In large scale production suppositories are wrapped individually or separately in foil packs. Candy wrapping is the more familiar aluminium foil or PVC polyethylene strip. Low melting point suppositories should be store in cool place and theobroma oil suppositories should be stored in refrigeration.

Mould Lubricant

Mould lubricants are used to remove theobroma suppositories without damaging their surfaces unless a lubricant is used. Lubrication is essential for glycero-gelatin bases because of their sticky nature. Following lubricants may be used for the preparation of theobroma oil suppositories.

Soft soap	10.0 g
Glycerin	10.0 g
Ethanol, (90%)	50.0 ml

Lubricant must be compatible with medicament or adjuncts. In industry silicone fluid is used as lubricant. Mould is lubricated using a pad of gauze or muslin or with a small fairly stiff brush. Cotton wool is not used because some fibers adhere to the mould. Excess of lubricant can be removed by inverting the mould on a clean white tile.

Example 01 : Prepare and dispense Compound Bismuth Subgallate Suppositories.

Rx

Bismuth subgallate	200.0 mg
Resorcinol	60.0 mg
Zinc oxide	120.0 mg
Castor oil	60.0 mg

Theobroma oil, sufficient to fill a mould

Method of Dispensing : Melt theobroma oil and add other additives and mix uniformly. Properly lubricate the suppository mould and pour the hot base in the moulds and cool immediately in ice bath. Excess of substance is scrapped off and re-used in next lot. Open the mould and remove the suppository carefully. Pack in butter paper and store in a well-closed container.

Uses : Astringent and antacid

Example 02 : Prepare and dispense Glycerol Suppositories.

Rx

Gelatin	14.0 g
Glycerol	70.0 g

Purified water, sufficient to produce 100.0 g

Method of Dispensing : Soak gelatin in purified water for about five minutes or until thoroughly softened. Drain well and add glycerin and heat on water bath. Evaporate excess quantity until the mixture weighs 100 g. Pour the products into suitable moulds.

Uses : Rectal evacuant.

Example 03 : Prepare and dispense Glycerin Suppositories

Rx

Glycerin	91.0 g
Sodium stearate	9.00 g
Purified water	5.00 g

Method of Dispensing : Heat the weighed amount of glycerin in a suitable container to about 120°C. Sodium stearate is dissolved in the heated glycerin with stirring. Add purified water and mix. Pour the hot mixture in the suitable mould.

Uses : Local application

Example 04 : Prepare and dispense Glycerinated Gelatin Suppositories.

Rx

Drug and purified water	10.0 g
Gelatin	20.0 g
Glycerin	70.0 g

Method of Dispensing : Dissolve the drug in purified water and moisten the gelatin. Heat the glycerin and add gelatin and drug solution. Mix uniformly and pour this mixture in a mould.

Uses : Antimicrobial.

Example 05 : Prepare and dispense Tannic Acid Suppositories.

Rx

Tannic acid	0.2 g

Theobroma oil, sufficient to produce qs

Method of Dispensing : Add lubricant in the mould and remove the excess of lubricant by draining and cool the lubricated mould over ice. Theobroma oil is heated in a porcelain dish over a water bath and avoid over heating. Remove dish from the water bath as soon as the mass is molten. Weighed amount of tannic acid is powdered and added in the molten theobroma oil. Mix the tannic acid by spatula (sometimes molten theobroma oil divided in two parts) and pour the mixture into the holes in the moulds. Place the mould on ice and remove excess mass carefully by sharp knife. When the suppositories have completely set hard, open the mould and remove the suppositories by slight pressure on the broad ends. Remove any lubricant on final product, by rolling on the filter papers.

Uses : Astringent.

11. OPHTHALMICS

Medication meant for the eye may be a liquid in the form of solution or suspension, or a semisolid in the form of an ointment or a cream. These preparations require special techniques, processes and theoretical considerations for compounding. Several factors have to be taken into account e.g. rendering the solution isotonic, adjusting it to proper pH and buffering if necessary, incorporating stabilizing agents, increasing the viscosity, adding preservatives etc. Further, all preparations for the eye have to be sterile. This requires considerable skill and caution on the part of the pharmacist.

Ophthalmic preparations are sterile products, essentially free from foreign particles, suitably formulated and packaged in suitable container for either topical application to the eyelids or instillation into the cul-de-sac between the eyeball and eyelids.

Following categories of drugs are used in and as ophthalmic preparations.

1. Anti-inflammatory agent

2. Anti-microbial drugs e.g. beta adrenergic blocking agent, cycloplegics, miotics, mydriatics and vasoconstrictors.
3. Anti-microbial drugs e.g. antibiotics, antiseptics, antivirals, fungicides and sulfonamides
4. Local anaesthetic
5. Others e.g. chelating agents, hyper osmolar agents, diagnostic products, lubricant ointments, artificial tears, eye washes, artificial eye solution and contact lens solution.

Drug from the ophthalmic preparation may be required to penetrate through the cornea or exert only local action. Drug absorption and permeability in the eye depends on the solubility of the drug in water. The extent of absorption is also dependent upon the quantity of the drug present and its concentration in the medication in the dosage form. Addition of buffers may be of assistance in stabilizing some of the preparations and adjustment of pH as well as in the absorption of the drug. This area however, concerns more the manufacturing pharmacist and has limited application in dispensing of extemporaneously prepared solutions for the eye. Some of the drugs are inherently irritating to the eye and initiate secretion of tears thus washing off the drug from the site of absorption and action.

Isotonic solutions

Solutions meant for the eye should be isotonic with the tear secretion to prevent irritation due to difference in the tonicity. If the concentration of the drug is not sufficient to yield an isotonic solution, addition of requisite amount of an inert substance compatible with drug is essential. The pharmacist is required to select the substance and calculate its quantity necessary to render the solution isotonic. A given solution, from tonicity considerations, may be either isotonic or paratonic in relation to the tear secretion. If the quantity of the drug(s) prescribed is just sufficient to produce, on appropriate dilution, the same tonicity as the tear secretion, no substance should be added. Such a solution is isotonic by itself. Some prescriptions direct that an isotonic solution of a drug be dispensed without stating the concentration of the drug in solution. In such cases a pharmacist may calculate the quantity of the drug required to dispense the volume of the solution but in case that concentration is too high, he may have to refer either to the physician or use the quantity normally prescribed in the conditions for which the prescription is meant. However, it is not infrequent that a pharmacist receives paratonic prescriptions. Such prescriptions may be of two types-hypertonic or hypotonic in relation to the tear secretion. Hypertonic solutions contain more quantity than required to have the same tonicity as the tear secretion. It is not possible to render a hypertonic solution isotonic unless the quantity of the medicament is reduced to tonicity level. Reducing the quantity of the medication amounts to altering the prescription. The pharmacist may have to consult the physician in such circumstances. However, a pharmacist adjusts the tonicity of the hypotonic solutions by adding appropriate quantity of soluble substances. The required quantities of such additive substances may be calculated by any one of the methods. In practice, by experience pharmacist prepares tables of the medication in different concentrations and the concentration of the adjusting substance for the drug for all generally prescribed solutions. Whereas it is desirable to make solutions isotonic with the tear secretion, it may be remembered that paratonic solutions within the range of 0.7 to 1.5% of sodium chloride or its equivalent in relation to other substances are easily tolerated by the eye.

Adjustment of pH, stabilization and preservation

Tonicity of a solution and pH appear to be independent but there is some bearing of one over the other. Drugs in solutions may ionize and dissociate at alkaline pH. Solutions having a pH value between 6.5 to 7.5 are very well tolerated by the eye. However, solutions having a pH as low as 4 and as high as 10 are known to be prescribed and instilled without extraordinary pain and irritation. Pain and irritation in the eye due to acidic drug solutions are immediately felt on instilling the solution and this results into tear secretion which is slightly alkaline. The alkaline tear fluid gradually neutralizes the acidity resulting in the reduction of irritation and pain. The degree of the tear secretion depends on the extent of acidic nature and the volume of the solution instilled. Buffer solutions are included in the eye solutions sometimes which serve many a purpose maximizing therapeutic activity of the medicament, bringing about stability of the solution, reducing pain etc. Lot of investigations has been recently carried out with regard to the choice of buffers to be included in eye drops and eye washes. However, this area relates more to the manufacturer than the practicing pharmacist as he faces lesser problems of stabilizing than the manufactured products. Sodium EDTA (Sodium ethylene diamine tetraacetate) in a concentration of 0.1% acts as a good preservative of eye solutions as it performs antibacterial action as well. Very often it is used in conjunction with boric acid. Salts of the alkaloid-pilocarpine are more stable in presence of phosphate buffer. Sodium borate is another substance employed for preservation of eye solutions.

Viscosity of the eye medication

For providing prolonged contact of the medication to the eye and reducing the possibility of being washed away, it may be desirable in certain cases to increase the viscosity of the preparation. However, it is imperative that the agent used to increase the viscosity should possess the properties of compatibility, inertness, clarity and refractive index, Polyethylene glycol, methyl cellulose, polyvinyl alcohol and polyvinylpyrollidone are the main additives employed for this purpose. Since sterility is an essential requirement for eye preparations, the additives employed ought to be sterilizable by the commonly used methods of sterilization. If heat is to be used for sterilization, the additive should not undergo any physical or chemical change in itself or bring about any coagulation or precipitation of the medication. Enhanced therapeutic action from a preparation with increased viscosity or reduction in the concentration of the drug in the presence of viscosity increasing agents is a subject which is receiving great attention of the investigators. However, this aspect has greater and deeper implications in ophthalmic formulations designed and manufactured by the industry.

Sterility aspects of eye preparations, aseptic processing and choice of preservatives

Preparations for the eye, till about 1953, were not required to be sterile which was a serious shortcoming in ophthalmic medication. However, in the present time sterility of eye medication has been prescribed officially by the Pharmacopoeias. This applied both to the manufactured preparations as well as to the dispensed preparations. In extemporaneous dispensing of prescriptions to sterilize a preparation may be time consuming and sometimes impractical. Thus medication for the eye is generally dispensed in manufacturer's sealed containers. It is essential, however, that a pharmacist though not very often required to compound and sterilize eye medication, must be familiar with every aspect of these preparations and their preservation. Facilities for dispensing such preparations must exist in the Pharmacy and a pharmacist must receive adequate training in the techniques associated with the compounding, sterilizing and filling the containers aseptically. Generally, a manufacturer's original package is a small sealed sterile container. A dropper may be an integral part of the closure device or may be supplied duly packed in the carton for instilling the solution in the eye. Once a sealed container is opened and the medication used, it becomes increasingly contaminated following each usage and therefore the supply is in a small container. Larger packages are also manufactured for clinics and hospitals where a large number of patients call for the treatment. However, in such institutions, a separate sterile dropper is used for each patient. In view of the unavoidable contamination, inclusion of chemical preservatives is essential in ophthalmic preparations. Common preservatives are listed below.

Table 13.5: Common Preservatives for Ophthalmic Preparations

Preservative	**Concentration**
Phenol	0.25-0.50%
p-chlorometaxylenol	0.03%
Phenylethyl alcohol	0.5%
Phenoxyethanol	0.3%
Chlorobutanol	0.5%
Nitromersal	1 in 2,500
Thiomersal	1 in 500
Phenylmercuric nitrate	1 in 1,00,000 to1 in 25,000
Polymyxin B sulphate	1000 units/ml
Benzalkonium chloride	1 in 1,00,000 to 1 in 10,000

Preparations for the eye can be sterilized by any method depending upon the nature of the drug and its stability under the conditions of sterilization. It is presumed that a pharmacist is familiar with the principles, methods and techniques of sterilization and the equipment to be used. The most common method for sterilizing aqueous liquid preparations is with the help of steam under pressure (autoclaving). For a Pharmacy a pressure cooker is good enough and sterilization can be brought about within half an hour at 121^0C and 15 lb per square inch pressure which is attainable in a pressure cooker. Thermolabile medication can be sterilized under aseptic condition by filtering the solution through bacteria-proof filters. It is desirable to have a few varieties of filters and candles available in the Pharmacy for this purpose.

A modern Pharmacy is expected to have an aseptic room to carry out aseptic operations. Even small Pharmacies must be equipped with a glass hood for aseptic work. Aseptic work is a specialized technique and a pharmacist is expected to master it during the period of his training so as to handle aseptic problems with confidence. A brief outline of the sources of likely contamination and aseptic operation is given below.

Two classes of pharmaceutical preparations are required to be sterile - injectables and preparations for the eye. The purpose of employing aseptic process is to eliminate the possibility of contamination with micro-organisms during preparation, packaging and testing of the medication. If the medicament is packed and sealed in such a container, which after sterlization, dose not permit contamination; there is no necessity of aseptic technique. In other words, the heat treatment at the end of the process and the sealed container safeguard the sterility of the product till the container is opened. But in cases there such terminal heat treatment is not possible; one has to resort to aseptic processing. Example of this type include thermo-labile drugs in solution and suspension form, thermo-labile drugs in powder form meant for dusting or for dilution just before use and thermo-labile substances to be mixed with the base as in case of eye ointments. In addition to the above requirements for preparation and packaging, aseptic handling is essential is testing the medication for sterility.

Aseptic technique precludes the possibility of contamination, which should ensure an aseptic operation. The biggest source of contamination is air. Although atmospheric air does not provide any nutrition to the micro-organisms and thus does not promote their growth, yet it acts as an effective agency for carrying micro-organisms in it. It carries in itself several substances on which micro organisms get conveniently deposited e.g. dust, droplets, and droplet nuclei. The air that one breathes can hold a considerable number of micro organisms. Other agencies that cause heavy contamination include hands, clothes, hair of the workers in the area, the working area and the equipment used.

From the above it is apparent that aseptic processing requires aseptic working condition and a good training in functioning of the pharmacist in a manner that will lead to minimal contamination. Working conditions embody the aseptic laboratory, its furniture, services and equipment needed therein. Functioning of the pharmacist requires a consciousness to the possibility of contamination and conducting oneself in a suitable manner.

DESIGN OF AN ASEPTIC LABORATORY

As long as a laboratory meets certain essential requirements, it is suitable for aseptic work. These requirements are given below.

The aseptic room

All openings except the openings for entry need perfect sealing and horizontal surfaces including windows should be eliminated. These surfaces may allow retention of dust and may create problems. The structure should be tight enough to prevent infiltration of uncontrolled air. All exposed surfaces should be smooth and impervious, easily cleanable and in no way prone to settling of dust upon them. The surfacing material should not be susceptible to hold dust, flaking or chalking under normal operative procedures. Uncoated smooth surfaces e.g. stainless steel, aluminium and chromium plating, plastic laminates and plastic films make satisfactory surfaces. Cement concrete is a very undesirable surface.

Air-conditioned atmosphere

In view of the sealed structure, preventing any source of entry of air, air conditioning is essential. Since no special requirement of temperature and humidity are prescribed, conventional air conditioning may be suitable enough. It is however preferable to have the humidity on the lower side to avoid contamination by the perspiration of the workers. Air cleaning part of the air conditioning is a critical factor as the nature of the atmospheric air may differ considerably from time to time. Cooling and heating coils, humidity control apparatus, reheat coils; blowers etc. are the equipment that should be of standard specifications. However, the fans selected should be such that can provide high pressure. The room has to be constantly maintained under positive pressure to prevent inlet of air from entry point whenever it is opened. Dust, temperature and humidity control are interdependent functions. Dust control is impossible without confining the area. Confined space is unlivable without air-conditioning. If temperature and humidity are controlled by air conditioning, dust control measures are automatically taken care of.

Cleaning of air

Cleaning of air is the key of the aseptic processing. The usual approach is a combination of the conventional cleaners e.g. regular filters or electronic air cleaners located within the system and some kind of super-interception or an ultra cleaner located down stream from all coils, blowers etc. Bactericidal equipment is incorporated in the assembly for providing sterile air in addition to be devices stated above. The air in the aseptic area should be free from fibers, dust and microbes. This can be conveniently achieved by the use of High Efficiency Particulate Air (HEPA) filters which can remove particles up to 0.3 μm with an efficiency of 99.7% or more. HEPA filters are made use of in Laminar Air Flow in which air moves with uniform velocity along parallel lines with minimum of eddies. The air flow can be either horizontal or vertical and 100 ± 10 ft/min. is considered to be the minimum effective air velocity. Such laminar flow stations and work benches are commercially available and should find immense use in compounding and dispensing practice.

Air distribution

Materials of construction for the air distribution system should be made of non-rusting and non-flaking materials (e.g. ducts, air outlets etc.). Duct insulation, if needed, should be applied on the outer side and only on the ducts that are located out of the clean area. Joints and other fittings, if any, should be sealed to prevent leakage and contamination. Air distribution is also employed for 'washing' the workers off dust who enter the sterile area. These are called air showers which are strictly blasts or air directed on the person to remove dust.

Controls

Conventional controls are used in the system for regulating humidity and temperature. Sometimes greater pressure may have to be maintained in critical areas and for this purpose additional controls may have to be installed. Interlocks may be required between the sterile area and the entrance or passing doors. In a highly elaborate system, alarm circuits are introduced to warn against the malfunctioning or inadvertent misuse of the air locks.

Instruments

Highly sophisticated instrumentation has to be installed which constantly or intermittently monitors and samples the clean atmosphere for analyzing its cleanliness. These devices immediately indicate the contamination, if any.

Furniture

Seating, work tables, racks etc. are essential requirements of furniture inside he clean area and have to be specially designed and built to meet certain rigid specifications. Adjusting mechanisms on the chairs should either not exist or ought to be sealed. These may be potential dust setting surfaces. Conventional upholstering of the chairs is completely out of question. Dust catching surfaces should be minimum and all parts should be readily cleanable and resistant to the action of the cleaning agents. Worker comfort is a very important factor in a confined area. The requirements of the job in a sterile room keep the workers chained to the work over long periods of time continuously without leisure and with minimum exits from the room and thus warrants high degree of comfort for carrying out the critical operations. Special jigs, fixtures and tools are developed for specific purposes but many operations need dust-free hoods-miniature aseptic rooms located on the working bench. Even when the aseptic hoods or chambers are located in dust free rooms, they may have to be provided with supply of pressurized air in each one of them. The air may be either super cleaned or an inert gas. Further these hoods have to be independently illuminated.

There are many several important factors to consider when called upon compounding a sterile ophthalmic preparation. Eyes are very sensitive to heat, light, drugs and chemicals. In many cases, the drugs involved have a narrow therapeutic range and even small errors when introduced have the potential to cause irreversible damage to the eye or loss of the eye sight. The following considerations are recommended whenever preparing such a product.

1. Ensure concentration is within the acceptable range or not before dispensing of the product.
2. Sterility of the final product is a must, strictly handled in aseptic area.
3. The pH of the final product must be within an acceptable range.
4. Stability of the final product must be known, as well as the recommended storage requirements.
5. Suitable knowledge of potential diluents or vehicles is required in order to ensure proper tonicity, viscosity, or dissolution of the final product.
6. Proper documentation of each step is an important consideration to reduce error.
7. If the preparation of a product requires the breaking of an ampoule or the reconstitution of a powder, it is recommended that the final product be made in sterile water for injection and free form particulate matter.
8. The preparation of intra-ocular products requires the use of preservative-free ingredients. Many preservatives have been found to be toxic to the inner ocular tissues.
9. Finally, before dispensing the finished product, always indicate the storage requirements, concentrations of ingredients, and the expected expiration date.

OPHTHALMIC PRODUCTS

(a) Eye drops (b) Eye ointments (c) Eye suspension

(d) Eye lotions (e) Contact lens solutions

EYE DROPS

Eye drops are sterile aqueous or oily solutions or suspension of one or more medicaments intended for instillation into the conjunctival sac for diagnostic or therapeutic purposes. Oily eye drops are less used but may nevertheless occasionally be requested. They are usually prepared with sterile castor oil and alkaloids incorporated in a vehicle suitable to be used in the form of the base (e.g. pilocarpine eye drops contains pilocarpine dissolved in sterile castor oil). Certain eye drops may be supplied in a drug, sterile form to be reconstituted in an appropriate sterile liquid immediately before use. In such cases the label should state clearly on the container 'Powder for Eye Drops' and should include direction for the use of eye drops.

Aqueous eye drops contain suitable antimicrobial preservatives at appropriate concentrations because it is intended for use on more than one occasion. The antimicrobial preservatives should be compatible with the other ingredients of the preparations and should remain effective throughout the shelf-life of the eye drops.

FORMULATION

Eye drops may contain the following ingredients:

1. Medicaments : anti-microbial agents, local anaesthetic, diagnostic agents, miotics, midriatic, sulfonamides etc.
2. Vehicle : sterile distilled water, sterile castor oil etc.
3. Viscosity : polyethylene glycol, polyvinyl alcohol, polyvinylpyrrolidone, hydroxypropyl methylcellulose, methylcellulose, carboxymethylcellulose and hydroxyethyl cellulose.
4. Surfactant : Benzthonium chloride, polysorbate-20 etc.
5. Hydrogen ion concentration : The greatest comfort for the patient is expected to be found at the normal pH approximately 7.4, of lachrymal fluid but usually adequate in the pH range of 6 to 8. Most of the active ingredients used in ophthalmic solution are salts of weak acids and have low buffer capacity e.g. sodium acid phosphate solution, sodium phosphate solution, sodium chloride solution etc.
6. Buffers : Monobasic sodium phosphate solution, dibasic sodium phosphate solution and sodium chloride solution.
7. Tonicity modifiers : sodium chloride and boric acid.
8. Antioxidant : Solution metabisulphite(0.1%) and sodium thiosulphite (0.1%)
9. Chelating agent : Disodium edetate
10. Antimicrobial : Benzylkonium chloride, chlorahedine acetate, chlorbutol, thromersal, phenylethyl alcohol, PMN and PMA.
11. Clarity : All solutions for the use in the eye should be clear and free from foreign particles.
12. Sterilization : Ophthalmic solution are required to be sterile when prepared and great care must be exercised subsequently to prevent contamination to use. The microbe must frequently found as a contaminant is Pseudomonas aeruginosa and the solution most often found contaminated is of sodium fluerescein. It is very dangerous and opportunistic organism that grows well on most culture media and produces both toxin and anti-bacterial products. This Gram (-)ve bacillus also grows readily in ophthalmic solutions which may become the source of extremely serious infections of the cornea. The common methods of sterilization are moist heat under pressure (autoclave), bacterial filtration (pore size 0.22 μm) and use of chemicals.

CONTAINERS

1. Single dose containers : It is minimum unit and consists of a disposable, pliable, tube-like applicator made from polypropylene by ultrasonic sealing. It has a nozzle protected by a cap. It is generally enclosed in a heat-sealed envelope.
2. Multiple application containers : The traditional container for eye drops is a glass bottle carrying in the cap a dropper fitted with a teat. e.g.
    a. Amber colored container to provide protection from light
    b. Hexagonal in cross-section and vertically ribbed on three adjacent faces, the ribs indicate that the contents must not be taken orally.
    c. Made from neutral or treated soda glass.
    d. Screw capped bottle with separate droppers.

LABELLING

Comply with the general requirements for labelling, following information is mentioned on the label clearly.

1. Name and concentration of medicaments.
2. Name and concentration of antimicrobial agent.
3. Date after which the product is not intended to be used.
4. Discard the contents at a specified time after opening (about one month).
5. If any discomfort or irritation discontinue use of the eye drop.
6. 'For External use Only'.

HOW TO USE EYE DROPS

1. Wash hands with soap
2. Pull lower eyelid down with one hand gently
3. If dropper is separate, squeeze rubber bulb once while dropper is in bottle to bring liquid into dropper.
4. Holding dropper above eye, drop medicine inside lower lid while looking up.
5. Do not touch dropper to eye or fingers.
6. Lift lower lid and try to keep eye open.
7. Do not blink for at least 30 seconds.
8. If dropper is separate, replace on bottle and tighten the cap.
9. Keep the dropper tip always down.
10. Never rinse the dropper.
11. Never use drops that have changed color

12. Open one bottle at a time if you have more than one.
13. If you are using more than one kind of drop at the same time, wait several minutes before using the other drop
14. After instillation of drops, do not close eyes tightly and try not to blink more often than usual.

EYE OINTMENTS

Ophthalmic ointments are ointments meant for application to the eye. It can be used to obtain the effect of a variety of medicaments on the outside and edges of the eyelids, the conjunctiva, the cornea and the iris. It contains sterilized ingredients packed under rigid aseptic conditions and meets the requirements of the official sterility tests. Ophthalmic ointments must contain a suitable substance or mixture of substances to prevent growth of or to destroy, microorganisms accidentally introduced when the container is opened during use. The medicinal agent is added to the ointment base either as a solution or as a micronized powder.

The finished ointment must be free from large particles. Most ophthalmic ointments are prepared with a base of white petroleum and mineral oil often with anhydrous lanolin.

CONTAINER

1. Ointments are packed in collapsible metal or plastic tubes or in single dose containers
2. Plastic tubes are used for some proprietary formulations of eye ointments
3. Certain proprietary formulations of eye ointments are available in single dose containers, elongated, flexible gelatin capsule with one end constructed and are opened by cutting off the constructed end with sterile scissors.

LABELING

The label on the tube or outer sealed envelop should state that the contents are sterile provided that the container has not been opened. Other information should be similar as discussed for eye drops.

EYE LOTIONS

Eye lotions are sterile aqueous solutions for first aid purposes over a maximum period of twenty four hours without bactericide. In another words, eye lotions are aqueous solutions for intermittent domiciliary administration for up to seven days having bactericide. Eye lotions are usually applied with an eye bath, for first aid purposes only hence it has limited use nowadays but may be prescribed e.g. sodium bicarbonate eye lotion is used for the emergency treatment of acid burns of the eye and is popular as **Factory eye drops No.2.** Sodium chloride is an isotonic solution which is occasionally used for irrigating the eye.

CONTAINERS

Eye lotions are dispensed in colored fluted bottle closed with a screw-cap. It is important to ensure that the liner of the screw cap is not covered by cork as it may be a source of microbial contamination. Rubber or plastics liners are suitable and the screw cap may be either of metal or plastics. Uncolored or non-fluted bottles may be used if a suitable colored, fluted bottle is not available.

LABELING

Following information is stated on the eye lotion label

1. 'For External use only'.
2. Discard any lotion remaining after use when the seal is first broken.

Eye lotions which are issued for domiciliary purposes should be labeled to indicate-

1. Not to be used more than 24 h. (without bactericide)
2. Not to be used more than 7 days (with bactericide)

12. INHALATIONS

The term inhalation is used commonly by the layman to describe preparations intended to be vaporized with the aid of heat, usually steam, and inhaled. Inhalations are solutions of medicaments administered by the nasal or oral respiratory route for local or systemic effect. Nebulizers are suitable for administration of inhalation solutions only if they give droplets sufficiently fine and uniform in size so that the mist reaches the bronchitis.

Another category of products also called insufflations consists of finely powdered or liquid drugs that are carried into the respiratory passages by the use of special delivery systems. Solutions may be nebulized by use of inert gases. Nebulized solutions may be breathed directly from the nebulizer or nebulizer may be attached to a plastic facemask or intermittent positive pressure breathing machines. Particle size is one of the important parameter for inhalation. The optimum particle size for penetration into the pulmonary cavity is 0.5 to 7.0 □m. Pressurized aerosols generate fine mists and hence posses basic advantages over the older nebulizers.

Example 01 : Prepare and dispense Aqueous Inhalation.

Rx	
Eucalyptus oil	6.0 ml
Menthol	3.0 g
Light magnesium carbonate	6.50 g
Purified water, sufficient to produce	100.0 ml

Method of Dispensing : Powder weighed amount of menthol in glass mortar and pestle, add eucalyptus oil and stir until the solid has dissolved and add other additives and mix well.

Example 02 : Prepare and dispense Benzoin Inhalation.

Rx	
Benzoin	10.0 g
Prepared storax	6.85 g
Specially denatured spirit, sufficient to produce	100.0 ml

Method of Dispensing : Benzoin and prepared storax should be macerated with 7.5 ml of specially denatured spirit for twenty four hours. Filter and add specially denatured spirit passed through filter to produce 100 ml.

Example 03 : Prepare and dispense Menthol Inhalation.

Rx	
Menthol	1.0 g
Specially denatured spirit, sufficient to produce	50.0 ml

Method of Dispensing : Mix menthol with specially denatured spirit in mortar and pestle. Add sufficient specially denatured spirit through filter and produce 50 ml.

13. THROAT PAINTS

Paints are solutions or dispersions of one or more medicaments intended for application to the skin or, in some cases, to the mucous membrane. They may contain volatile solvent that evaporates quickly to leave a dry or resinous film of medicament. Throat paints are more viscous due to high content of glycerin. Paints are sticky and adheres to the affected site and prolong the action of the medicaments. Common examples of pastes are : 1. Brilliant green and crystal violet paint, 2. Crystal violet paint, 3. Coal tar paint, 4. Compound mastric paint 5. Mandl's paint 6. Tannic acid glycerin paints

STORAGE : Paints should be kept in airtight containers.

LABELLING

Comply with the general requirements for labeling. In addition it should states 'For External Use Only'.

CONTAINER : Wide mouth screw capped colored bottles.

Example 01 : Prepare and dispense Brilliant Green and Crystal Violet Paint.

Rx	
Brilliant green	0.5 g
Crystal violet	0.5 g
Ethanol (90%)	50.0 ml
Purified water, sufficient to produce	100.0 ml

Method of Dispensing : Dissolve the brilliant green and crystal violet in ethanol (90%). Add sufficient water to produce 100 ml.

Example 02 : Prepare and dispense Crystal Violet Paint.

Rx	
Crystal violet	0.1 g
Purified water, sufficient to produce	100.0 ml

Method of Dispensing : Dissolve crystal violet in purified water. Add sufficient purified water to produce 100 ml.

Example 03 : Prepare and dispense **C**oal Tar Paint.

Rx	
Coal Tar	10.0 g
Acetone, sufficient to produce	100.0 ml

Method of Dispensing : Disperse the coal tar in 70 ml of acetone and allow to stand for one hour. Filter if necessary and dilute with acetone to 100 ml.

Example 04 : Prepare and dispense Iodine paint (Syn. : Mandl's paint)

In this preparation Iodine acts as antiseptic and potassium iodide dissolves the iodine, peppermint oil acts as flavoring agent and produce cooling effect, alcohol is used as a solubilizing agent for the peppermint oil. This preparation contains iodine, hence should be prepared in glass apparatus. It should not be prepared in mortar and pestle because porcelain contains pores and iodine enters in these pores. It is difficult to washout the iodine and this entangled iodine can change the color of other preparations.

Rx	
Potassium iodide	2.5 g
Iodine	1.25 g
Ethanol (90%)	4.0 ml
Peppermint oil	0.4 ml
Purified water	2.5 ml
Glycerin, sufficient to produce	100.0 ml

Method of Dispensing : Dissolve potassium iodide and iodine in purified water in glass mortar and pestle with small portion of glycerin. Add peppermint oil dissolve in ethanol and mix. Add sufficient glycerin to produce 100 ml.

14. SPRAYS (NASAL)

Sprays are solutions of various drugs in aqueous vehicles and are applied to the mucous membrane of the nose and the throat by means of an atomizer or nebulizer. Spray devices should produce relatively coarse droplets if the therapeutic action of the medicaments is to be restricted to the upper respiratory tract. Very fine droplets penetrate into the respiratory tract. Initially the sprays were prepared by dissolving various medicaments in light liquid petrolatum. It may damage the normal ciliary activity of the nasal mucosa and, if drops of oil enter the trachea it can cause lipoid pneumonia. Because of this problem, aqueous sprays that are isotonic with nasal secretions and of approximately the same pH are preferred. Sprays contain substances such as antibiotics, antihistamines, vasoconstrictors, alcohol, solubilizers, and wetting agents.

Example 01 : Prepare and dispense Isoprenaline Compound Spray.

Rx	
Isoprenaline	0.250 g
Papaverine hydrochloride	0.625 g
Atropine methonitrate	50.0 mg
Propylene glycol	1.25 ml
Sodium metabisulphite	25.0 mg
Purified water, sufficient to produce	25.0 ml

Method of Dispensing : Mix isoprenaline, atropine methonitrate and papaverine hydrochloride and dissolve in purified water. Dissolve sodium metabisulphite and add in the solution. Add other additives and add sufficient purified water to produce 25 ml.

Example 02 : Prepare and dispense Compound Adrenaline and Atropine Spray.

Rx	
Adrenaline acid tartrate	0.80 g
Atropine methonitrate	0.10 g
Papaverine hydrochloride	0.80 g
Sodium metabisulphite	0.10 g
Chlorbutanol	0.50 g
Propylene glycol	5.00 ml
Purified water, sufficient to produce	100.0 ml

Method of Dispensing : Boil purified water for about 10 minutes, to remove oxygen and destroy vegetative bacteria and mould spores. Cool the water and use for the preparation of sprays. Prepare solution of adrenaline acid tartrate, atropine methonitrate and sodium metabisulphite in separate containers, respectively using small proportion of purified water. Mix three solutions and add papaverine hydrochloride in the mixture. Dissolve weighed amount of chlorbutanol in propylene glycol and mix in the mixture. Filter, if necessary and add sufficient purified water to adjust the volume 100 ml through the filter.

CHAPTER 14

EXTRACTION AND GLANICAL PRODUCTS

EXTRACTION PROCESSES

Extraction may be defined as the process of removal of desirable soluble constituents from a substance, leaving out those which are undesirable, with the aid of solvents and standardized processes. Plant and animal tissues contain chemical substances some of which provide relief and treatment in a variety of diseased conditions. In many cases the medicinal value of a natural drug, whether of plant or animal origin, is due to a single constituent. However, the isolation of active agent may be an extremely difficult and expensive process. If the other constituents have no undesirable effect, the administration of the unprocessed drug or its partially purified extract may provide the desired therapeutic effect. At times, the presence of other constituents may beneficially modify the effect of the active principle(s) and hence the removal of such other constituents may not be desirable.

Glanicals : Following preparations are still used in pharmaceutical practice are known glanicals products such as –

- Decoctions
- Fluid extracts
- Infusions
- Solid (dry) and semisolid (soft) extracts and
- Tinctures

In recent years active principles from both plants and animals have been isolated or obtained as purified products of precisely known potency and stability and therefore extractives are less frequently prescribed. But the trend is reverting back due to increasing popularity of polyherbal formulations and herbal formulary.

Menstuum : means the solvent used for the extraction process

Marc : The un-dissolved residue left behind is known as marc.

Expression : means extraction accomplished by mechanical process.

PRINCIPLE OF DRUG EXTRACTION

The general procedure employed in extraction of organized drugs those built up of natural cells and tissues) differs from that employed in extraction of unorganized drugs (mere exudates like gums, resins, gum resins, or oleogum-resins). Extraction implies that the desirable constituents should dissolve in the menstruum leaving behind the marc. Thus all the factors which help in accomplishing, facilitating, or enhancing the solubility of desired constituents in the menstruum explain the theory of extraction. In case of organized drugs, the cells forming the tissues contain various plant constituents in the fluid called 'the cell' sap either in solution form or dispersed in a colloidal state. On drying the drug, such dissolved or colloidally dispersed matter is either precipitated, crystallized or deposited in an amorphous form in the cell structure. The drying or dehydration of natural drugs affects the strength of 'the cell wall but the contents of the dried cell sap are enclosed within and therefore prevented from being directly exposed to the solvent action of the menstruum. Thus it is often necessary to comminute the drug prior to extraction so as to rupture it and expose the cell contents to the menstruum.

The cell walls consist essentially of cellulose and these molecules being polar, there is natural affinity for polar solvents such as water, alcohol etc. Therefore, in presence of a polar solvent, the cellulose walls get hydrated or solvated, and swell. This is why moistening of the drug with the menstruum is an important stage in extraction. Swelling or **imbibition** is maximum in polar solvents. Thus water causes considerable swelling, while there is lesser swelling with ethanol.

Endosmosis : Mobility of liquids through a crude drug is generally diffusion controlled, which may be termed endosmosis. The process is faster if the system is agitated.

Exosmosis : As the solution within the cell wall becomes stronger, a differential concentration is set up within and outside the cell. This causes the stronger solution to diffuse out of the cell until equilibrium in reached. This phenomenon is called exosmosis.

Equilibrium is attained faster by agitation.

The movement of liquid through the pores and capillaries present in natural systems is influenced by -

- the surface tension
- wetting properties of the liquid and
- the displacement of air entrapped in capillaries facilitates the diffusion of liquid inside the cell.

This displacement of air can be aided by employing a vacuum pump. In absence of agitation, a significant stagnant diffusion layer exists around a given particle, which acts as a barrier to diffusion away from the site. The entire process of drug extraction can summarily be divided into four essential steps:

1. Penetration of the solvent into the drug;
2. Dissolution of constituents;
3. Outward diffusion of the solution from the cells; and
4. Separation of dissolved p0l1ion and the exhausted drug.

The efficiency of drug extraction depends therefore, upon the following:

1. Nature and properties of the drug and its extractable constituents;
2. The particle size of the powdered drug;
3. The nature of the solvent; and
4. The state of contact between the solvent and the drug particles.

Following physical factors are influencing drug extraction such as gravitation, diffusion, osmosis, adhesion, capillarity, convection, solubility and surface tension. The optimum particle size of the crude drug powder will depend upon the botanical structure of the drug. Treatment of the powdered drug with the menstruum at high temperature under pressure or passing a suspension of the drug powder in the menstruum through a colloid mill, can alter the permeability of cell walls. Wetting property of a solvent can be improved by displacing the air entrapped in the capillaries and also by using surface-active agent. A surfactant can also increase the solubility of cellular contents in the menstruum by solubilization. Agitation brings about a faster equilibrium of the contents outside and inside the cell thus facilitating rapid dissolution of the desired constituents in the menstruum.

Extraction at elevated temperatures, whenever feasible, has many more advantages *e.g.*

(i) decrease in viscosity reduces the boundary layers;

(ii) convection currents have an effect similar to agitation during extraction;

(iii) diffusion coefficients being directly proportional to absolute temperature and inversely proportional to viscosity, rate of diffusion is moderately influenced by raising the temperature; and

(iv) in general, the solubility of the constituents in the menstruum increases as the temperature is raised.

The solvent (menstruum) used for extracting drugs should be chemically and physically inert, non-toxic, inexpensive and selective, i.e. it should dissolve the desired active constituents with a minimum of the inert material. Based on these considerations, water, ethanol and their mixtures are most commonly used. Extraction implies separation of soluble matter from insoluble substances and thus differs from dissolution although the object of both the processes in the same.

EXTRACTION PROCESSES

1. Maceration :

The word maceration means softening. The maceration process is employed in the production of a number of preparations such as tinctures, extracts and concentrated infusions. It is the simplest method of crude drug extraction and was official in IP 1966. The process consists of keeping the crude drug in intimate contact with whole of the menstruum in a closed vessel with occasional shaking for seven days, straining, pressing the marc, mixing the liquids, and finally clarifying by subsidence or filtration. The drug should be properly comminuted. The cellular structure gets penetrated and the soluble portions are softened and dissolved. Occasional shaking brings about a rapid equilibrium between the intra- and extra-cellular fluids. A closed vessel is recommended so as to prevent loss of the menstruum. As the degree of pressing the marc may vary, the final product is not adjusted to any fixed volume. The process may take upto 14 days in some cases for complete extraction. The drug: menstruum ratio should normally be 1: 10 .

A sediment may form on standing; the fluid product should therefore be allowed to stand for a few days before use. Maceration process is very simple and does not require a skilled operator. Simple maceration may not be suitable for all drugs and therefore other maceration processes may have to be employed. E.g. Tincture of Myrrh and Compound Tincture of Benzoin are prepared by this method.

(a) **Modified maceration :** It is essentially used for extracting unorganized drugs, which have no cellular or tissue structure *e.g.* gums, resins, gum-resins and oleogum-resins. In case of unorganized drugs, the marc left behind forms a compact mass and does not retain any appreciable amount of the macerate and hence pressing the marc is neither desirable nor convenient. Unlike simple maceration, in modified maceration process the final product is adjusted to a definite volume. This is done for extracting unorganized drugs because more or less complete extraction of the constituents takes place in a short time.

A typical modified maceration process may be described as follows :

(i) Properly comminuted unorganized drug with the menstruum equal to 80% of the bulk of the finished preparation is placed in a closed vessel for 2 to 7 days.

(ii) The mixture is agitated occasionally.

(iii) The mixture is strained and the strained liquid is filtered.

(iv) Marc is washed with fresh menstruum (less than 20% of the finished bulk) and the washings are passed through the same strainer and filter.

(v) Sufficient menstruum is passed through the filter to make up the desired volume.

The filtrate should be collected in a dry receiver or in receiver which has been rinsed with the menstruum. This is necessary because the resinous matter present in most of the unorganized drugs are insoluble in water and hence get precipitated, adversely affecting the clarity of the finished preparation.

Tincture of Opium IP is prepared by method is as follows –

Pour 500 ml of boiling purified water on to the opium and set aside for six hours, add 500 ml of alcohol (90%), mix thoroughly and set aside in a covered vessel for 24 hours; strain, press the marc, mix the liquids and set aside for not less then 24 hours, filter.

The opium latex is not pulverizable and the morphine contained in it is one of the water-soluble alkaloids. The preliminary treatment with hot water disintegrates the latex and facilitates extraction. Further addition of 90% alcohol stabilizes the preparation and undesirable inert matter present in opium is also precipitated.

(b) Multiple maceration : Multiple maceration is aimed at achieving maximum extraction by using portions of the total volume of the menstruum for successive maceration. However, allowance is made for the volume of menstruum retained by the marc at the conclusion of the process. The drug menstruum ratio is low. The volume of menstruum for each maceration can be calculated as follows:

Double Maceration :

The equation for double maceration is -

$$\text{Volume for first maceration} = \frac{\text{Total volume - volume retained}}{2} + \text{Volume retained}$$

Note : This formula is true only when the whole of the soluble matter dissolves during the first maceration.

Example :

200 g of drug is to be extracted by double maceration. The total volume of menstruum to be used 1100 ml. It showed that after pressing each 2 g of drug retains 1 ml of menstruum.

$$\text{Volume of menstruum for first maceration} = \frac{1100 - 100}{2} + 100 = 600 \text{ ml}$$

Calculation Double Maceration :

a. First maceration :

600 ml added to 200 g of drug. 100 ml of menstruum retained by drug. Volume of combined strained and expressed liquid is 500 ml.

$$\text{Soluble matter} = \frac{500}{600} \times 100 = 83.3 \text{ percent}$$

b. Second maceration :

Remaining 500 ml of menstruum added to marc already containing 100 ml of menstruum. Volume of combined strained and expressed liquid is again 500 ml.

$$\text{Soluble matter} = \frac{500}{600} \times 16.7 = 13.9 \text{ percent}$$

Therefore, total soluble matter extracted = 83.3 + 13.9 = 97.2 percent

Calculation single maceration :

1100 ml menstruum added to 200 g of drug. The volume of combined strained and expressed liquid is 1000 ml (as 2 g drug retained 1 ml menstruum).

$$\text{Soluble matter} = \frac{1000}{1100} \times 100 = 90.9 \text{ percent}$$

Double maceration extractred more as compare to single =

$$\frac{97.2 - 90.9}{90.9} \times 100 = 6.93 \text{ percent}$$

A. TRIPLE MACERATION

The equation for triple maceration is –

$$\text{Volume for first maceration} = \frac{\text{Total volume - Volume retained}}{3} + \text{Volume retained}$$

The volume for the second and third maceration is half of the remaining menstruum. It is only true when the whole of the soluble mater of the drug dissolves during the first maceration.

Example

1000 g of drug is to be extracted by triple maceration. The total volume of menstruum to be used is 9000 ml. The marc is not be pressed until the conclusion of the third maceration.

- Experiment showed that each 1 g of unpressed drug retains 3 ml of menstruum.
- At the marc is lightly pressed, 1 g of drug retains 1 ml of menstruum.

$$\text{Volume for first maceration} = \frac{9000 - 3000}{3} + 3000 = 5000 \text{ ml}$$

$$\text{Volume for second and third maceration} = \frac{9000 - 5000}{2} = 2000 \text{ ml}$$

a. First maceration **:** 5000 ml added to 1000g of drug. Menstruum retained by drug 3000 ml. The volume of strained liquid is 2000 ml.

$$\text{Soluble matter} = \frac{2000}{5000} \times 100 = 40 \text{ percent}$$

b. Second maceration ; 2000 ml added to marc already containing 3000 ml of menstruum. Volume of strained liquid is again 2000 ml.

$$\text{Soluble matter} = \frac{2000}{5000} \times 60 = 24 \text{ percent}$$

c. Third maceration : 2000 ml menstruum added to marc already containing 3000 ml of menstruum. After slightly the marc is pressed. The volume of combined strained and expressed liquid is 4000 ml.

$$\text{Soluble matter} = \frac{4000}{5000} \times 36 = 28.8 \text{ percent}$$

The total soluble matter expressed by

triple maceration = 40 + 24+ 28.8 = **92.8** percent

B. DOUBLE MACERATION

$$\text{Volume for first maceration} = \frac{9000 - 3000}{2} + 3000 = 6000 \text{ ml}$$

a. First maceration : 6000 ml added to 1000 g of drug. 3000 ml of menstruum retained by drug.

$$\text{Soluble matter} = \frac{3000}{6000} \times 100 = 50 \text{ percent}$$

b. Second maceration : 3000 ml added to marc already containing 3000 ml of menstruum. The marc is slightly pressed, each 1g of drug retained 1 ml of menstruum .

$$\text{Soluble matter} = \frac{5000}{6000} \times 50 = 41.66 \text{ percent}$$

The soluble matter extracted by

double maceration = 50.00 + 41.66 = **91.66** percent

C. SINGLE MACERATION

9000 ml of menstruum added to 1000 ml of drug and marc pressed at conclusion, the combined volume of strained and expressed is 8000 ml.

$$\text{Soluble matter} = \frac{8000}{9000} \times 100 = 88.88 \text{ percent}$$

Table 14.1 : Comparative study of maceration process

S.No.	Maceration	Total soluble matter in percent
01	Triple maceration	92.80
02	Second maceration	91.66
03	Single maceration	88.88

c. **Vacuum extraction:** This is another modification of maceration process and employs a specially designed maceration vessel with arrangement for connecting it to a vacuum line. Basically this modification increases the permeability of the cell walls considerably and facilitates extraction in a much shorter time.

2. Digestion : This is a modified maceration process in which extraction is accomplished at a higher temperature at which the active ingredients are not adversely affected. Use of higher temperatures provides for enhanced solvent action of menstruum and constant mechanical agitation of the system accelerates establishment of equilibrium in a short time. If the solvent or menstruum is readily volatilized at the temperature employed, it is necessary to attach a reflux condenser to the vessel in which the digestion is being carried out so that the solvent may get condensed, recovered and returned to the container.

3. Percolation : In Greek, the word 'percolare' means 'to pass through'. It is also known as lixivation. It is the extraction process in which granulated or powdered drug is deprived of its constituents by the descent of a suitable menstruum through it. The process implies a slow passage of the menstruum under the influence of gravity through a column of the drug. During this movement, the menstruum goes on extracting the drug particles layer-wise, it being replaced by other layers above as it moves downwards. It is an important method for complete extraction.

Principle: Percolation may be defined as 'short successive maceration' or 'extraction by the method of displacement'. The powdered 'drug is placed in a cylindrical or conical vessel called percolator, with a diaphragm at the base. The menstruum is allowed to pass through a column of the drug at a regulated rate, which allows the menstruum to dissolve the active constituents and get saturated. The combined forces of gravity and that of the column of liquid above, impel the saturated menstruum downward. This movement is opposed by capillarity force. The physical forces which play an important role in percolation include gravitation, viscosity, adhesion, friction, osmosis, capillarity, surface tension and dissolution rate.

The percolation process as described in IP (1966) is given below. "Moisten the solid materials with a sufficient quantity of the menstruum, allow to stand for four hours in a well-closed vessel, pack in a percolator and add sufficient of the menstruum to saturate the materials. When the liquid commences to drip from. the percolator, close the outlet, add sufficient of the menstruum to leave a layer above the drug, and allow to macerate for twenty-four hours. Allow percolation to proceed slowly until the percolate measures about three-quarters of the volume required for the finished tincture. Press the marc, mix the expressed liquid with the percolate, and add sufficient of the menstruum to produce the required volume. Clarify by subsidence or filtration" The entire process of percolation can conveniently be explained by dividing it into the following steps:

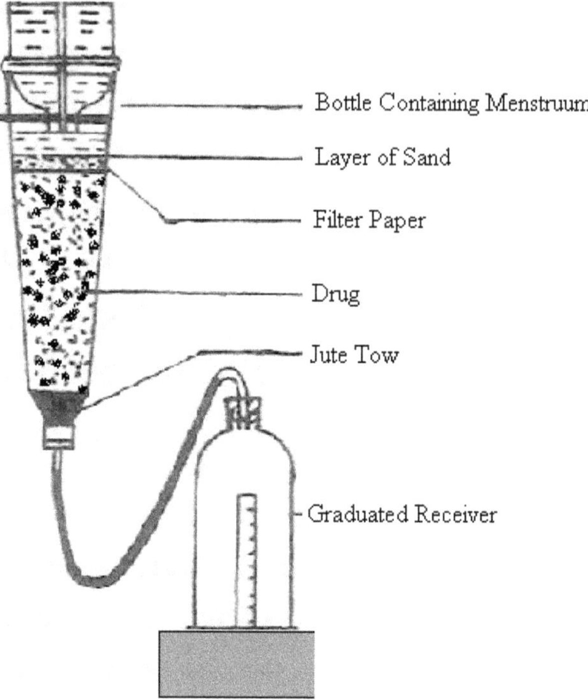

Fig. 14.1 Packing arrangement in a percolator

(a) Size reduction of the drug to a suitable degree : The degree of size reduction of the drug to be extracted should be established by experimentation. The golden rule 'finer the powder better the extraction' does not always hold true. Sometimes it is the optimum and not the finest grade of the powdered drug that gives most efficient extraction.

(b) Moistening or imbibition : Preliminary moistening helps the removal of air contained within the cells and facilitates the penetration of the menstruum. If the dry drug powder is packed in a percolator and menstruum added, packing would not be uniform and on adding the menstruum the drug particles will swell and ultimately choke the column and hamper the extraction process. Menstruum used for moistening should be sufficient for the drug to swell before it is packed in the percolator. However, preliminary moistening may also adversely affect the extraction process in certain unorganized drugs like oleogum-resins and in the so-called cold percolation of sugar in making syrups. Four hours are ordinarily quite enough for preliminary imbibition.

(c) Packing: The moistened drug should be packed carefully in the percolator in layers. Each successive layer should be packed moderately or firmly as the requirement may be. Whether moderate or firm, packing should always be uniform. Non-uniformity in packing will hinder complete extraction because the menstruum will mostly flow through the loosely packed portion leaving the tightly packed part of the drug incompletely extracted. If the column is too tightly packed, it will not allow adequate flow of the menstruum and lead to slow extraction rate. Similarly, too loose packing will allow free passage to the menstruum requiring unduly large quantity to affect complete extraction. The exit of the percolator is plugged with jute tow. The drug occupies almost two thirds of the column and a layer of washed sand is spread at the top. The layer of sand prevents the drug from being disturbed when the menstruum is poured on it.

(d) ***Maceration*** **:** Sufficient menstruum is now poured into the percolator to saturate the column and leave at least 2 cm layer at the top. While adding the menstruum, it is necessary to open the stopcock at the exit (not shown in figure) so as to allow the displacement of air by the menstruum otherwise air will force its way upwards in the column and disturb the packing. Again, enough of menstruum is poured to leave a layer at the top to prevent the drying of the upper layers of the drug. The percolator is then closed for 24 hours. During this time preliminary maceration takes place and the menstruum gets enough time to penetrate into the cells and dissolve the soluble constituents. This preliminary maceration prior to the commencement of actual percolation enables the drug to be exhausted by a small volume of the menstruum.

(e) Percolation : At the end of maceration, percolation is commenced by opening the lower stopcock. The rate of percolation should neither be too fast nor too slow. In case of the former a lot of menstruum will be required and in the latter it will take a long time to complete the process. During the process, the column should never be dry. This is conveniently achieved by inverting a bottle full of menstruum carrying a delivery tube to the percolator so that the delivery tube dips into menstruum layer upon the drug column in the percolator thus avoiding the necessity of constantly watching the percolation process. This process is continued until three quarters of the volume of the finished product has been collected. Complete extraction can be ascertained by chemical tests for active ingredients in a few drops collected towards the end of percolation.

(f) Pressing the marc : The marc is removed from the percolator and pressed in a tincture press or a hydraulic press. This expression is aimed at recovering the liquid, which still remains in the marc. However, complete removal of menstruum by expressing the marc may not be possible in which case it can be subjected to distillation in specially designed solvent recovery stills.

(g) **Adjustment of volume:** Expressed liquid and the percolate are mixed together and more menstruum is added to make up the desired volume. In case of standardized preparations, the volume to be added is governed by the result of the assay of the mixed percolates.

(h) **Clarification :** Clarification by subsidence or filtration gives a brilliantly clear preparation.

Intermittent percolation : In this process percolation is preceded and followed by maceration so that the menstruum is allowed more time to remain in contact with the drug particles. This provides greater extraction with smaller quantity of the menstruum.

Repercolation : It is a process of percolation employing the same volume of menstruum, for extracting the drug, in divided quantities. Thus the menstruum is allowed to extract the active principles by the first portion of the menstruum completely and the percolate from the first lot becomes the menstruum for the second lot and so on. The whole drug powder is divided into 4 or 5 lots. The intention is to obtain maximum extraction of constituents with the minimum of the menstruum. However, the method is not very successful as the drug in the last percolator in the series remains incompletely extracted by the time the prescribed volume of the final percolate is obtained.

Hot percolation : The efficiency of extraction can be improved by applying higher temperatures provided the active constituents and the menstruum can withstand such temperature without affecting the product adversely. Hot percolation is based on this principle and carried out by using a hot water jacketed percolator instead of an ordinary one and percolation is allowed to proceed at a higher temperature. In this method, complete extraction is possible with lesser volume of the menstruum. However, the method is not applicable if the active ingredients are thermolabile or if the menstruum is volatile. Obviously, water alone can be used as menstruum in hot percolation.

Reserved percolation : As the name implies, the method consists of reserving the first part of the percolate measuring equal to almost three quarters of the finished preparation and continuing the percolation till complete extraction is affected. The first percolate is more concentrated and contains maximum quantity of soluble ingredients. The subsequent percolates are less concentrated although the menstruum is fresh having maximum solvent action, but the drug is quite exhausted and contains very small quantity of ingredients. The process is used when the drug's preparation ratio is 1 : 1 or 2 : 1 and the product is fluid. After the extraction is complete, the marc is pressed and the liquid is combined with the subsequent percolate and the whole liquid is concentrated by distillation, if necessary; at reduced pressure, to a volume less than one fourth of the finished preparation. The concentrate is mixed with the first portion, the reserved percolate, and the final volume is adjusted with fresh menstruum after assay, if necessary.

Advantages of percolation

1. The reserved percolate which contains major quantity of ingredients is not subjected to heat treatment.
2. As the entire percolate is not to be distilled, the process is more economic.
3. There is no precipitation from the reserved percolate due to fractionation of the solvent which would take place if the entire percolate was distilled.

Hot continuous extraction (soxhelation) :

This is another modification of simple percolation in which percolation is affected by the use of a Soxhlet extractor whereby a small volume of hot liquid is made to percolate through a column of the drug again and again by evaporation and subsequent condensation. A soxhlet extractor as shown in Fig. 7.2 consists of a flask holding the menstruum, the extractor or a cylindrical percolator provided with an attached siphon called the soxhlet extractor and a reflux condenser fitted at the top of the soxhlet. The material to be extracted is usually placed in a thimble made of filter paper and then inserted into the extractor. The menstruum is placed in the flask and boiled. The vapours arising from the flask Fig 7.2 Soxhlet extractor pass by the side tube into the condenser. The vapour is condensed and drips into the body of the extractor as pure menstruum. It percolates through the drug to be extracted dissolving the soluble substance(s). As soon as the level of the menstruum in the main extractor rises above the siphon bend, the extract is drained out flowing through the siphon into the flask. This alternate filling and emptying of the body of the extractor goes on continuously and in the cycle the distillate obtained from the extract (pure menstruum) gets delivered upon the drug, extracts its soluble constituents and flows into the flask where it is evaporated leaving behind the extracted matter. Thus the same quantity of menstruum is recycled every time and complete extraction is achieved with a very small volume of the menstruum. Extraction process (maceration and percolation) and the preparation obtained by these process (tinctures and extracts) are no more official in IP.

OTHER EXTRACTION METHODS

1. **Infusion and decoction :** Both the methods are now obsolete. Infusions were usually prepared from vegetable drugs containing water soluble and easily extractable principles. The process consisted of moistening the drug with water, macerating it with boiling water, straining and making up the volume. Decoction process was also employed previously for extracting vegetable drugs containing water-soluble and heat-soluble constituents. The process consisted of boiling the drug with water, cooling, expressing, straining the liquid, and finally making up the volume. Concentrated Chirata Infusion and Compound Chirata Infusion were official in IP 1966.

2. **Pressure cooker extraction :** The method involves preliminary maceration of the drug with the menstruum and then holding it in a pressure cooker at 15 lb/sq inch pressure for 5 to 15 minutes. The cooker is then allowed to cool and the extract is removed by straining and pressing the marc. The method is claimed to yield almost complete extraction of a drug in lesser time but it is not applicable to drugs containing heat-labile constituents.

3. **Extraction by passage through a colloid mill :** In this method a suspension of the drug in the menstruum, after maceration, is passed through a colloid mill running at a speed of 1500 r.p.m. Recirculation through the mill yields efficient extraction. Passage of the drug particles through the colloid mill does not enhance the direct dissolution of drug constituents but is attributed to increased permeability of the cell walls when they are passed through narrow clearance of a colloid mill.

4. **Ultrasonic extraction :** The speed of drug extraction is enhanced by application of ultrasonic vibrations. The mixture of the drug and the menstruum is subjected to ultrasonic waves of 20 to 450 kilocycles/second followed by extraction in a soxhlet extractor. The treatment with ultrasonic vibrations provides rapid and superior extraction.

5. **Use of surface active agents in drug extraction:** Small quantities of surface-active agents (surfactants) or wetting agents like PEG 400-monooleate, PEG 600-monolaurate, PEG 400-dilaurate, sorbitol laurate and polyoxyethylene sorbitol monolaurate are reported to enhance the extraction of ingredients from some drugs like cinchona, hyoscyamous and belladonna. The surfactant is incorporated in the total menstruum, which is then added to drug powder and the entire mixture is agitated in a mechanical shaker and the extract is separated from the marc.

6. **Expression :** Expression as applied in the preparation of fruit juices can be employed as an extraction process. Extraction by expression can be carried out by using a screw press on a small scale and a hydraulic press for large scale operations. Pressures up to 30 tons can be applied with a hydraulic press.

7. **Diacolatiori :** In diacolation the menstruum is made to flow from the bottom of the drug-charged cylinder by positive pressure of compressed air. Some drugs offer resistance to upward flow of the menstruum under hydraulic pressure and diacolation is designed mainly for extraction of such drugs.

TYPES OF EXTRACTS

Mainly three forms of extracts are recognized

1. LIQUID EXTRACTS

Liquid extracts are liquid preparations of which, in general, 1 part by mass or volume is equivalent to 1 part by mass of the dried herbal drug or animal matter. These preparations are adjusted, if necessary, so that they satisfy the requirements for content of solvent, and, where applicable, for constituents.

Production

Liquid extracts are prepared by using ethanol of suitable concentration or water to extract the herbal drug or animal matter, or by dissolving a soft or dry extract (which has been produced using the same strength of extraction solvent as is used in preparing the liquid extract by direct extraction) of the herbal drug or animal matter in either ethanol of suitable concentration or water. Liquid extracts may be filtered, if necessary. A slight sediment may form on standing, which is acceptable as long as the composition of the liquid extract is not changed significantly.

Tests

Relative density : The liquid extract complies with the limits prescribed in the standard monograph.

Ethanol : In liquid extracts, alcoholic strength carry out the determination of ethanol content. The ethanol content complies with that prescribed.

Methanol and 2-propanol : 0.05 per cent V/V of methanol and maximum 0.05 per cent V/V of 2-propanol for alcoholic liquid extracts prescribed.

Dry residue : The liquid extract complies with the limits prescribed in the standard monograph corrected if necessary using prescribed any excipient.

Storage : Protected from light.

Labelling : On the label states in addition to the requirements content of ethanol in final extract.

2. SEMISOLID/ SOFT EXTRACTS

Soft extracts are semi-solid preparations obtained by evaporation or partial evaporation of the solvent used for extraction. For the preparation of soft extracts, suitable concentration are used as prescribed in the standard monograph.

TESTS

Dry residue : The soft extract complies with the limits prescribed in the standard monograph.

Storage : Protected from light.

3. DRY EXTRACTS

Dry extracts are solid preparations obtained by evaporation of the solvent used for their reduction. Dry extracts usually have a loss on drying or a water content of not greater than 5 per cent.

TESTS

Water content : The dry extract complies with the limits prescribed in the standard monograph, not more than 5.0 percent.

Loss on drying : The dry extract complies with the limits prescribed in the standard monograph.

Solvents : A dry extract prescribes a limit test for the solvent used for extraction.

Storage : In an airtight container, protected from light

TINCTURES

Tinctures, according to the Pharmacopoeia of India, are defined as alcoholic or hydroalcoholic solutions usually containing, in comparatively dilute proportions, the active principles of vegetable or animal drugs. Thus solutions of chemical substances are not included in the IP definition of tinctures. However, in USP, solutions of chemical substances are included under tinctures. For example, a hydroalcoholic solution of iodine is termed as Strong Iodine Solution or Weak Iodine Solution in IF but according to USP it is Iodine Tincture.

Definition

Tinctures are liquid preparations which are usually obtained using either 1 part of herbal drug or animal matter and 10 parts of extraction solvent or 1 part of herbal drug or animal matter and 5 parts of extraction solvent.

Internally tinctures are used as –

- Cardiotonics - Digitalis Tincture
- Anticholinergics - Belladonna Tincture
- Parasympatholytics - Datura Tincture
- Emetics - Ipecacuanha Tincture
- Flavouring agents - Orange Tincture IP or Sweet Orange Peel Tincture USP

Compound Tincture : contains more than one vegetable or animal drugs. Official tinctures vary greatly in their methods of preparation, the active ingredients and alcoholic content, and the intended use. Usually the proportion of the drugs required to make 100 ml of the finished product is as follows –

a. Potent drug : 10 g *(e.g.* Belladonna Leaf)
b. Non-potent drug : 20 g *(e.g.* Tolu Balsam)
c. Undried fresh fruit peel : 50 g *(e.g.* Sweet Orange Peel).

The ratio of the drug to the finished tincture is usually constant for the same type of drugs but the actual concentration of the active principles varies from one to another drug because the amount of soluble active constituents varies in different drugs. In order to adjust the potency of the tincture as prescribed in the Pharmacopoeia, many tinctures are to be assayed before completion of the finished product. Alcoholic strength of the tinctures may also vary greatly, for example

- Compound Cardamom Tincture IP contains 24 to 28% alcohol
- Strong Ginger Tincture IP contains 80 to 88% alcohol;
- other IP tinctures contain intermediate alcoholic strengths

Tinctures are therefore generally considered to be stable preparations provided the proportion of alcohol and water is not so disturbed that the dissolved solutes separate out as upon mixing or dilution with other preparations or vehicles in compounding practice. Tinctures should be kept in tightly-closed containers to prevent loss of alcohol, which may result in change of concentration of the active constituents either by precipitation or concentration of the latter. Storage in a cool place would also minimize the evaporation of alcohol.

Storage : Some of the active constituents of tinctures may be light-sensitive. Therefore the Pharmacopoeia of India recommends that the tinctures should be kept in tightly-closed containers, protected from light and stored in a cool place. It also recommends that the tinctures whose active principles changed with time - Aconite Tincture, Belladonna Tincture, Hyoscyamous Tincture, should be discarded after one year.

METHODS OF PREPARATION

1. **Maceration :** This method is suitable for drugs, which either contain a large proportion of soluble constituents or cannot be packed uniformly in a percolator and hence are not suited to the percolation process. General method is as follows : Place the solid materials with the whole of the menstruum in a closed vessel and allow to stand for seven days, shaking occasionally. Strain, press the marc, and mix the liquids obtained. Clarify by subsidence or filtration.

   Examples - Capsicum Tincture and Compound Cinchona Tincture

2. **Percolation** : This process is most commonly employed in the preparation of official tinctures. General process is as follows : Moisten the solid materials with a sufficient quantity of the menstruum, allow to stand for four hours in a closed vessel, pack in a percolator, and add sufficient of the menstruum to saturate the materials. When the liquid commences to drip from the percolator, close the outlet, add sufficient of the menstruum to leave a layer above the drug, and allow macerating for twenty-four hours. Allow percolation to proceed slowly until the percolate measures about three-quarters of the volume required for the finished tincture. Press the marc, mix the

expressed liquid with the percolate, and add sufficient of the menstruum to produce the required volume. Clarify by subsidence or filtration.

Examples - Aconite Tincture, Belladonna Tincture and Compound Cardamom Tincture

3. **Dissolution :** It involves the dissolution of soluble chemical agents in the solvents employed, generally varying proportions of alcohol and water. The following USP and NF tinctures are made by dissolution or dilution of active medicaments.

   Examples - Iodine USP, Strong Iodine NF XI, Nitromersol NF, Thimerosal NF, Ferric Chloride NF XI and Ferric Citrochloride NF XI.

   Some tinctures as Camphorated Opium Tincture IP' are combinations of vegetable extractive with additional agents added and hence they are prepared by a combination of methods as percolation and dissolution.

Compound Cardamom Tincture

Ingredients: Cardamom seeds, in moderately coarse powder : 14 g

Caraway, in moderately coarse powder : 14 g

Cinnamon, in moderately coarse powder : 28 g

Amaranth : 5 g

Glycerin : 50 ml

Alcohol (45%), sufficient quantity. : 1000 ml

Mixed powders are moistened with a sufficient quantity of alcohol and the tincture is prepared by percolation to make about 9/10th of the volume of finished product. Glycerin and amaranth are added and the final volume is made up with alcohol. Glycerin prevents the precipitation of tannins from the final product and renders it more stable. It may be filtered if necessary. It contains 38 to 43% of alcohol.

Dose : 2 to 4 ml. Use : Carminative.

Camphorated Opium Tincture IP

Ingredients : Opium tincture : 50 ml

Benzoic acid : 5 g

Camphor : 3 g

Anise oil : 3 ml

Alcohol (60%) : sufficient quantity to 1000 ml

It is prepared by dissolving benzoic acid, camphor and anise oil in alcohol, opium tincture is added and required volume is made up with sufficient alcohol. It may be filtered if necessary. It contains 0.05% *w/v* of morphine calculated as anhydrous morphine and 56 to 61 % alcohol.

Storage : It should be stored in tightly-closed containers, protected from light, and in a cool place.

Dose : 2 to 8 ml.   Use: Hypnotic, sedative.

Compound Benzoin Tincture

Synonym: Friar's balsam

Ingredients: Benzoin crushed	: 100 g
Prepared storax	: 75 g
Balsam of Tolu	: 25 g
Aloes	: 20 g
Alcohol (90 percent) sufficient to produce	: 1000 ml

Procedure : It is prepared by macerating the benzoin, prepared storax, tolu balsam and aloes with 800 ml of ethanol (90%) in a closed vessel for not less than 48 hours with occasional shaking. After filtration the volume is made up with ethanol (90%).

Alcohol content : the ethanol content should be between 70 to 77% vlv

Total solids : Total solids should be not less than 13.5% wlv

Total balsamic acids : 4.5% wlv of total balsamic acids, calculated as cinnamic acid and., determined on 1 ml by drying at 105^0 C for 4 hours.

Label : The label states that it is flammable.

Storage: Store in tightly-closed, light resistant containers and avoid exposure to direct sunlight and to excessive heat.

Use: Topical protective, expectorant and comforting by steam inhalation in acute laryngitis.

INFUSION

Concentrated Compound Chirata Infusion

Ingredients: Chirata cut small	: 1000 g
Dried orange peel thinly sliced	: 100 g
Lemon Peel, thinly sliced	: 200 g
Alcohol (25 percent)	: 1200 ml

Preparation : Macerate, in a covered vessel for forty-eight hours, the Chirata, the Dried Orange Peel and the Lemon Peel with 800 ml of Alcohol (25 percent). Pressed the marc and add alcohol, macerate and left for twenty-four hours. Press, add the liquid to the product of the first pressing. Set aside for not less than fourteen days if required filter it.

Alcohol : 20-24 percent v/v

Category : Bitter and tonic

Preparation : Compound Chirata Infusion

Dose : 2 to 4 ml

Compound Chirata Infusion

Ingredients: Concentrated Compound Chirata Infusion : 125 ml g

Purified water, sufficient to produce : 1000 ml

Category : Bitter and tonic

Dose : 152 to 30 ml

For dispensing purposes Compound Chirata Infusion should be used within twelve hours of its preparation.

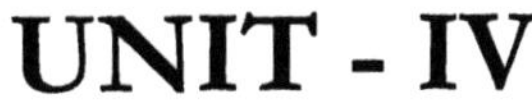

UNIT - IV

CHAPTER 15

INCOMPATIBILITY

Incompatibility signifies the problems arising when two or more ingredients prescribed, result into undesirable changes in the appearance, safety or therapeutic purpose of the product. Interaction of a drug with another drug, or of a drug with additives or adjuvants, dosage errors, omissions etc. also fall under incompatibility. Incompatibility may occur in compounding and dispensing of prescriptions so also at any stage during formulation, manufacturing, packaging, storage or administration of drugs. Contrary to expectations, the importance of incompatibility has increased in modern pharmaceutical practice mainly due to the introduction of large number of newer and more complex drugs as well as the indiscriminate use of combination therapy. In present day dispensing practice since the pharmacist invariably reviews each and every prescription, he should be in a position to detect and overcome the incompatibilities. This calls for the ingenuity of a pharmacist who is knowledgeable in pharmacy, pharmacology and chemistry. The problem of incompatibility is to be solved mainly through two angles firstly the detection or prediction of possible occurrence, and secondly, the correction which comprises of preventing or minimizing the incompatibility.

Incompatibility may be classified as physical, chemical and therapeutic.

I. PHYSICAL INCOMPATIBILITY

Physical incompatibility is mostly due to insolubility. However, liquefaction and physical complexation are not uncommon. Such incompatibilities are easier to predict, detect and correct by applying proper technique, mixing, selection of additives etc. Physical incompatibilities are commonly manifested by non-uniform, unsightly or unpalatable products. Physical incompatibilities may be classified as follows:

(A) Insolubility

Insolubility or immiscibility results in non-homogeneous product when two or more substances are combined. Separation of two phases when oil and water are shaken together (i.e. emulsion) is the classical example of such incompatibility but it is corrected by the use of an emulsifying agent whereby a uniform dispersion of one phase into the other is obtained. Gums are insoluble in alcohol and resins are insoluble in water. Insoluble substances like phenacetin, salol, precipitated sulphur etc. in mixtures require the use of a thickening agent. Use of another solvent or a cosolvent usually resolves the problem of insolubility.

Example 1.

Rx

Terpin hydrate		3.0 g
Simple Syrup q.s.	ad	120.0 ml

M. Ft. Sol.

In this preparation terpin hydrate is not soluble in syrup and hence half of the vehicle may be replaced by alcohol or isoalcoholic elixir. Alternate remedy would be to use any suspending agent (acacia, tragacanth or methocel) and dispense the product with a `shake well' label.

Example 2.

Rx

Phenobarbital	250.0 mg
Elixir Phenobarbital q.s. ad	30.0 ml

M. Ft. Sol.

Sig : Teaspoonful at bedtime

In this preparation phenobarbital is in excess and hence all of it is not soluble in the elixir. 10 ml of the elixir should be replaced by alcohol and 40 mg more of phenobarbital added to compensate the loss in phenobarbital (10 ml of the elixir).

Sometimes the prescriber may intend for reasons of stability or for therapeutic efficacy that insoluble compound be suspended rather that solubilized. Thus it is recommended that the intention of the prescriber should be held supreme.

Example 3.

Rx

Aspirin		gr V
Cherry syrup	q.s. ad	oz i.

D.T.D. ≠ 24

Here a suspension is prepared because of better stability of aspirin in suspension than in a solution.

Example 4.

Rx

Zinc sulphate	4.0
Sulphurated potash	4.0
Rose water q.s. ad	60.0

Again a suspension is intended because the active ingredients are the insoluble polysulphides formed by the reaction of the two compounds employed. A suitable suspending agent is to be included.

(B) Precipitation

A drug in solution may be precipitated upon addition of a solvent in which it is insoluble. Thus resins are precipitated from alcoholic solution on addition of water. Mucilaginous and albuminous substances may be precipitated from aqueous solution on addition of alcohol.

Precipitation from a saturated solution is often referred to as salting out.

- Camphor and volatile oils may get salted out of aromatic waters when salts of metals are dissolved in the liquid.
- Addition of electrolytes to colloidal solutions often results into precipitation.
- Addition of tragacanth is responsible for precipitation of boric acid from a saturated solution.

(C) Separation of immiscible liquids

A prescription containing ethyl nitrite spirit and substantial amount of potassium citrate will separate out and a layer of spirit will float.

Example 5.

Rx

Chloral hydrate	15.00 g
Sodium bromide	11.25 g
Elixir aromatic q.s. ad	60.00 ml

Soluble bromide is responsible for separating an immiscible layer consisting of chloral alcoholate, chloral and alcohol. In order to obtain a clear solution the alcoholic strength of the prescription should be above 50% or below 10%. A simple remedy would therefore be to dilute it with water to bring alcohol concentration to below 10% and inform the physician.

(D) Liquefaction of Solid

Liquefaction of dry solid materials may result from eutexia, release of water of hydration or absorption of water. Many drugs containing a phenol, aldehyde, or ketone group possess this tendency. Phenol, menthol, thymol and salol when mixed with one another, form eutectic mixtures. Liquefaction occurring at room temperature due to depression in melting point of a solid in contact with certain other components is known as eutexia. Eutectic forming ingredients may be dispensed separately or if a pasty mass has already resulted, the eutectic may be absorbed on sufficient inert diluent such as kaolin, talc, starch, magnesium carbonate, light magnesium carbonate, light magnesium oxide; and suitably dispensed.

Example 6.

Rx

Menthol	5.0
Camphor	5.0
Ammonium chloride	30.0
Magnesium carbonate, light	60.0

Make insufflation, send 4 oz.

Menthol, Camphor and ammonium chloride can be diluted separately with light magnesium carbonate and then mixed with gentle trituration in ascending order of weights.

Example 7.

Rx

Aminopyrine	0.3 g
Codeine sulphate	15.0 mg
Belladonna extract	10.0 mg
Acetyl salicylic acid	0.2 g

M.ft. Caps. ≠1. DTD ≠ 12.

Aminopyrine and acetyl salicylic acid form eutectic mixture. The resultant wetting of belladonna extract is further responsible for intensification of its green colour. 65 mg of light magnesium oxide per capsule should be included as diluent. One half of the quantity of the diluent is mixed with aminopyrine and the other half with acetyl salicylic acid and both are combined with gentle trituration. The remaining ingredients are then incorporated as usual.

(E) Physical complexation

Preparations containing carbowax and phenols, salicylic acid, or tannic acid are known to show loss in elegance and acceptability due to physical complexation. Their complexation is attributed to hydrogen bonding between the hydroxyl groups of the active ingredient and the ether oxygen of the polyether chain. Complexation of benzoic acid, salicylic acid, sulphonamides and barbiturates with urea is also reported.

Example 8.

Rx

Phenol		1.0 g
Polyethylene glycol 400		10.0 ml
Zinc oxide		15.0 g
Purified Water q.s.	ad	100.0 ml

M.ft. lotion.

Unsatisfactory suspension is produced due to complexation of phenol and PEG, and phenol is inactivated. PEG may be substituted by bentonite magma. Physical complexation may not be physically evident and hence prediction may be difficult. But it may result in therapeutic incompatibility.

(F) Miscellaneous

Drugs insoluble in water are not uniformly distributed in the bulk of the preparation and these results in non-uniform dose delivery. The problem is solved by i.) increasing the viscosity of the vehicle, and ii.) using suspending agents. In fact the suspending agents also act by enhancing the viscosity of the vehicle thus minimizing the settling of the solids. Suspending agents which are commonly used include acacia, tragacanth, methylcellulose derivatives; clays like bentonite; glycerin and syrups.

II. CHEMICAL INCOMPATIBILITY

This term signifies the chemical changes which occur due to the interaction of the prescribed substances leading to the formation of a harmful or dangerous product. Chemical incompatibilities often occur due to oxidation-reduction, hydrolysis or combination reactions. A chemical incompatibility, which is visualized rapidly by effervescence, precipitation or colour change, is called **immediate** incompatibility. An incompatibility without immediate and visible physical change is known as **delayed** incompatibility and may or may not result in loss of therapeutic activity.

Unintentional incompatibility may be **tolerated** i.e. interaction is minimized but composition of the prescription is not altered; or **adjusted** i.e. interaction is prevented by addition or substitution of constituents without affecting the medicinal action of the preparation. It is recommended that the pharmacist must consult or notify the prescriber about the suggested modification in the prescription while overcoming the incompatibility. However, this should be done in such a manner as not to raise any doubt in the mind of the patient.

Chemical incompatibilities may be classified as follows:

(A) Oxidation-reduction

Oxidation refers to the loss of electrons and reduction to the gain of electrons. Prescription mixtures are usually oxidized on exposure to air, higher storage temperatures, light, over dilution, incorrect pH adjustment or in presence of catalysis. Use of antioxidants such as ascorbic acid, sodium sulphite or sodium metabisulphite is often helpful. Trace metal ion catalysis may be counteracted by complexing agents such as disodium edetate and sodium calcium edetate. Auto-oxidation in fats and oils, phenolic substances, aldehydes and vitamins is controlled by agents such as propyl gallate, thymol, butylated hydroxyanisole (BHA), butylated hydroxytoluene (BHT), and hydroquinone etc. Silver, mercury and gold salts may be reduced by light to the metallic form although such reactions are rare in prescriptions.

Example 9.

Rx

Sodium salicylate	8.0 g
Sodium bicarbonate	16.0 g
Peppermint water q.s. ad	180.0 ml
M.ft. sol.	

The solution darkens on standing due to alkali catalysed oxidation of salicylate to quinoid form. Sodium bisulphite (0.1%) may be used as antoxidant to prevent the development of colour.

Example 10.

Rx

Potassium chlorate	4.0 g
Syrup ferric iodide	15.0 ml
Purified Water q.s.	ad 180.0 ml

The probable reaction is $KClO_3 + 3FeI_2 = 3\ FeOI + KCI + 3I$

Ferric oxide is oxidized with potassium chlorate. This mixture remains quite clear when fresh but on standing for some time, crystals of iodine are deposited. For solving this problem, the two reacting substances must be dispensed separately.

Example 11.

Rx

Mild mercurous chloride	gr XVIII
Potassium bromide	gr XXX
Sucrose	gr XXIV

M. Ft. powders = 12

The incompatibility occurs in the presence of moisture. Mercurous chloride reacts with potassium bromide, resulting in simultaneous oxidation and reduction of the mercurous salt to mercuric bromide and free mercury. The prescription should not be dispensed.

(B) Acid-base reactions

Such reactions result into precipitation, gas formation, colour development or colour change.

Precipitation

Except for the alkali metals, soluble inorganic salts react with hydroxides to yield water-insoluble compounds. Soluble salts of phenols, carboxylic acids and barbituric acids also yield free acid in the presence of relatively strong acids. Similarly, soluble salts of amine drugs liberate free base in the presence of relatively strong bases. Correction of acid-base incompatibilities requires thorough knowledge relating to acid-base strengths and solubilities of the acidic and basic forms of the particular compounds in question.

Example 12.

Rx

Cocaine HCl		0.3 g
Boric acid		0.3 g
Sodium borate	aa	1.2 g
Purified water q.s.	ad	60.0 ml

Sodium borate imparts alkalinity and the water-insoluble cocaine base is precipitated. Elimination of sodium borate would solve the problem.

Evolution of gas

Gas may be evolved due to a chemical reaction between ingredients. Evolution of carbon dioxide resulting from the reaction of carbonates and acids in aqueous media, and decomposition of syrups of p-amino salicylic acid, are common examples. Boric acid in the presence of glycerin forms glyceroboric acid that reacts with bicarbonates and gas is evolved.

Example 13.

Rx

Sodium bicarbonate	1.50
Borax	1.50
Phenol	0.75
Glycerin	25.00
Purified Water q.s. ad	100.00

Make a spray.

The substances should be mixed with water in an open vessel until effervescence ceases.

Change in or development of colour

Most of the dyes employed in pharmaceutical practice and their colour are influenced by their ionization depending on pH of the solution. Laxative phenolphethalein is colourless in acid solution but red in alkaline mixtures. Gentian violet is a basic purple compound but on addition of acid, the compound changes the colour through green to yellow. Such incompatibilities are corrected by the addition of a buffer or change of the vehicle to prevent formation of free acid or base from the salt.

(C) Hydrolysis

Many substances hydrolyse in water and their reaction may be facilitated by heat catalysts, hydrogen ions and hydroxyl ions. Esters, amides and metals like Zn and Fe etc. are common examples. Soluble salts of barbituric acid derivatives and sulphonamides hydrolyze in water and yield insoluble free acids. Phenyl salicylate hydrolyses in basic media to salicylic acid and phenol. Addition of any of the species formed as a result of hydrolysis is a common method employed to prevent or reverse the ionic hydrolysis. Examples of drug substances which may undergo hydrolytic decomposition include procaine, sulphonamides, chlorothiazide, barbituric acid derivatives, aspirin, some alkaloids, and penicillin. Similarly gelatin, sucrose, sodium acetate, flavouring oils and chlorobutanol; some of the common ingredients in prescriptions; are also liable to decomposition by hydrolysis.

Example 14.

Rx

Sodium salicylate	8.0 g
Phenobarbital sodium	5.4 g
Vitamin B complex elixir	240 ml

The alkalinity of salts causes decomposition by hydrolysis of the B vitamins of the acidic vitamin B complex elixir and precipitation of the acids of the sodium salts. To overcome the problem the salts should be dispensed separately.

Example 15

Rx

Penicillin G sodium 1,000,000 u

Syrup of cherry q.s. ad 30 ml

M.ft. sol.

Penicillin salt is hydrolyzed in acidic medium and penicillin is precipitated as free acid. Rate of hydrolysis can be slowed down by employing a neutral vehicle.

(D) Explosive combinations

Oxidizing agents are chemically reactive with reducing agents and some of these combinations may be potentially explosive.

Example 16

Rx

Potassium chlorate 0.6 g

Tannic acid 0.3 g

Sucrose aa 0.3 g

Make a powder. DTD $\neq$ 20

Ingredients of this prescription can be compounded with minimum rubbing. Tumbling the powders on a sheet of paper is also satisfactory. Alternately, each ingredient powdered individually, can be dispensed separately with adequate directions to the user. Explosion may take place if the ingredients are mixed by simple trituration in a pestle and mortar.

(E) Racemization

It is the conversion of an optically active form of a drug substance to an optically inactive form without a change in chemical constitution but is usually associated with a reduction in pharmacological activity. Examples of substances undergoing racemization are adrenaline, ephedrine, norephedrine etc. In alkaline solution but not in acid solutions, l-hyoscyamine may undergo racemization to form atropine.

(F) Other changes

Other types of chemical incompatibility may occur as a result of cementation (due to formation of hydrates e.g. plaster of Paris, polymerization, or conversion to new crystal habits), development of heat or lowering in temperature, polymerization, double decomposition, substitution, addition etc.

III. THERAPEUTIC INCOMPATIBILITY

When the response to one or more drugs in the patient is of a nature or intensity different from that intended, it is known as therapeutic incompatibility. It is within the realm of the physician and mainly concerned with prescribing errors and post-administration effect. Some of the adverse drug reactions may be considered as examples of therapeutic incompatibilities. Drug interactions have been dealt with in a separate chapter in this book. Common types of therapeutic incompatibilities are due to:

(A) Dosage errors

Dispensing of an overdose of a prescription constitutes the most serious type of dosage errors. Any experienced pharmacist should be able to detect such an error while checking the prescription.

Example 17.

Rx

Atropine sulphate	0.006
Phenobarbital	0.015
Aspirin	0.300

M.ft. cap. 1. Disp.≠12.

Sig : One capsule t.i.d.

The quantity of atropine sulphate for a single capsule is more than the recommended maximum dose. The physician should be contacted.

(B) Wrong dose or dosage form

As many drugs have confusingly similar names, there is always a possibility of dispensing the wrong drug e.g. prednisone and prednisolone, protamine and protamide, digoxin and digitoxin. Similarly many dugs are available in different dosage forms and hence if the dosage form is not mentioned clearly on the prescription, the pharmacist must seek clarification from the prescriber. It is highly desirable that the pharmacist should be aware of the potential hazard of such errors.

(C) Contraindicated drugs

Certain drugs may be contraindicated in a particular disease or when a particular patient is allergic to it. Thus corticosteroids are contraindicated in patients having an active peptic ulcer. Morphine, barbiturates, and related drugs may be dangerous in severe asthma. Vasoconstrictors should not be given to any hypertensive patient.

Example 18.

Rx

Sulphadiazine	0.25 g
Sulphamerazine	0.25 g
Ammonium chloride	0.5 g

M.cap. DTD ≠ 36.

Sig : 2 caps. q 4h for cough.

Ammonium chloride being a urinary acidifier, would cause deposition of sulphonamide crystals in the kidney. It being a contraindicated combination, the physician should be contacted.

(E) Synergistic or antagonistic drugs

Prescribing of synergistic or antagonistic drugs may be either deliberate or by mistake. The activity of penicillin derivatives may be prolonged by the use of probenecid and hence this combination is advantageous therapeutically as well as economically. Prescribing an amphetamine with a babiturate is apparently antagonistic combination but has been accepted in modern therapeutic practice to help in weight control. Some other antagonistic combinations would result in prescribing stimulants with sedatives, cholinergic drug with anticholinergic drug, purgatives with antidiarrhoeals etc. Concurrent use of an antacid with tetracycline will lead to decreased absorption of the antibiotic.

In conclusion it must be emphasized that although incompatibility continues to pose a serious problem in drug therapy, an experienced pharmacist should be able to detect and reasonably correct the same through his professional knowledge, skill and common sense. Drug interactions also lead to incompatibility.

SECTION - B
HOSPITAL PHARMACY

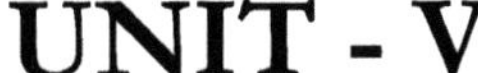

CHAPTER 16

ORGANIZATION OF A HOSPITAL PHARMACY

ORGANIZATION OF A HOSPITAL AND HOSPITAL PHARMACY

The four fundamental functions of hospitals are patient care, teaching, research and public health. The hospital pharmacy must be considered as one of the many departments of a hospital and as such it has several general functions. Several universities in India have included hospital pharmacy in their B.Pharm syllabi while few universities offer Clinical Pharmacy specialization at M.Pharm level. In USA there is a trend toward specialization within hospital pharmacy, such as nuclear pharmacy, drug information specialist, pharmacy administration specialist, clinical pharmacy etc.

Definition

Hospital pharmacy may be broadly defined as the practice of pharmacy in a hospital. A hospital pharmacy caters for the drug needs and other relevant services. It is also the area where prescriptions are filled for in-patients and out-patients, pharmaceuticals are manufactured in bulk and packaged, narcotics and other dangerous drugs are dispensed, biologicals are stored and dispensed and injectable preparations are prepared and sterilized. Thus hospital pharmacy is a department in which the drugs are procured, preserved, stored, compounded, assayed, dispensed, manufactured, packaged and distributed to in-patients and out-patients; by professionally competent and legally qualified pharmacists. In a general way, hospital pharmacy and a hospital pharmacist do not differ from pharmacy and a pharmacist. In addition to the common functions of a pharmacist, a hospital pharmacist is expected to have a thorough knowledge of various systems of drug distribution, economics and drug budgeting, apart from a specialized knowledge of all dosage forms. A hospital pharmacist should also be aware of the concepts of unit dose dispensing, prepackaging and radio-pharmaceuticals. An emerging field allied to hospital pharmacy practice is clinical pharmacy. A hospital pharmacist is expected to provide up-to-date drug information to all concerned.

A unique feature of hospital pharmacy as compared to the traditional physician-pharmacist-patient relationship in private practice of pharmacy and medicine, is a physician-pharmacist-nurse-patient relationship.

Jonathan Roberts in colonial America is claimed to be the first hospital pharmacist who was attached to Pennsylvania hospital in 1752. There is no record of the first hospital pharmacist in India. Mr. S.H. Merchant was appointed as hospital pharmacist at K.E.M. Hospital, Bombay in 1941. Significant advances in hospital pharmacy took place in 1940's in America and in 1960's in India. The credit for developing hospital pharmacy in America and India goes to the American Hospital Pharmacists' Association and the Indian Hospital Pharmacists' Association, respectively.

Functions of Hospital Pharmacy

The functions of a hospital pharmacy are regulated by the Governing Board of that hospital. Following are the functions in general:

1. To provide and support medical care to the patients and to implement the departmental services according to the objectives, policies and standards of the hospital.
2. Dispensing of drugs, chemicals and other pharmaceutical preparations, alcoholic and narcotic preparations; and maintaining a running stock account of the same.
3. Preparation and sterilization of injectable medication required to be produced in the hospital.
4. Filling and labelling of all containers issued to services from which medicines are to be administered.
5. Inspection of all pharmaceutical supplies.
6. Maintenance of stocks of approved drugs, antidotes and other emergency requirements.
7. Maintaining correct specifications as to the quality of all purchases.
8. To plan departmental administration and fix the responsibilities and duties of each category of personnel.
9. To coordinate it's functions with other departments and services in the hospital.

10. Ascertaining the requirements of the department and establishing procedures to maintain adequate and competent staff.
11. Developing and maintaining an effective system of clinical and administrative records and reports.
12. Ascertaining needs for facilities, supplies and equipment, and implementing a system for evaluation, control and maintenance.
13. To initiate and participate in studies or research projects designed for the improvement of patient care and improvement of other administrative and hospital services.
14. To initiate/implement a programme of continuing education for all personnel.
15. To supply information concerning medicines to the hospital staff.
16. Maintenance of correct costing to the value chargeable to patients, if applicable.
17. Preparation of periodical and annual reports about working of the pharmacy.

Classification of Hospital

In these days variety of hospitals are available. Hospitals may be classified on the basis of system of medicine, on clinical basis and on the basis of bed size.

A. Classification on the basis of system of medicine

   a. Allopathic hospitals
   b. Ayurvedic hospitals
   c. Homoepathic hospitals
   d. TB Hospitals
   e. Unani hospital
   f. Naturopathy hospitals

B. On the basis of beds

   a. More than 1000 bed hospital
   b. 500 bed hospitals
   c. 300 bed hospitals
   d. 100 bed hospitals
   e. 50 bed hospitals

C. On the Clinical basis

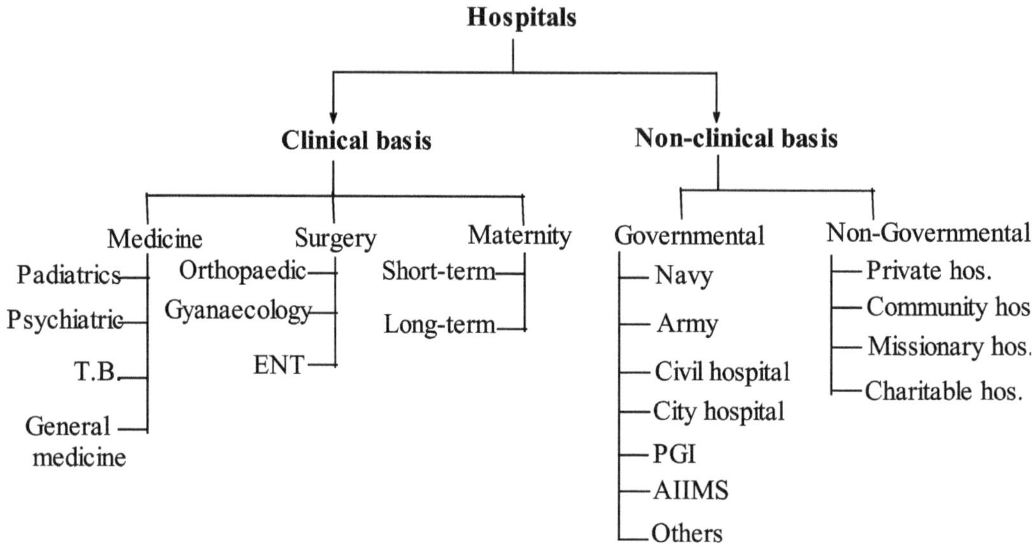

Chart : Classification of Hospitals on Clinical basis

ORGANIZATION

It is important that a hospital pharmacy should be under the direction of a professionally competent and legally qualified pharmacist. **Hathi Committee** has also recommended that a Chief Pharmacist possessing adequate educational qualification, preferably a post-graduate in pharmacy and having adequate practical experience (about three years) should be in overall charge of the –

(i) medical stores

(ii) dispensary

(iii) hospital pharmacy (transfusion solutions) and central sterilization; and

(iv) quality control.

In India hospital pharmacy is not well developed but serious efforts are being made to organize it on sound basis. In order to provide efficient hospital pharmacy services it is essential that it is treated as a full-fledged, self contained department. Hathi Committee has recommended that the Chief Pharmacist should be treated on par with the senior cadre officers in the hospitals and offered a suitable pay scale so that he may command respect not only from his staff members but also from the medical staff in the hospital. For an average daily attendance of 60 patients, one registered pharmacist is recommended.

Location and Layout

Hospital pharmacy should be located in a place easily accessible from all clinics and nearer to the natural exit of the hospital. Preferably it should be located on the ground floor so as to avoid inconvenience to the persons availing the services of the pharmacy. The sub-departments like in-patient and out-patient dispensing units, manufacturing unit, preparation unit, store etc., should be continuous as far as possible. If these departments are separated, then they should be in a direct vertical relationship. Pharmacy and other divisions of hospital should also be related in a direct vertical relationship. Using basement for storage of drugs is not recommended because of difficulties in controlling the optimum conditions for storage. Out-patient pharmacy should be well-furnished, airy, well-lit and giving a pleasant look, and provided with comfortable seats. Work benches and furniture etc. should be so arranged as not to give a congested look. The waiting room of the out-patient pharmacy should reflect a professional look. It is a good place for educating the general public on health matters. Family planning literature and general information on drugs, health and hygiene can also be displayed at appropriate place. Anybody visiting the pharmacy must carry a good impression about the pharmacy and it's service.

Planning

Planning of a hospital pharmacy requires a thorough knowledge of hospital's objectives, plan of operations and operational policies. It calls for the cooperation of the hospital administrator; the Chief Pharmacist, and the building committee. The overall planning consists of *(i)* a master programme; *(ii)* functional programming; and *(iii)* equipment planning and architectural design. The following points must be considered:

1. The objectives of the pharmacy and plan of operations.
2. The functions to be performed.
3. Determination of work flow and procedures; the estimated workload and personnel to be accommodated.
4. The space, shape, furniture, equipment and service needs of each work area.
5. The inter-relationship between work areas of the pharmacy and other departments.
6. Designing of one or more schematic floor plans and their evaluation till an optimal design is arrived at.
7. Legal aspects

An effective planning always provides for future growth and expansion and hospital pharmacy is no exception. Thus, apart from the present activities like compounding, dispensing and manufacturing of various dosage forms etc. while planning; one should also keep in mind that in future the number of in-patients as well as out-patients may increase, the pharmacy unit may have to establish a research laboratory and a radiopharmaceutical laboratory etc. Besides the area, equipment, and personnel; the planner must also take into consideration the communication and transport *e.g.,* conveyor and pneumatic tubes; electrical and gas fittings; water supply, ventilation, plumbing etc.

Staff

The staff requirements for a hospital pharmacy depend on –

(i) Number of beds in the hospital
(ii) average number of inpatients and outpatients
(iii) activities of the unit, and
(iv) whether the pharmacy also stocks and dispenses surgical and laboratory supplies.

In order to facilitate this, it becomes necessary to prepare the **Activity Chart** and the **Flow Process Chart** of the pharmacy. These help in evaluating the time and motion involved in the performance of various jobs *e.g.,* the average time required in dispensing an out-patient prescription etc. This constitutes **job evaluation** study. Answering a few questions like what is the purpose of a job, why is it necessary, where and when would it be done, who should do the job, and how should it be done; helps in utilizing more efficiently the time of each personnel in the department. According to an estimate the average time required for dispensing of a non-compounded prescription is 8 minutes while dispensing of a compounded prescription requires 14 minutes. Thus the total work load is calculated and accordingly the number of personnel is determined.

General guidelines for the determination of staff of pharmacy are:

(i) One Chief Pharmacist.
(ii) One registered pharmacist for an average daily attendance of 60 patients (inpatients + out-patients) with a *minimum* of 4 pharmacists for smaller hospitals.
(iii) Adequate number of assistants, attendants and sweepers.
(iv) One typist-cum-clerk.
(v) For a hospital pharmacy involved in manufacturing of drugs and formulation; in addition to compounding, dispensing, distribution and storage of medicines:
    (a) A deputy to the Chief Pharmacist designated as manufacturing pharmacist preferably having a post-graduate degree in pharmacy and relevant manufacturing experience.
    (b) One analytical pharmacist having a degree in pharmacy and possessing adequate experience.
(vi) In general, hospitals having a bed strength of upto 50, 100, 200, 300 and 500 beds, require 3, 5, 8,10 and 15 pharmacists, respectively.
(vii) For large hospital one pharmacist should be appointed for every 133 patients.

Space

Space requirements of a hospital pharmacy depend on the number of beds, number and types of sections in pharmacy unit, number and types of out-patients, and location of the hospital. The requirements relating to manufacture of tablets, parenterals, ophthalmic preparations under aseptic conditions, filling of hard gelatin capsules and repacking operations are laid down in schedule M of Drugs and Cosmetics Act and Rules, which should be considered as a minimum. Dispensing department should not be less than 6 sq. metres for one pharmacist and additional 2 sq. metres for each additional pharmacist. A modern hospital pharmacy should provide an adequate area for –

(i) waiting room and some magazines with toilets,
(ii) office of the Chief Pharmacist including a Library and Drug Information Centre
(iii) office for the clerk-cum-typist,
(iv) inpatient dispensing laboratory,
(v) outpatient dispensing laboratory,
(vi) manufacturing laboratory,
(vii) sterile products laboratory,
(viii) product formulation, control and research laboratory,
(ix) pharmacy storeroom;
(x) alcohol and volatile liquids vault or room,
(xi) narcotics, investigational drugs and other dangerous drugs vault or room,
(xii) additional bulk storage facilities, and
(xiii) a radiopharmaceutical laboratory if the hospital is to provide this service.

Minimum space requirements depending on bed strength of a hospital are given in Table 16.1. This space requirement includes accommodation for staff amenities and duty room for pharmacist on night duty and duty on holidays.

Table 16.1 Minimum Space Requirements of a Hospital

Facilities	**Area required in sq. meters for**		
	100 beds	**300 beds**	**700 beds**
Compounding and dispensing laboratory	350	500	800
Preparation room	100	400	650
Store	450	1000	2400
Office	110	150	200
Filling of hard gelatin capsules			200

Table 16.1 *Contd....*

Manufacture of pills and compressed, tablets including hypodermic tablets			900
Manufacture of eye lotions, eye-drops, eye ointments and other preparations for, external use; under aseptic conditions		250	250
Repacking operations			300
Parenteral preparations laboratory		600	600
Total Area	1010	2900	6300
Average Area per bed	10	9.7	9.0

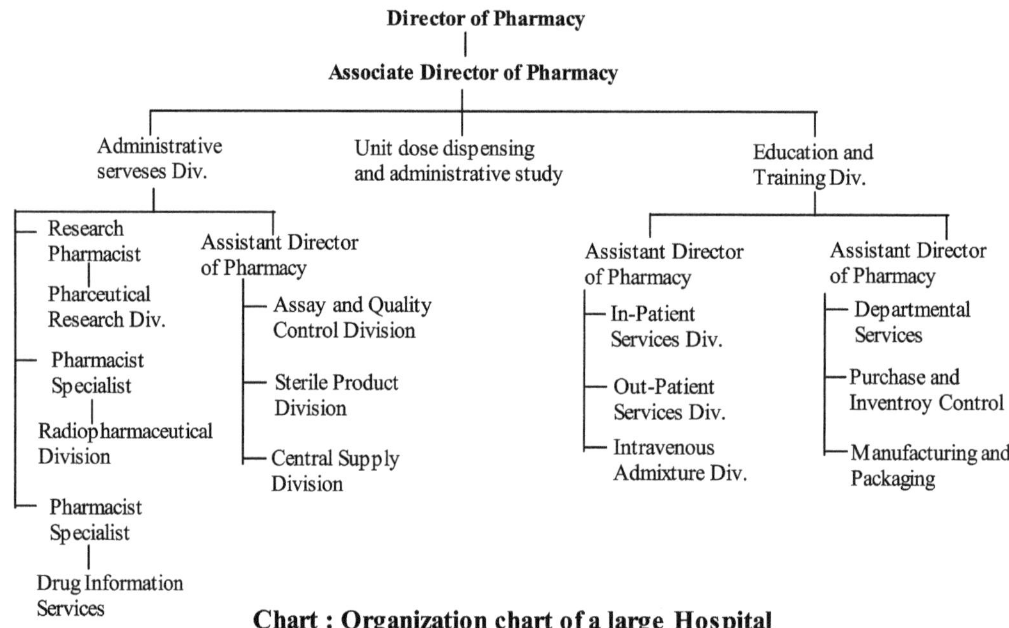

Chart : Organization chart of a large Hospital

HOSPITAL PHARMACY

Hospital pharmacy is one of the most important sections among several departments of a hospital. Hospital pharmacy may be defined as that department of the hospital, which deals with procurement, compounding, dispensing, manufacturing, testing, distribution, storage and packaging of drugs. Hospital pharmacy also provides other pharmaceutical services and education. It is controlled by a professionally knowledgeable and a trained pharmacist. In these days, Hospital pharmacy provides clinical pharmacy services of drug monitoring and drug information system.

Functions and Objectives of Hospital Pharmacy

Pharmacy is accepted as an essential hospital service in all hospitals. It is managed by qualified pharmacists. Qualified and experienced pharmacists are the most desirable professionals for purchasing, handling of prescription, dispensing and storage of medications. Pharmacist is playing important role in hospital and also as a good communicator between physician and the patient. Pharmacist has many other responsibilities in the hospital as given below:

1. As a guide of patient and provide correct information with specifications for purchase of drugs, chemicals, and biologicals.
2. Maintain drugs in proper place as per the requirement of storage.
3. Some parenteral products dispense in the hospital, need very skilled person (Pharmacist) for sterilization and storage.
4. Manufacturing of medicaments such as solid, liquid and semisolid dosage form.
5. Distribution of medicaments in the hospital
6. Dispensing of drugs as per the prescriptions of the medical staff of the hospital.
7. Filling all drug containers from which medicines are to be administered.
8. Maintaining proper labeling of medicines
9. Management of records of purchase of drugs etc.
10. Establishment of Drug Information Centre for necessary information to physician, nurses or any other competent person who deals in drugs.
11. Patient counseling for out-patient department.
12. Maintaining liasion among medical staff, nursing staff and patients.
13. Removing expired drugs and containers and also remove missing labels containers

RESPONSIBILITIES OF HOSPITAL PHARMACISTS

Hospital pharmacy may be broadly defined as the practice of pharmacy in a hospital. A hospital pharmacy caters for the drug needs and other pertinent services. It is also the area where prescriptions are filled for inpatients and outpatients, pharmaceuticals are manufactured in bulk and packaged, narcotics and other dangerous drugs are dispensed, biologicals are stored and dispensed and injectable preparations are prepared and sterilized. Way back in 1975 Hathi committee had recommended that the parenteral formulation (IV formulation) should be formulated under the supervision of qualified person by graduate/diploma holder in pharmacy. Pharmacist is highly responsible person in hospital that plays a key role in hospital services and management.

1. Technical Ability

Pharmacist should have technical ability because of they have thorough knowledge of all basics of pharmaceutics, pharmacology, pharmacognosy, Pharmaceutical chemistry, toxicology, route of administration, drug interaction, stability and pharmaceutical analysis. A pharmacist in hospital should provide information regarding handling, storage and distribution of drugs.

2. Development of Manufacturing Section

Manufacturing section in a hospital is very important to control quality, quantity, supply and costing of material commonly used in hospital. Hospital pharmacist is no doubt qualified pharmacist and have capability to analysied the things in the benefit of hospital.

3. Administrative Ability

The hospital pharmacist should be able to control various functions of hospital pharmacy. He should prepare work schedule, policies and procedure of various activities. Chief Hospital Pharmacist is also responsible for selecting staff members. He should interact with the staff daily and also solve their problems.

4. Ability to Control Inventory

Chief Pharmacist has responsibility to control inventory of drugs and managing at nursing stations, supply rooms and clinical units.

5. Ability to Conduct Teaching Programmes

Pharmacist trains nursing staff and other supporting staff for storage of drugs, proper use of drugs, dosage forms, pharmaceutical calculation, conversions and calculations of dosages forms.

6. Ability to Participate in Research

The pharmacist is required to maintain latest information about drugs by using pharmaceutical journals, bulletins, internet literacy and tune with the technology. Pharmacist has capability to maintain all latest literature and technology for maintaining all the drugs, storage and proper labeling.

PHARMACY AND THERAPEUTIC COMMITTEE

In these days of modern medicine when many agents are available for the management of disease, the careful selection of drugs for use in the hospital has become an important administrative and therapeutic tool. It is essential to establish definite rules, standards for improving drug therapy, guide manufacturers, as well as physicians for proper use of medicine. The Pharmacy and Therapeutic Committee or its equivalent is the organizational keystone of the program for maximizing rational drug use. According to the American Society of Hospital Pharmacists (ASHP) this committee is an advisory group of the medical staff and serves as the organizational line of communication between the pharmacy department and the medical staff. It is policy recommending body to the administration and medical staff of the hospital on all matters related to the therapeutic use of drugs. The committee is composed of physicians, pharmacists, and other health professionals selected with the guidance of the medical staff. The Council on Pharmacy and Chemistry of the American Medical Association had been well established and was successfully operating when we were suddenly push into the modern era of therapeutics. It was considered as a result of the discovery of the sulfa compounds and was rapidly followed by the discovery of penicillin, streptomycin and the other antibiotics. In the 1950s, there was a flood of new substances with high potency and activity in many fields of medicine. This flood of new therapeutic agents made very difficult task for the doctor to become knowledgeable about more than a relatively few products. It was found that some excellent, some not so good, and some practically useless, it was necessary for the hospital to establish a method or system to bring the best medicinal agents to the staff, and thus assist them in the proper selection of therapeutic substances for the treatment of the hospitalized patient. In view of this, Pharmacy and Therapeutics Committee was constituted whose responsibility was to include –

- publishing of a pharmacy educational bulletin,
- preparations of a hospital formulary
- establishment of automatic stop orders for dangerous drugs,
- preparation of emergency *kits*
- supervision of investigational use drugs,
- development of a program for reporting, and
- investigating adverse drug reactions

The Pharmacy and Therapeutics Committee in a hospital is a tool for maintaining medical staff self-government. It is responsible to the medical staff as a whole and its recommendations are subject to medical staff approval. The Pharmacy and Therapeutics Committee is a mandatory committee under the Conditions of Participation of the

Hospital Insurance Program-Medicare. Composed of physicians and the pharmacist, it serves as the organizational line of communication of liaison between the medical staff and the Pharmacy Department. This committee assists in the formulation of broad professional policies regarding the evaluation, selection, procurement, distribution, use, safety procedures and other matters relating to drugs in hospitals. This Committee is also known as Drug Therapeutic Committee, Pharmacy Committee, Formulary Committee, Therapeutics Committee and sometime abbreviated as P&T Committee.

Purposes

The main purposes of the pharmacy and therapeutics committee are as specified in the following.

a. Advisory : The committee recommends the adoption of, or assists in the formulation of, policies regarding evaluation, selection, and therapeutic use of drugs in hospitals.

b. Educational : The committee recommends or assists in the formulation of programs designed to meet the needs of staff -physicians, nurses, pharmacists, and other health-care practitioners for complete current knowledge on matters related to drugs and drug use.

ORGANIZATION AND OPERATION

The composition and operation of the Pharmacy and Therapeutics Committee may vary from hospital to hospital. Some common rules will apply :

1. In Pharmacy and Therapeutics Committee should consist of at least three physicians, a pharmacist, a nurse, and an administrator. All members are appointed by a governing unit or elected official of the organized medical staff.
2. A Chairman of the committee among the physician will be appointed and a pharmacist shall work as its Secretary.
3. The Committee should meet regularly, at least six times per year. If required the Committee can meet more often when necessary.
4. The Committee should also invite persons from within or outside, who can contribute specialized or unique information, skills, and judgments.
5. An agenda with minutes of the previous meeting should be prepared by the Secretary and submitted to the committee members in advance before the meeting.
6. Minutes should be prepared by the Secretary and maintained in the permanent records of the hospital.
7. Any new recommendations, policies, rules framed by committee shall be presented to the medical staff for adoption or recommendation.

8. Liaison should be maintained with other hospital committees concerned with drug use e.g., infection control, medical audit etc.

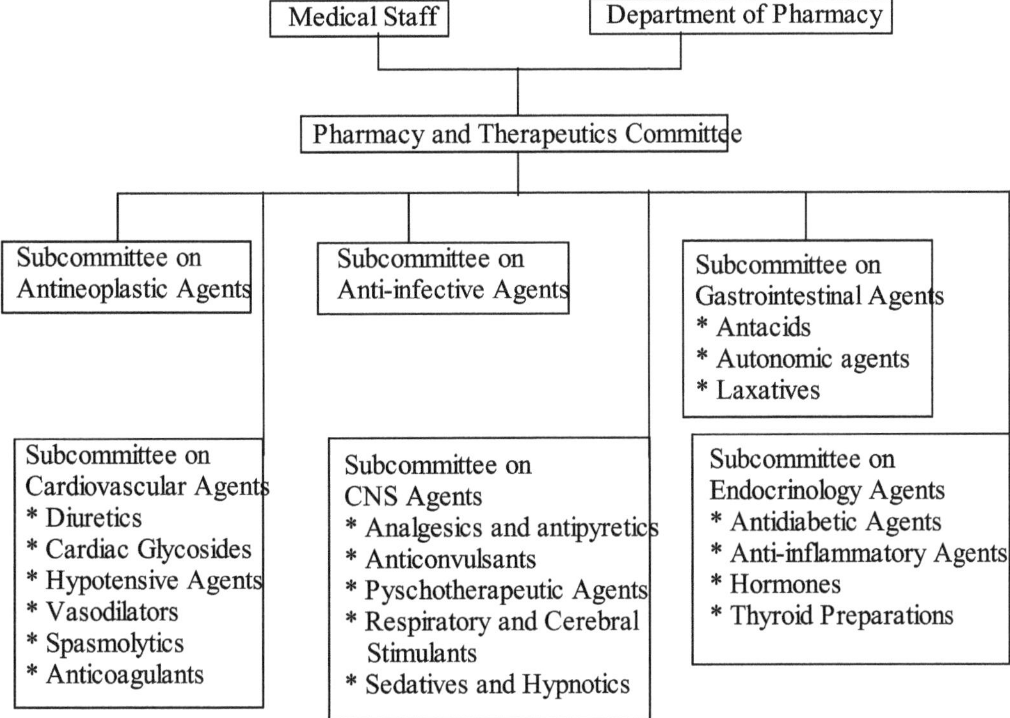

Fig. 16.1: Organization of a Pharmacy and Therapeutic Committee

SCOPE OF COMMITTEE

The functions and scope of the Pharmacy and Therapeutics Committee are determined by the basic organization of the hospital and medical staff. The scope of Pharmacy and Therapeutic Committee is given below:

1. To develop a Formulary of drugs approved for use in the hospital and keep it up to date by for its constant revision. Formulary items are selected on the basis of their relative therapeutic merits, safety and cost.
2. To act as advisor to the medical staff and hospital administration in all matters pertaining to the use of drugs in the hospital. Investigational drugs are included.
3. To minimize duplication of the same basic drug type, drug entity, or drug product.
4. To make recommendations concerning stocking of drugs in hospital patient-care areas.

5. To advise the pharmacy in the implementation of effective drug distribution and control procedures.
6. To establish programs and procedures that help in cost-effective drug therapy.
7. To establish and disseminate relevant educational materials and programs for the professional staff (medical, nursing etc) of the hospital on matters related to drugs.
8. To participate in quality-assurance activities related to the use, administration and distribution of medications.
9. To review from time to time the adverse drug reactions occurring in the hospital.
10. To diret and/or initiate drug-use review programs and studies and review the results of such activities.

FUNCTIONS OF COMMITTEE

The guidelines of the Pharmacy and Therapeutic Committee given below are essential for its functioning within the realm of a hospital. These functions do not constitute the activities of the Committee :

1 To help the Pharmacy Department in the development and review of policies, rules, and regulations regarding the use of drugs in the hospital in accordance with local, state, and national regulatory agencies.
2. To act as advisor to the Pharmacy Department Medical Staff and hospital administration in all matters pertaining to the use of drugs in the hospital. Investigational drugs are included.
3. To evaluate, approve, or reject drugs proposed for inclusion in or deletion from the Hospital Formulary.
4. To develop and organize suitable educational programs and materials related to drug to the members of Nursing and Medical staff.
5. To specify categories of drugs used in the hospital and also to assign drugs to different categories
6. To promote optimum standards for rational drug therapy by evaluating drug utilization in the hospital.
7. To collect and review reports on adverse drug reactions reported in the hospital.

Frequency of Meetings

Size of the hospital as well as volume and types of drugs used dictate the number and frequency of meetings of the Committee. The Committee should meet as often as necessary but at least once is a fortnight and in the busier institutions at least monthly. Notices of the meeting, date, venue, time and accompanying agenda should be circulated by the secretary (Pharmacist) of the Committee. The Secretary also insures the attendance and knowledgeable participation in the discussion of the agenda items.

The Committee's Role in Drug Safety

For each new class of therapeutic agents, the scope, knowledge and responsibility of the hospital pharmacist increases commensurately. This is the moral, legal, and professional obligation of insuring safety in the handling and administration of drugs in hospital. Unfortunately, too many pharmacists and physicians take drug safety for granted and false state of complacency by the fact that pharmacy "accidents" resulting in serious injury or some times death of patients are rare. In the first press release telling a tragic drug "accident" in a neighboring hospital, every trustee, administrator, physician, and pharmacist suddenly awakens to the fact that their policies governing the pharmacy ought to be reviewed in the light of modern dispensing and prescribing trends. The Pharmacy and Therapeutics Committee may serve as a guide for the safeness of the hospital pharmacy as mentioned below :

1. Does the hospital employ a qualified registered pharmacist to supervise the pharmacy?
2. Does the hospital employ an adequate number of trained personnel to permit for adequate coverage of the pharmacy seven days per week?
3. Does the hospital employ employees commensurate with the pharmacy work load?
4. Does the hospital permit non-pharmacist personnel to dispense drugs and allied materials?
5. Does the hospital provide adequate, safe work space, and safe storage facilities for the pharmacy?
6. Does the hospital have an automatic stop order regulation for dangerous drugs such as hypnotics, narcotics and anticoagulants?
7. Does the pharmacy have the equipment essential to safely and sufficiently carry out the modern practice of pharmacy?
8. Does the hospital have a drug formulary?
9. Does the drug formulary periodically revised and kept up-to-date?
10. Does the hospital have a solid policy regarding the use of research drugs in the hospital and its clinics?
11. Does the hospital permit anybody other than a licensed pharmacist into the pharmacy "after hours"?
12. Are poisonous materials adequately segregated from non-poisonous materials in the pharmacy and on the nursing stations?
13. Are external use preparations separated from internal use medications in the pharmacy and on the nursing stations?
14. Does the pharmacy manufacture products for patient's use and checked for accuracy and asepsis by chemical and bacteriologic means?
15. Does the hospital allow the pharmacist sufficient help to permit him to engage in a teaching program to acquaint the nursing and resident staff with new drugs?

16. Does the pharmacy have a suitable reference section which has latest texts on pharmacology, toxicology and posology?
17. Are all nursing stations periodically verified for the purpose of removing deteriorated and outdated drugs?

Committee's Role in the Adverse Drug Reaction Program

Recent advances in drug therapy are the proportionate increase in drug reactions. In order to increase an understanding of these troubles are required to formulate competent opinions for prevention and treatment. The Pharmacy and Therapeutics Committee must assume the responsibility for developing and instituting a procedure for the timely reporting of an adverse drug reaction.

An adverse drug reaction defined by the Food and Drug Administration as follows:

"An adverse drug reaction includes any pathological condition precipitated by a drug regardless of its nature or the circumstances of its occurrence, *i.e.,* toxicity caused by overdosage (therapeutic, accidental, homicidal); hypersensitivity; allergy; or injury from improper technique of administration, use of the wrong drug, error in compounding, labeling, or packaging, or from other error in the manufacture of the drug, or in its preparation for use in the hospital. Reactions caused by blood and plasma products need not be reported unless a chemical agent other than the basic substance is responsible."

An Adverse Drug Reaction Report Form prepared by the Committee is made available on every nursing station. Adverse drug reaction may be followed using the following criteria :

- Every case of adverse drug reaction must be reported by the attending physician to the clinical pharmacologist
- If staff is not available, it is advised to report the Chairman of the Pharmacy and Therapeutics Committee.
- The attending physician should complete an Adverse Drug Reaction Report Form on any patient having an adverse reaction.
- The Medical Record Room will, upon the patient's discharge, remove the Adverse Drug Reaction Form from the medical record and forward it to the clinical pharmacologist.
- Adverse drug reactions should be listed in the medical record as a diagnosis.

Automatic Stop Order for Dangerous Drugs

The Pharmacy and Therapeutics Committee should devise a mechanism so that dangerous drugs may be properly used under qualified and responsible medical staff control. All drug orders for narcotics, sedatives, hypnotics, anticoagulants, and antibiotics administered orally or parenterally shall be automatically discontinued after 48 hours. These types of drugs are continued or prescribed unless –

1. the order indicates an exact number of doses to be administered,

2. exact period of time for the medication is specified, or
3. the attending physician reorders the medication.

The second example of an automatic stop order is :

- It is advised for all orders for narcotics, sedatives and hypnotics must be rewritten every 24 hours.
- It is also advised that a PRN (pro re nata) and standing orders for all medications except narcotics, sedatives and hypnotics shall expire at 10:00 a.m. on the seventh day unless renewed.

For maintaining quality of hospital, the Joint Commission on Accreditation of Hospitals specifically determines whether or not the hospital has an automatic stop order in force.

Committee's Role in Developing Emergency Drug Lists

It is imperative that emergency drug or "Stat" boxes containing drugs and supplies be readily available for use by the bedside. The Pharmacy and Therapeutics Committee should make a list of supplies and drugs which ought to be in an emergency box and instruct the pharmacist and nursing service supervisors of their joint responsibility to have the box ready for use at all times. The emergency kit/box placed in the clinic, in the emergency ward and in the special procedures room of the department of radiology. It is mandatory to check daily either by the hospital pharmacist or by the nursing supervisor responsible for the ward. An emergency box contains following items.

1. Syringes and needles

Syringes	Needles
4- 2 ml	2 #16
4- 5 ml	2 #18
1-20 ml	2 #20
1 insulin	2 #23
	2 cardiac, #20. 4"

2. Files. ampul. Airway and Tourniquets
3. Drugs in emergency box

Aminophylline 0.25 gm/l0 ml	Metaraminol Bitartrate 10 mg/ml
Amphetamine Sulfate 20 mg/ml	Mannitol Injection 25%
Amyl Nitrite Inhalation	Nalorphine HCl10 mg/2 ml
Atropine Sulfate 0.4 mg/ml	Neostigmine Methylfulfate 0.25mg/ml

Contd…

Caffeine Sodium Benzoate 0.5 gm/2 ml Calcium Gluconate 1 gm/l0 ml	Nor-epinephrine Injection 0.2%
Chloroprophenpyrimadine Maleate 50mg/ml	Pentobarbital 50 mg/ml
Digoxin 0.25 mg/ml	Pentylenetetrazol Injection 0. 1 gm/ml
Diphenylhydantoin Sodium 50 mg/ml	Phenobarbital 120 mg/ml
Epinephrine HCl 1: 1 000	Phenylephrine HCl10 mg/ml
Heparin 10,000 Units/ml	Phytonadione Injection 50 mg/ml
Hydrocortisone 100 mg	Picrotoxin Injection 3 mg/ml
Isoproterenol 1: 1 00	Procaine Amide 100 mg/ml
Magnesium Sulfate Injection 10% and 50%	Protamine Sulfate 10 mg/ml
Sodium Molar Lactate Solution	Saline for Injection 30 ml
Water for Injection 50 ml	

4. Supplies for Cabinet Utility Room

1 Venous cannulization set	3 Sterile suction catheters
2 each-#14 and #17 venous catheters	1 Sengstachen-Blakemore tube
2 6" shock blocks	1 Razor with blades
2 Oxygen catheters	1 pkg. sterile gelatin sponge
1 Resuscitation tube	

5. Other Emergency supplies

Resuscitation carts	Tracheostomy sets
Phlebotomy sets	Dextran and tubing
Oxygen equipment	Burn sheets

As hospitals enter the era of cost containment and prospective payment systems, the pharmacy and therapeutic committee assumes added responsibility to promote rational and cost effective drug therapy and procedures. Both the clinical pharmacy staff and drug information pharmacist will play an ever-increasing role in committee recommendations. The popularity of medical insurance (e.g. MediClaim) in India will further boost the importance of pharmacy and therapeutic committee in hospitals.

UNIT - VI

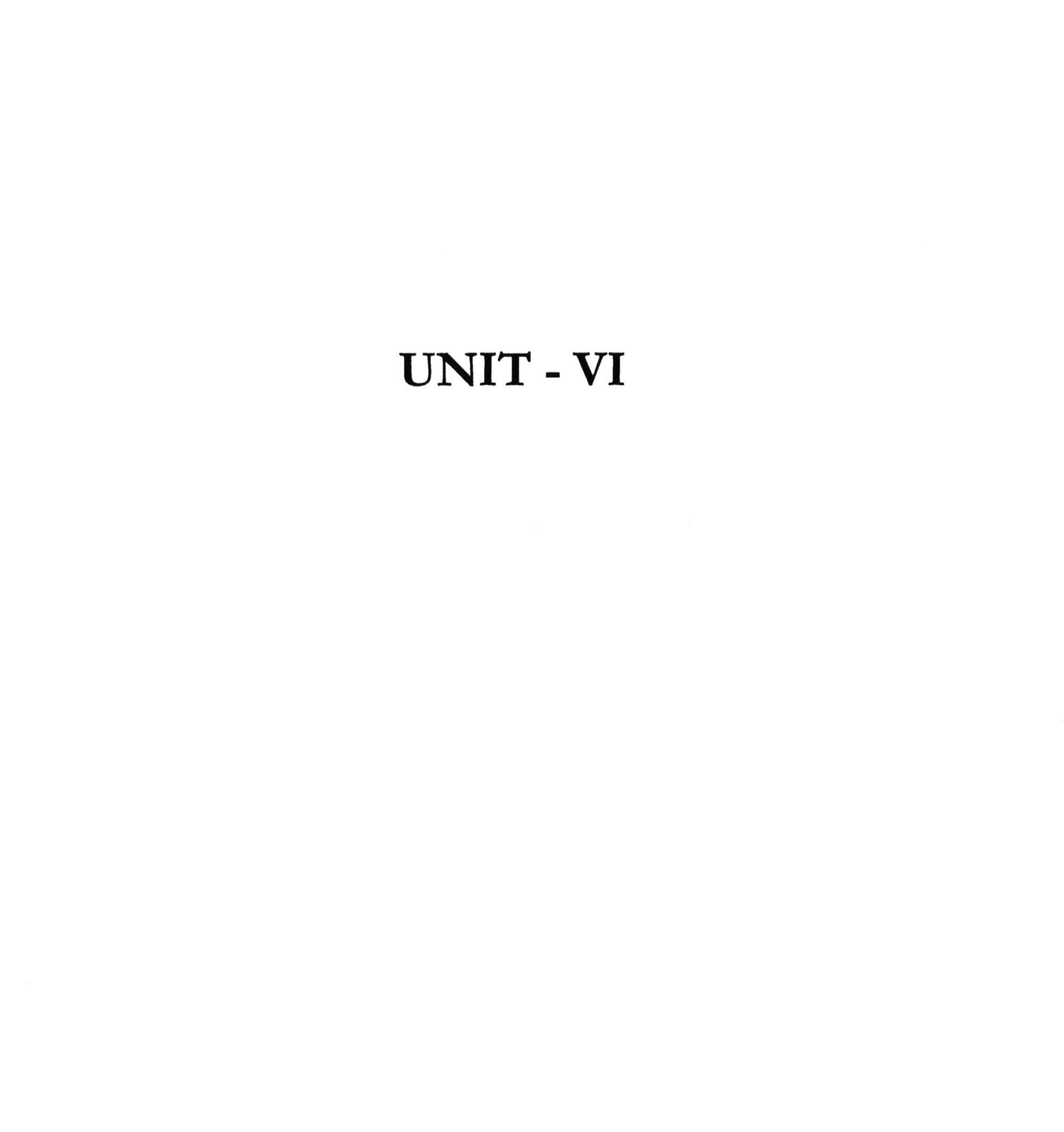

CHAPTER 17

DRUG DISTRIBUTION

PROCEDURAL MANUAL

Procedural manual is a book that gives instructions about how to use a procedure.

In general the hospital and pharmacy should have written policies for a number of reasons:

- They work as a guide for educating the new employees.
- They remove difficulties or problems from the verbal transmission of the policy.
- They try to apply the same policy in all like situations.
- They work as a organizer to ensure all procedure for performing his job and avoid waste of materials.
- The supervisor should evaluate job performance, errors and carelessness.
- Legally, they may serve as an important part in the hospital's defense in an action.

The management of the department of pharmacy in the hospital apply the same concepts which are generally used in industry. The pharmacist-in-chief works as the manager or supervisor. They must coordinate people, supplies and equipment in such a manner so that all activities are worked properly and efficiently.

DEFINITION

A procedural manual may be defined as a sequence of administrative and professional policies which may prove as guide to the hospital pharmacist in the development and execution of effective and proficient pharmaceutical services in the hospital.

The operational manual of any pharmacy department must contain –

1. The detail record of development,
2. The operation of the department
3. Its objectives

4. Description of the department
5. Organizational plan and chart, floor plans and plot plans
6. Description of its Formulary System and Pharmacy and Therapeutics Committee
7. Motivation, policies, and regulations
8. Departmental procedures
9. Staffing pattern
10. Specifications of Job
11. Listing of physical facilities and library holdings
12. Intradepartmental and interdepartmental relationships, and
13. Guidance manual for Internship and/or Residency Program in Hospital Pharmacy

Organization of administrative and professional policy needs a smooth planning and complete homework otherwise it will create many types of problem and complication.

The procedural manual can be divided into four general sections :

1. Organization
2. Facilities
3. Personnel and
4. Services and Activities (Administrative and a Professional division)

1. ORGANIZATION

- Organization of the hospital
- Organization of the pharmacy
- Services offered by the department
- Relationship among departments
- The Pharmacy and Therapeutics Committee
- The Antibiotics Committee

2. FACILITIES (Equipment and physical plant)

a. General policies

- The distilled water still
- Ointment mill
- High speed mixer
- Variable speed mixer
- Homogenizer
- Miscellaneous

b. Policy and procedure for pharmacy equipment

c. Maintenance department and services

d. Services of engineering department for the pharmacy.

e. Policy for Central Sterile Supply Department autoclaves and sterilizers.

f. Policy governing for controlling laboratory equipment procedures.

3. PERSONNEL POLICIES

a. Job descriptions

b. Fringe benefits-General Policy

Sick leave

- Vacation
- Holidays
- Jury duty
- Attending institutes, seminars or conventions etc.

c. Hospital Employee Relations

d. Discipline-Criteria for Warning, Probation and Dismissal

4. SERVICES and ACTIVITIES

(a) ADMINISTRATIVE

- Hours of operation
- Purchasing procedure
- Pricing policy
- Refund policy
- Handling of cash receipts
- Requisitioning of charge floor stock
- Requisitioning of non-charge floor stock
- Requisitioning of special patient charge drugs
- Requisitioning of ancillary surgical and medical supplies
- Alcohol records and controls
- Controlled substances records and controls
- Inventory taking and its records
- Compounding records
- The monthly and annual report
- Drug Recall Program

- Capital Expenditure Budget
- Competitive Bid Policy
- Policies regarding (i) Pharmaceutical Company Representatives, (ii) After Hours Procurement of Drugs, (iii) Drug Defects, (iv) Prescriptions-New and Discharge, (v) Prescription Refills, (vi) Forged or Altered Prescriptions, (vii) Nursing Responsibilities for the Management of Narcotics and Other Controlled Substances
- Use of Approved Abbreviations in the Hospital

(b) PROFESSIONAL

- Narcotic regulations
- Use of research drugs
- Automatic stop orders
- The Formulary System
- Policy governing drugs brought to the hospital by patients
- Labels and labeling
- Use of the metric system
- Prepackaging of bulk drugs
- Dispensing policies
- On-call service
- Bulk compounding (Formula, procedure. etc. for each product.)
- Sterile compounding (Formula. procedure, etc. for each product.)
- The residency training program in the hospital pharmacy
- Poison Control Center
- Information Services
  - (i) Pharmacy Library
  - (ii) Pharmacy Bulletin
  - (iii) Lecture Service
  - (iv) Drug Displays
- The addition of drugs to intravenous solutions by nurses.
- Patient Counseling
- Medication Quality Assurance Rounds
- Pharmacist's Notations in the Medical Record
- Policies regarding (i) Radiopharmaceutical Procedures, (ii) The company should not have a history of returning product recalls.

- Medication Errors, (iii) Confidentiality and Conduct in Patient Areas, (iv) Regional Poison Control Center, (v) Pharmacy and Therapeutics Committee, (vi) Patient's Self-administration of Drugs, and (vii) Prescription Blank Control
- Large volume Admixture Program and Policy
- Hyperalimentation Program and Policy
- Clinical Pharmacy Activities
- SAMPLE BULLETINS FOR A MANUAL

The method of procedural manual writing need not be restricted. It may be in text style format and language should be very clear, simple and direct.

A. Requisitions for Pharmacy Supplies

Proper and accurately distribution of Pharmacy supplies issued to the various hospital departments need proper requisition application must be completed. The ward stock Medications and surgical supplies must be requisitioned in the prescribed form specified by the hospital authority. The prescription drugs for personal use must be requisitioned in separate prescribed form. All request forms must be filled completely and clearly mentioning all the required items with proper code numbers.

B. Hospital Prescriptions

Hospital policy needs that a prescription be written for any drug, prescribed for clinic patients, discharge patients, or employees regardless of its nature, which is to be issued from the Hospital Pharmacy. White forms are used for prescriptions of discharge patients and yellow for clinic patients and employees.

C. Automatic Stop Order for Dangerous Drugs

1. *Controlled Substances:* Orders are automatically cancelled after 72 hours.
2. *Anticoagulants:* Low dose subcutaneous heparin for primary prophylaxis of deep vein thrombosis is discontinued after 7 days. All other orders of anticoagulants are discontinued after 24 hours unless the physician indicates otherwise.
3. *Parenteral drugs:* are routinely discontinued after 24 hours unless physician indicates otherwise and oral drugs after 72 hours.
4. *Post-operative medications:* During the surgery of patient, *a*ll standing orders are cancelled and must be reordered postoperatively.

All other drug orders are cancelled after seven days unless the physician indicates otherwise.

D. Separation of Internal and External use preparations

Poisons and medications for external use must be kept in a separate compartment and labelled properly with all relevant instructions.

E. Pharmacy Hours

For the convenience of patient, it is essential to display timing of hospital. The following hours are commonly for use by both clinic and house patients.

Monday- Friday	8:00 A.M.-9:00 P.M.
Saturday and Holidays	9:00 A.M.-2:00 P.M.

For house patients requiring special medications after these hours, it may be dispensed by the Pharmacist available during the emergency duty. The Nursing Supervisor may not mix or compound medications. The Nursing Supervisor shall not dispense the prescription. A list of the "on call" pharmacists is maintained by the switchboard operator.

F. Intravenous Solutions

1. The addition of drugs for intravenous administration to intravenous solutions is performed by the Nursing Service and may thereby facilitate patient care.
2. It may be performed only under specific written order in the order book by the doctor responsible for the patient's care.
3. This addition may be performed under supervision of a graduate nurse or senior nurses.
4. Medication may not be given by the Nursing Service directly intravenously, *i.e.,* without proper instruction and specified volume of intravenous fluid.
5. For intravenous dilution factor should be considered. Some testing drugs and solutions commonly used without dilution, and experimental drugs and solutions not yet accepted for routine use by the Pharmacy and Therapeutics Committee, e.g., phenolsulfonaphthalein (PSP) and sulfobromophthalein sodium (Bromsulphalein, BSP),
6. The following medications and solutions in intravenous preparations may be added under the rules-
   - Antibiotics
   - Electrolyte solutions, *e.g.,* sodium bicarbonate, potassium chloride, sodium lactate, sodium iodide, sodium chloride and all other intravenous electrolyte solutions
   - Vasopressors, *e.g.,* Phenylephrine, Levophed and other such agents
   - Vitamins

- Aminophylline
- Barbiturates
- Diphenylhydantoin (Dilantin)
- Hormonal preparations for intravenous use, *e.g.,* hydrocortisone

7. Heparin and 5-fluouracil drugs may be administered by a graduate nurse provided that the initial dose has been administered by a physician and its dilution are specifically written in the Doctor's Order Book.

G. Medications, Preparation and Administration

Purpose : To prepare and administer medications as ordered by the physician safely, accurately and efficiently.

Responsibilities of the Nurse

1. The nurse must know the properties of the drug, the pharmaceutical effect, the average dose, the toxic symptoms, calculation of dose, the method of preparation and administration and the antidote before administering of any medication.
2. The nurse must prepare a list of those medications which she herself has prepared.
3. The nurse must clearly know all medication orders before carrying them out.
4. Medications poured must be discarded and may not be returned to the drug bottle.
5. Nurse must know adverse drug reactions, drug intoxication, emergency drugs and reporting process.
6. Storage condition of internal and external preparations should be maintained

Regulations Concerning Narcotics

All narcotics received from the Pharmacy are to be counted and signed for by a professional nurse. Any discrepancy is to be reported to the pharmacist at once. All narcotics must be counted after change of shift at least by two nurses. Both nurses those are responsible for storage and counting must sign any errors found in the count must be reported to the supervisor or senior officers.

Medication at Bedside

a. No medication other than nitroglycerin is maintained or left at the bedside of any patient during the hospitalization.
b. Nitroglycerin tablets may be left at the bedside if so ordered by the doctor. The tablets are to be counted at 7 A.M. and 7 P.M. and the number used by the patient recorded and additional tablets added to the bedside (total not more than ten tablets).

c. Medication with the patient is not kept at the bedside and returned to a responsible family member after showing to the physician. If this is not possible, the medication is labelled with the patient's name, placed in medication cabinet. These medications are sent home with the patient at the time of his discharge with the permission of the physician.

Administration of Medications

1. Policies

a. Medication cards of patients are made out by the nurse in-charge and signed it with the following information - patient's name, full name of the drug, dose, route of administration, frequency of administration.

b. The medicine card is checked against Doctor's Order Book for drug, route, patient's name, date and time.

c. The drug label is verified carefully with the medication card at least three times –
   - before removing the bottle from the shelf,
   - before pouring, and
   - while placing the bottle in shelf.

d. Before administration of medication the patient must be identified and confirmed –
   - by checking the medication with card
   - by the name on the wrist band
   - by the name on the bed card, and
   - by asking name of patient if he is able to do so.

e. The nurse reside at the bedside until the patient has taken the medication.

f. Medication is never left at the bedside or near to patient except emergency medication. The medication chart is maintained immediately after administration.

g. If any troublesome situation such as –
   - patient refuses to take medication
   - absent on bed

2. Intravenous medication

No medication may be given intravenously by nurses at any hospital.

3. Liquid Medications

a. Containers must be kept tightly capped since the strength of the drug increases as the solvent evaporates i.e. spirits and tinctures or other alcoholic preparation.

b. Iodine preparations are to be given with milk or well diluted with water or fruit juice.

c. Acidic formulations are to be given through a straw to avoid discoloration of the teeth.

4. Rectal Medications

a. Rectal medications may be administered by suppository or by retention enema.

b. Before administration of medication rectally, it is explained to the patient and assisted to cooperate for administration.

c. The nurse puts on a glove or finger cot, lubricates the tapered end of the suppository and inserts it well beyond the sphincter.

d. If medication is given by retention enema. The safe dilution is used and the solution is allowed to run in slowly.

e. After administration, the patient remains gently on the left side for a few minutes to aid in retention.

5. Parenteral Medications

a. Policies [Graduate Nurses]

Trained Nurses may give subcutaneous, intramuscular and intradermal parenteral medications. No more than 5 ml of medication may be injected intramuscularly into one site at anyone time.

b. Policies [Student Nurses]

Nurses in training period may not administer narcotics, medication intravenously or into the Large Volume tubing without first obtaining the permission of the head nurse. The nurse must prepare following information about patient :

- patient's full name,
- medication and dose ordered,
- frequency of medication
- Administration time
- Pulse and respiration of the patient.

c. Administration of Parenteral Medications

The cup and syringe with needle protected by a needle guard are carried to the bedside. Disposable needles are bent after use to prevent re-use and discarded *only* in the container provided for needles.

Injection sites and methods:

(i) *Subcutaneous* : Injected at a 45^0 angle into the lateral aspect of the upper arm.

(ii) *Intramuscular* Injected at a 90^0 angle. The injection is administered in the upper portion of the upper outer quadrant of the buttocks, two inches below the crest of the ileum. The deltoid or the lateral aspect of the thigh may also be used. Sites of injection should be changed.

(iii) *Intradermal* Injected as nearly parallel as possible in the skin of the anterior forearm. Only the tip of the needle should be inserted in the skin and a wheal should come into sight as soon as the medication is injected.

DRUG DISTRIBUTION

Drug distribution systems:

Dispensing for inpatients comprises of removing two or more doses from a bulk drug container and placing them in another container by a pharmacist for subsequent use.

Drug distribution systems are divided into following classes:

1. Individual prescription medication for each patient;
2. Complete floor stock system;
3. Combination of (i) and *(ii);*
4. Unit-dose dispensing, either centralized or decentralized; and
5. Pharmacy coordinated unit-dose dispensing and drug administration system.

The last two systems are considered to be superior.

1. Individual prescription medication for each patient

The drugs are compounded and dispensed in the usual manner and the name and strength of each drug is stated on the label. Generally medication is stored in a nursing-unit cabinet under the custody of the nurse-in-charge. In such a case, pre-packaging is quite useful. The medication is administered by the nurse-in-charge or her assistant. Hence they should observe the patient for untoward reactions and adverse drug reactions, which should be reported to the physician. The nurses should also be aware about the proper storage, labelling and accounting of the drugs.

2. Complete floor stock system

The drugs under this system are classified as free floor stock drugs or charge floor drugs. **Free floor stock** consists of a predetermined list of medication available on every nursing unit of the hospital for use of the patients for which they *do not pay* charge. Usually the nurse submits a requisition and a pharmacist dispenses them in a drug basket. Orders from each nursing unit are received daily. In a modification of this system, the pharmacy is made responsible for maintaining a proper inventory of free floor stock drugs called **automatic free floor stock replacement system**. In the **basket system**, the requisition for medication along with empty containers are kept in a basket at night and the pharmacist puts the supply next morning in the same basket when the pharmacy opens. **Charge floor stock** drugs are those for which the patient is charged for every single dose administered to him. Patients are charged mostly because of the high cost of such drugs. Such drugs include injections or other single dose forms. Under **envelope system**, pre-labelled envelopes are filled with specific drugs and a predetermined quantity is placed at the disposal of the nursing unit. When the drug is administered, the patient's name and room number are entered on the envelope and placed in the out basket.

3. **A combination of (1) and (2)**

   In this system, free floor stock drugs are charged against the nursing service and the patient pays for the drugs as a part of nursing service.

4. **Unit-dose dispensing system**

   In this system, the pharmacist prepares every dose of the medication ready for administration. Solid medication is labelled for each patient, liquids are pre-measured and injections are accurately measured into sterile syringes etc. Thus unit dose dispensing becomes the sole responsibility of the pharmacist. Such system may be centralized in the pharmacy or decentralized at the nursing unit level.

5. **Pharmacy coordinated unit-dose dispensing and administration system:**

   This system calls for coordination in between drug distribution and drug administration. The system is better operated under the supervision of a pharmacist even during the drug administration phase. **Pharmacy technicians** may also be trained to administer drugs. In this way pharmacist shall be working with physician on the nursing unit to carry out the function of safe and appropriate use of drugs for inpatients. Besides these well recognized systems, drugs may also be distributed in modern hospital through Mobile Dispensing Units and Mechanical Dispensing.

Unit-dose dispensing

Unit dose medication is ordered, packaged. handled, administered and charged in multiples of single dose units sufficient for one regular dose, application or use. Strip packaged tablets and capsules are examples of unit-dose medication. Drugs are mostly purchased from the manufacturers in bulk and hence supplying the same as unit-dose is an important function in dispensing in hospital pharmacy practice both for inpatients and outpatients.

Advantages

1. Pilferage and drug wastage are eliminated.
2. Unit-dose medications are prepared by the pharmacist and hence medication errors are minimized because the pharmacist himself checks each medication order.
3. It provides improved pharmaceutical services round the clock.

1.Excessive duplication of orders and paper work at nursing stations and pharmacy are avoided. Patients are charged only for the doses administered to them.

4. Automation is feasible, which saves on cost and time.
5. Credits are eliminated and revenue losses are reduced.
6. Drug accounting is facilitated.

The concept of unit-dose dispensing can be introduced either as **Centralized Unit-Dose Distribution System (CUDD)** or **Decentralized Unit-Dose Distribution System (DUDD)**. In CUDD all in-patient drugs are dispensed in unit-doses and all the drugs are stored in a certain place in pharmacy. DUDD operates by setting up satellite pharmacies on each floor of the hospital.

The system can be introduced initially for injections, tablets and capsules, and liquid preparations. Injections can be supplied as unit dose solutions filled in sterile syringes. Tablets and capsules are strip packaged and liquids are generally filled in unit-dose container bottles measuring 15, 30, 45 ml etc. Unused pre-packaged drugs *cannot* be returned to the pharmacy if the package has been opened or not stored properly. Such problems usually do not occur in unit-dose dispensing. Drug manufacturers are also adopting single application or single use systems in supplying ointments and cosmetic preparations.

Before adopting the unit-dose dispensing system in practice, the cost factor must be considered critically.

Maintenance of Records for Narcotic and Dangerous Drugs

Drugs falling under schedule X of the Drugs & Cosmetics Act are designated as prescription drugs. Dangerous drugs are dealt separately under the Narcotic Drugs & Psychotropic Substances Act. These drugs warrant stricter controls and hence their issue and use are to be accounted properly. Prescription for these drugs must include *(a)* patient's full name, age, and address; *(b)* date; *(c)* name and strength of the drug product; *(d)* quantity of drug product to be dispensed; in addition to other information. These drugs are prescribed on a special requisition form by placing a checkmark against name, strength, form of the narcotic or dangerous drug. This requisition form should be accompanied with another form showing the consumption and balance of narcotic and dangerous drug in the inpatient department. This is helpful in inventory control. A dose of a drug lost or wasted must be reported by using a special report form. The prescriptions should be written in triplicate. One copy is to be retained in the pharmacy department. The quantity of drugs received by the department should be checked and entered in record meant for this purpose. A daily usage record is maintained based on which a monthly usage record can also be prepared.

Ward stock medicines

This type of medicines is mostly obtained as a stock of drugs commonly required in a ward or a number of wards. The ward nurse prepares the requisitions and sends it to the pharmacy store along with the containers etc. On receipt of the supply, she checks it and enters the quantity in the record meant for the purpose. Every time the drugs are issued for the use to the patient, a note is made on the sheet showing the daily consumption of ward stock medicines. This further helps when a duty nurse is handing over charge to another nurse.

Emergency drugs

Emergency drugs are usually stocked in an emergency box or **Stat Box** which is kept at a suitable location, easily accessible and ready for use round the clock. A list of emergency drugs can be obtained from the reference books. An emergency box inventory and control card shows inventory of each emergency medicine and its monthly usage. The pharmacist is responsible for the stock of emergency box. Besides boxes, emergency drugs can also be kept in emergency medicine carts, kits or night drug cabinets.

Routine inspection of drugs stock in wards

An inspection visit is the best opportunity for a pharmacist to educate the nurse on all the aspects of proper stocking of the drug products. The pharmacist going on the routine inspection of ward stock medicines should also check the prescriptions dealt or to be dealt.

For reducing wastage and ensuring that only drugs in good condition are used, pharmacist must devise a method of routine inspection of drugs stocks in wards. Stocks should be decided in consultation with the ward sister. The time and frequency of inspection of a ward by the pharmacist should be decided jointly by the pharmacist and the ward sister. During the inspection the pharmacist must check the stocks, stock arrangement, labelling, records etc., of all ward stock drugs. He must also check whether the drugs are arranged alphabetically, whether expiry dated drugs are arranged systematically, whether the stock is rotating adequately, the containers have been labelled properly or not, and whether investigational drugs have been stocked separately. In addition the pharmacist must also ensure that drugs requiring special storage conditions are stocked under desired conditions like temperature, humidity light etc.

Medical stores

More than 50% of the total budget of any medium size hospital in India is spent only on drugs. Hence, a properly maintained store occupies a very important position in the general administration of the hospital. Inefficient running of a medical store may lead to serious losses. Following points are important for efficient functioning of a medical store:

1. Proper control of all issues from the stores.
2. Foolproof storage facilities to prevent the stocks from theft, deterioration, evaporation, pilferage etc.
3. Safety measures to meet any emergency like fire etc.
4. Maintaining the stocks by regulating the receipts and issues at fixed hours.
5. Storing the items in packages so that stocks can be easily checked periodically.
5. Periodical check-up for expiry dates for timely return of stocks, and
6. Careful handling of narcotics with utmost care and control.

Medical stores in a hospital should not be confused with commercial drug stores or pharmacies.

Types

1. **Centralized store :** In centralized store the stocks of drugs are procured from outside and the same are issued directly against the indent from any authorized person of the hospital.
2. **Decentralized store :** Decentralized store is attached to every department carrying on the function of procuring the drugs with the approval of purchasing authority and issuing the same against the indents from the authorized persons from the concerned department of the hospital.
3. **Mixed *i.e.,* a centralized store with sub-stores.**

Objectives: The three broad general objectives of medical stores are summarized as utility, amenity and expression. The primary function of the medical store is to store the drugs under condition, which ensure pharmacological activity, clinical safety and stability of drugs and drug formulations.

Medical store in a hospital must be under the supervision of the Chief Pharmacist possessing adequate educational qualifications and practical experience. Drugs must be stored under proper conditions of sanitation, temperature, light, moisture, ventilation, segregation and security.

Location : The medical store may be located on the ground floor (not basement) of a multi storey building, well away from autoclaves, heating apparatus, laundry etc. It should be well lit and ventilated. It should be situated in such a place, which is easily accessible to all concerned departments.

There should be sufficient space and enough shelves for storage, fireproof room for storage of inflammable items and refrigeration facilities for the storage of sera, vaccines, biological etc.

Layout : In order that a pharmacist may properly supervise the storage of drugs, the drugs should be stored in an area directly under his control. Facilities and equipment should be so designed that the drugs are accessible only to medical practitioners authorized to prescribe, pharmacists authorized to dispense or nurses authorized to administer such drugs. It should also facilitate the routine inspection of the drugs prior to the time of administration.

Facilities : Adequate space should be provided for storage of drugs. Separate space should be allocated for internal medication, narcotics, barbiturates and amphetamines, poisons and external use drugs, emergency drugs, ampoules and investigational drugs. The space should be well lit. Adequate ventilation, work space free from noise and dust, hot and cold running water, sufficient equipment and supplies in readily usable form, refrigerator, interlocking narcotic cabinet, and adequate means for security should also be provided. Effective messenger and delivery service for medical store should also be provided when required. Drugs that require storage between 2 to 10^0 C *e.g.* sera, vaccines and glandular products and other thermolabile products should be kept in cold room.

Procurement of Drugs

1. **From medical stores depot:** Medical Stores Organization started as a part of the Army Organization in India during pre-war period. During the post-war years it became civil institution and presently it works. as a public utility service on no-profit no-loss basis. It is obligatory for Central, State, Municipal Corporation or other government hospitals to purchase drugs from Medical Stores Depot. Annual indent is sent in the prescribed proforma. Indent may be for drugs, pharmaceuticals, laboratory chemicals and stains, surgical instruments and other items stocked by the Medical Stores Depot. To facilitate the indenting job, Medical Stores Organization publishes Vocabulary of Medical Stores (Civil) (VMS). This book contains particulars like VMS number, nomenclature, specifications, catalogue number, and accounting unit for various items. At the time of supply, the quadruplicate copy of the indent is sent to the indenter. The supply should be checked immediately after opening in the presence of a gazette or responsible officer of the hospital. Discrepancies, if any, should be reported within a week. On the quadruplicate copy, the page number and stock register number are entered against each item; duly signed at the back and sent back to the depot as a proof of receipt of correct supply. On receipt of this document, the Depot sends the priced copy of the indent in duplicate, out of which one copy is verified and sent back so that necessary adjustment of the amount involved can be affected. The drugs are procured from the market only when they are not supplied against the indent by the Medical Stores Depot.

   For procuring any single item costing Rs 25000/- or more in Government hospitals, the indent should be sent in quadruplicate to the Directorate General of Supplies and Disposals (DGS&D).

2. **From manufacturers, distributors, local market :**

   Drugs from these sources are procured usually by inviting quotations or tenders. A requisition list is prepared embodying the names of the items, their specifications, quantity needed etc., and sent to the approved manufacturers, distributors and their local representatives. Medical stores normally keep a list of reputed manufacturers, distributors and their local dealers along with their addresses, telephone numbers etc. A due date for receiving the sealed quotations in the medical store is specified. All the quotations received by the due date are opened by any gazette or responsible officer and signed by at least two officers. A comparative statement is prepared and usually the lowest rates are accepted. Orders are then placed with the suppliers. The purchase of drugs in a private drug store is much simpler because most of the proprietary drugs and formulations are ordered directly with the respective manufacturer or distributor and there is no need of inviting quotations or tenders.

   In hospitals, the purchasing may be centralized or decentralized. The disadvantage of **centralized purchasing** is that the drugs are also dealt with like any other items such as a bed-sheet or a blanket. **Decentralized purchasing** has the advantages that the whole process of purchasing is under the direct supervision of a qualified person *i.e.,* a pharmacist. Even in case of centralized purchasing, the pharmacist in charge should be a member of the purchase committee and he should also prepare the specifications for drugs and other related supplies.

Laying down specifications for drugs and related supplies is best done by a pharmacist as he is expert on drug.

Emergency Purchases

1. **By inviting local tenders :** If the item is not on rate contract and is not supplied by the DGS&D and the same is required in huge quantity, costing more than *Rs.1000/-,* the tenders are invited for the item and finalized immediately. This purchase should not constitute more than 10% of the total grant.
2. **By inviting local quotations:** Any item required in emergency costing not more than *Rs.1000/-* can be purchased by inviting local quotations and finalizing them immediately.
3. **Purchase from government :** Some items can be purchased directly from the Government institutions or undertakings like Hindustan Antibiotics Limited, Pimpri, Pune; IDPL etc.
4. **Direct purchase in emergency:** In emergency the items may be purchased from the manufacturer if such items are not manufactured by any other manufacturer. In such cases the permission of the Purchase Committee is necessary.
5. **Miscellaneous :** Miscellaneous purchases without inviting quotations are permitted up to Rs *25/-*.

Licensing Procedure for Procuring and Stocking of Alcohol and Narcotics

The control in respect of purchase, stocking and sale of excisable items is a State subject and is regulated by the Excise Act of the respective State. The procedure in respect of narcotics is prescribed under the Narcotic Drugs and Psychotropic Substances Act. Tax free alcohol is the most used item in hospitals, especially in operating theatres and in surgical and allied complexes. Besides, it is also widely used in the manufacture of pharmaceutical preparations. Alcohol being excisable item, necessary stocking permits is issued by the Excise Commissioner of the State in the prescribed Form. On the basis of this permit, request has to be made to the Excise Department to issue permit for the storage every now and then and for the purchase of alcohol whenever necessary. Permits for the possession of denatured spirit and rectified spirit are also issued in the prescribed

Denatured Spirit	Rectified Spirit
The exemption extends only to the possession and use and not to the sale of spirit rendered effectually and permanently unfit for human consumption	The permit holder is authorized to possess rectified spirit for use in the manufacture of drugs, medicines and chemicals, except in the case of educational institutions where rectified spirit shall be kept for teaching and research purposes
The permit holder may purchase denatured spirit from a licensed distillery after obtaining the permit in the prescribed form.	The permit holder shall not have in his posession more than gallons of rectified spirit.

forms by the Excise Commissioner, prescribing the maximum quantity of the spirit that can be possessed at a time. In addition to the general conditions, these permits are also subject to the above special conditions. However, the permit holder can also keep in his possession supplies exceeding specified number of gallons after obtaining the sanction of the Excise Commissioner.

If the supply of rectified and methylated spirit is received from other States, the information is to be submitted in writing to the Excise Officer. The supply can be opened only after a prior intimation of 10 days to Excise Officer so that he may inspect the same. Excise Officer is authorized to check the physical stock, maintenance of accounts and licenses. Duty free alcohol is issued to the hospitals, teaching and research institutions. Proper accounts have to be maintained for each lot received and issued for ultimate consumption in a hospital for which the pharmacist is responsible.

Sampling for quality control: This is applicable to the manufacturing of drugs containing alcohol in hospital pharmacies. Ideally, samples should be chosen at random from any point in a batch. Truly random sampling will give an overall picture of the average contents of ingredients in a batch. Usually one unit from each batch or, when unit size is small *e.g.,* ampoules and tablets, a sufficient number of units are taken by the authorized person from the quality control department. Samples of biologicals should be taken according to the procedure prescribed in the IP. It is advisable that a check sample of each batch is also reserved for future reference.

Samples should be taken by a person who understands the principles of sampling. A sample must be a true representative of a batch. Adequate quantity of the material should be withdrawn so that there will be enough for duplicate testing and a similar quantity left over for filing after completion of the test. Samples are subjected to testing for specifications laid down for a drug. These specifications are laid down by the quality control department of the hospital pharmacy unit.

Depending upon the positive or negative results of the quality control tests a sample is approved or rejected.

Methods to avoid duplication

If proper procedures are not followed in stocking, duplication is likely to take place. Thus it is essential that detailed procedures are laid down for the procurement, stocking and disposal of the materials. It is also necessary to take physical inventory at appropriate intervals of time. Duplication of the stock can also be avoided by proper accounting of the stock and maintenance of relevant records. The stock should be arranged properly so that the material received first is used first and the one received last is used last. Before placing a subsequent order, the balance of the material on hand must be ascertained and it is helpful to determine the **reorder quantity level (RQL)**for each item. To summarize, following guidelines can avoid duplication of stock in a hospital pharmacy unit or a medical store:

1. The stock should be properly arranged.
2. The stock should be properly accounted for and suitable inventory control measures must be exercised and reflected in the relevant records.
3. It is advisable to work out the reorder quantity level (RQL) for each item being stocked.
4. Stocks should be frequently inspected to ensure proper rotation of each item.
5. Requisition form for the procurement of all items must carry statement on the stock on hand of each item separately.

Disposal of slow moving items and dead stock

These problems may often be faced in any medical store. If proper care is taken, dead stock and slow moving items will not exit. Slow moving items should be purchased in smaller quantity, and if anyone bears expiry date then the same should be monitored carefully. Slow moving items having expiry date should be removed well before expiry date and sent for credit to the supplier or disposed off as per the prevailing practice. It is better to have a separate list of slow moving expiry dated drugs, indicating the month and year of the expiry date. A precise list of such slow moving items can be prepared by experience.

Dead stock may result due to overstocking, improper stocking, faulty inventory control programme and also due to obsolescence. Dead stock, particularly of drugs and pharmaceuticals is to be discarded from time to time. Dead stock items should be removed from the storage place but may be kept in a separate space till disposed off. If the dead stock material is to be destroyed, proper procedures must be followed and the destruction and the disposal of destroyed material be ensured. After disposing off the dead stock, adequate entries should be made in the relevant records and books of account, mentioning the details of the material being written off. Drug substances do not have any depreciation value and hence the cost of the material written off amounts to a financial loss or reduction in the net profit of the hospital..

Stock arrangement

Proper stock arrangement shows the efficiency and foresight of the store keeper. Stock can be arranged into the following areas:

- Chemicals
- Gallon goods
- Alcohol and liquors
- Capsules and tablets
- Narcotic drugs
- Ointments
- Sutures
- Laboratory supplies
- Surgical instruments
- Rubber goods
- Biological and other cold room inventory
- Surgical and medical supplies

The stock should be arranged alphabetically. Test reagents, general disinfectants and antiseptics should be arranged separately. Inflammable explosive liquids like ether and acetone should be kept in as small supply as possible and in accordance with the applicable fire regulations. Stock should be so arranged that all container labels are clearly visible and read. Under the Drugs and Cosmetics Act, it should be kept in mind that a Drugs Inspector is fully authorized to inspect the premises of a hospital stores in order to ensure the compliance of the statutory provisions. Due to the implementation of Section 42 of the Pharmacy Act, 1948 from 1st September 1984, no one except a registered pharmacist can undertake compounding and dispensing of drugs.

DISPENSING TO OUT-PATIENTS

Outpatients are those who do not occupy beds in hospitals or clinics. They are also referred to as ambulatory patients. Outpatinets mostly need primary care. Out-patient dispensing is one of the basic functions of the pharmacy department in any hospital. Out-patient departments in Indian hospitals are usually over crowded due to paucity of space in such units as compared to the population they are expected to cater for. The conditions in outpatient dispensing units in India are far from satisfactory.

Location

It is always preferable to have a separate outpatient pharmacy. When this is not feasible, in-patient and outpatient units are combined and the services provided from the same window or from separate windows. A separate outpatient dispensing unit is desirable when it is separated geographically from the main pharmacy. There is no general rule regarding location of outpatient pharmacy but it should be so located that minimum disturbance is caused to the inpatients and the routine working of the hospital and it's pharmacy. It should be located in such a place that it is easily accessible to the out-patients.

Layout

Layout of the outpatient pharmacy is important because the outpatients can carry a good or a bad impression about the hospital depending on the services they get. The unit should be provided with a prescription receiving window and a delivery window. Mostly while the prescriptions are being compounded, patients have to wait and hence a waiting area should be provided. The waiting area should be elegant, clean, well-lit and ventilated and provided with comfortable seats. Some general publications relating to pharmacy and medicine as well as news papers and magazines can be provided. Patients can also be made familiar with family planning projects, general hygiene etc., through display of wall posters. Thus the waiting area of an outpatient dispensing unit can be a good place for educating the people on matters related to health and hygiene. It is essential that the patient's waiting period is kept to a minimum so as to avoid overcrowding.

Receipt and issue systems

As per the common practice the outpatients have to get themselves registered at the registration counter when they visit the hospital for the first time. Depending on the symptoms, the patients are directed to a particular department. The physician diagnoses the disease and writes the prescription, which bears the name, age, registration number and diagnosis of the patient. This prescription is to be produced before the pharmacist at the prescription receiving counter. Prescriptions should always be received by a pharmacist only. The prescription should be received without raising any doubt in the mind of the patient. In case the pharmacist needs any clarification about the prescription, he should contact the physician without the knowledge of the patient. The pharmacist checks the prescription and assembles the materials required for compounding. Most of the modern prescriptions are sort of 'pour' and 'count' the tablets or capsules. The compounded prescriptions should be filled in the container and labelled to include details like patient's name and registration number, age and directions for use and storage, if necessary. The pharmacist should maintain a register for the purpose of accounting but prescriptions in respect of supply of mixtures, lotions, ointments and powders are usually not recorded. Sometimes a separate chit may be issued by the physician for tablets and capsules, which is retained by the pharmacist. Costly drugs *e.g.,* injections and antibiotics etc., are issued to poor outpatients and such drugs are issued in restricted quantities on Special Drug Form.

Pharmacist can employ a call check system for delivering the filled prescription and he should ensure that it is delivered to the correct patient. For this purpose, a system of issuing a token (as is done in banks) may be introduced. The prescription is usually given back to the patient so that the same can be produced by him during his next visit. In some of the hospitals the outpatients are given only an identity slip carrying a registration number. Prescriptions relating to Schedule G, H and X drugs are to be written and dealt with according to the provisions of the Drugs and Cosmetics, Act and the Rules thereunder. All the procedures regarding receipt and issue systems are greatly improved by using computers.

Recovery and service charges

The prescription laboratory contributes to the net profit of most pharmacies and hence the pharmacist must be well versed with the business aspects of his practice. Unless it be a charitable institution the patients have to pay the charge for the medication and services rendered to them in the hospital. Three important methods of pricing are based on (i) arbitrary fee depending on dosage form and number of doses supplied, as per the prevalent practice; (ii) a simple mark-up procedure, depending on the cost of the drug; and (iii) a professional fee system. Any pricing system, to be meaningful and realistic, must take into consideration the cost of the ingredients, containers, time required for dispensing and compounding, professional services, overhead expenses; and a guaranteed profit. American Pharmaceutical Association recommends mark-up on cost. However, the professional fee concept is most widely used.

The professional fee (service charges)

The concept is not new. It represents an amount that covers the cost of providing services and overheads and a reasonable profit for the pharmacist. Combination of Ingredient cost and professional fee system of pricing is based on the following considerations:

1. A prescribed drug is not an ordinary article of commerce capable of being bought and sold by anyone; it requires professional expertise of a pharmacist.
2. Dispensing of medication requires a specialized knowledge and judgment and a degree of responsibility greater than that associated with mere commercial transactions, and
3. The cost of providing prescription service is not a function of the cost of ingredients.

Thus, the true professional fee is same for all types of prescriptions irrespective of the cost of the ingredients used but the basic fee for a prescription requiring more time for compounding may be higher.

Prescription prices can be calculated by the following formula :

Prescription price = Drug cost + Professional fee

Professional fee may vary depending on the practitioner's environment.

Thus, $PF_i = COD_i + \text{Profit}$

Where "i" is the practice environment, PF is the professional fee, and COD is the Cost of Dispensing.

COD can be calculated as:

CODi = (professional services rendered + overhead)

or CODi = $[(\text{Total expenses} - \text{Drug cost})/\text{Number of medication orders dispensed}]_i$

Professional fee based on operating expenses can be calculated as –

Professional fee = A + (B x C) / D + E

Where A stands for proprietor's or manager's salary; B stands for prescription sales to total sales; C stands for expenses minus proprietor's or manager's salary; D stands for total number of prescriptions; and E stand for net profit per prescription (desired or actual)

Professional fee can also be calculated in the following manner :

Professional fee =(Expected net income + Prescription laboratory expenses)/ No of prescriptions dispensed

Pharmacist works out a satisfactory pricing by trial and error. Whatever be the mode in which price is computed, it must be realistic.

Pre-packaging

Pre-packaging is a very convenient method of improving the standard of dispensing in hospital pharmacies. It can be employed for fast moving items or for those, which take too much time in packaging before dispensing. It requires accurate procedures, controls, and records in order to trace the identity of the drug. Pre-packaging policy is based on the following considerations:

1. Demand for the product.
2. Size of unit to be packaged and numbers in each unit.
3. Type of containers and closure to be used.
4. Special labelling required, if any.
5. Packaging facilities available *i.e.* mechanical or manual.
6. Stability of the product and expiry date, and
7. Unit cost of pre-packaging

Advantages

1. Improves standard of dispensing.
2. Cuts down patient's waiting time in receiving the dispensed medicine.
3. It can be employed for both inpatient and outpatient dispensing.
4. Operations can be undertaken at off-peak hours thus curtailing provision for over-time and staff.
5. Usually no special equipment is necessary.

(a) ***Package size*** **:** The package size can best be ascertained by consulting the nursing service as well as Pharmacy and Therapeutic Committee. The data concerning the quantities and rate of use of such items as ward stock hypnotics, sedatives, antitussives, antiseptics, mouth–washes etc., can be obtained from the nursing service. Pharmacy and Therapeutic Committee can help establish a quota concerning the number of tablets and capsules or volume of liquid preparations, which can be sent to the pavilions. Some of the hospital formularies also publish the quantity to be prescribed and is based on permitting a therapy for not more than a specific number of days on single drug order. Thus in most hospitals 20 or 25 tablets or capsules is considered to be an adequate pre-package size for in-patients. Pre-package size for outpatients is mostly based on the cycle for obtaining subsequent appointments *i.e.,* whether the patient shall be visiting after 15, 30,45 or 60 days; and the quantity of the drug supplied should be sufficient to lost until the date of the subsequent appointment. For outpatients 50, 75 or 100 units are considered to be an adequate pre-package size.

However, if the pre-packaged drug is to be discontinued, it will amount to a total loss to the hospital once the package has been dispensed to the patient and opened.

(b) ***Pre-packaging operation:*** In a small pharmacy, pre-packaging is managed by a pharmacist with the assistance of a part time helper and usually undertaken during off-peak periods. The hospitals undertaking pre-packaging operation at a large scale may establish a separate unit for the purpose. It should be under the supervision of a pharmacist and may employ automatic or semi-automatic filling machines for liquid preparations, capsule and tablet counters, and labeling machines. In a medium size hospital pharmacy unit, the responsibility for maintaining a supply of pre-packaged drugs is rotated within the pharmacy staff and assisted by lay personnel, other pharmacists during off-peak hours, or members of the volunteer group in the hospital.

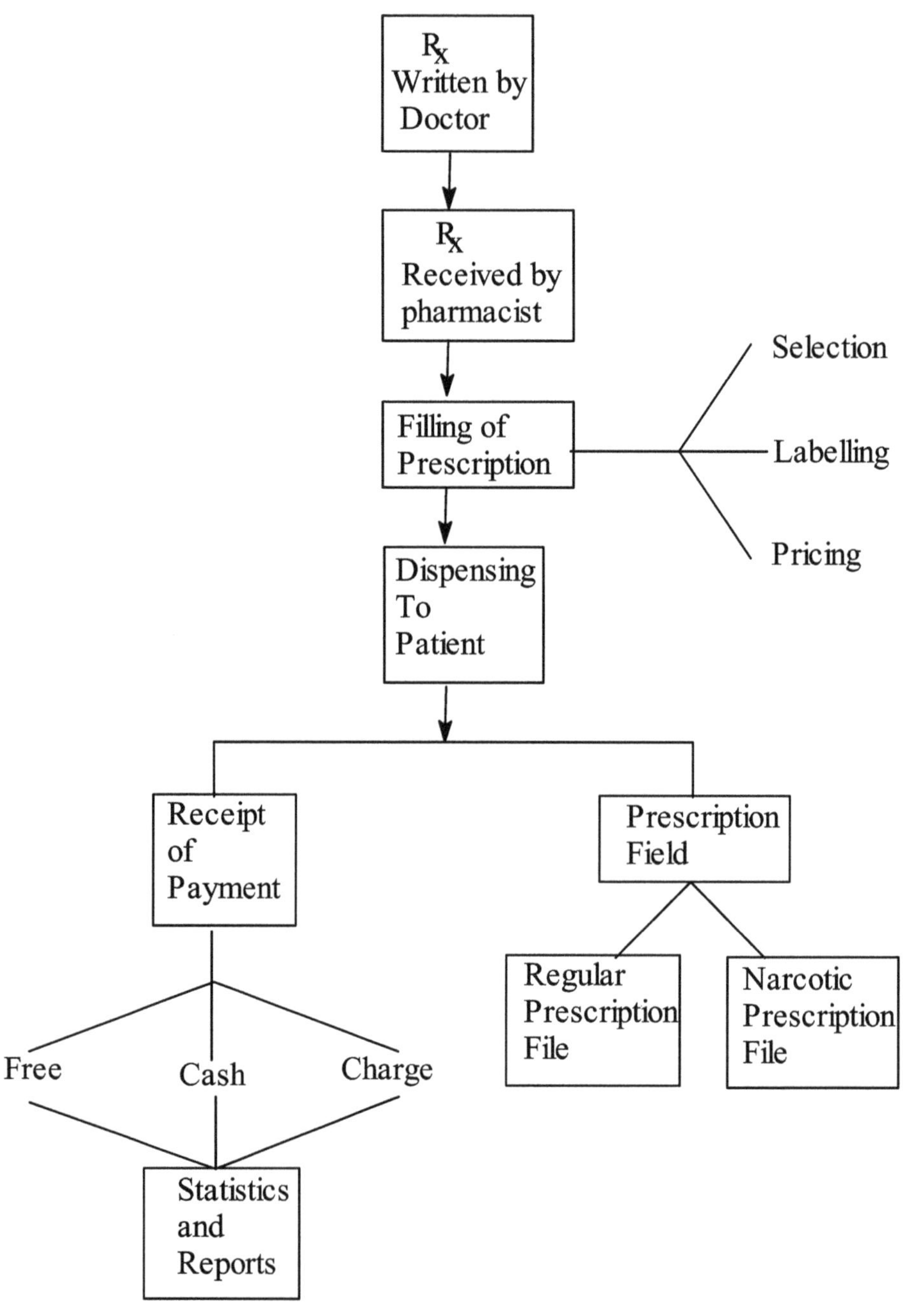

Chart 17.1 Outpatient acitivity`

INPATIENTS DISPENSING

Dispensing to hospitalized or in-patients is another important activity of a pharmacy department. All hospitals usually have provision for pharmaceutical services to in-patients but not necessarily for outpatients.

Location and layout

If a hospital provides outpatient services in addition to inpatient services, the two services may be combined. Depending on the feasibility, it is preferable to have a separate inpatient pharmacy department. This unit should be located in a place easily accessible to all wards and free from disturbances as far as possible. All sections of the in-patients pharmacy *e.g.,* storage, dispensing, manufacturing, parenteral solutions etc., should be continuous as far as possible. These sections should be in a direct vertical relationship and this concept of direct vertical relationship should be extended to other divisions of the hospital utilizing pharmaceutical services. The unit should be well equipped to render the desired pharmaceutical services. In some modern hospitals, satellite pharmacies are operated to cater to the needs of pharmaceutical services under the supervision of a qualified pharmacist. Physical plant of the inpatient pharmacy should be well planned, in order to avoid frequent modifications in the building and equipment etc., keeping in view the future growth of the hospital.

Personnel

There are no standard rules regarding the requirements of personnel for inpatient pharmacy department and it is the nature and quantum of services to be provided that governs the personnel requirement.

As mentioned under the staff of hospital pharmacy department, hospitals having a bed strength of upto 50, 100, 200, 300 and 500 beds may require, 3, 5, 8, 10 and 15 pharmacists, respectively. It is emphasized that these pharmacists must possess adequate qualifications and experience and the overall charge of the inpatients unit should remain with the Chief Pharmacist. However, depending on whether the pharmacy is also involved in the manufacture of drugs and the extent of this activity as well as other activities, an adequate number of pharmacy technicians, assistants, orderlies, peons etc., may be recruited. In brief, both measurable and non-measurable workload should be taken into account for determining the personnel requirement of an inpatient pharmacy department.

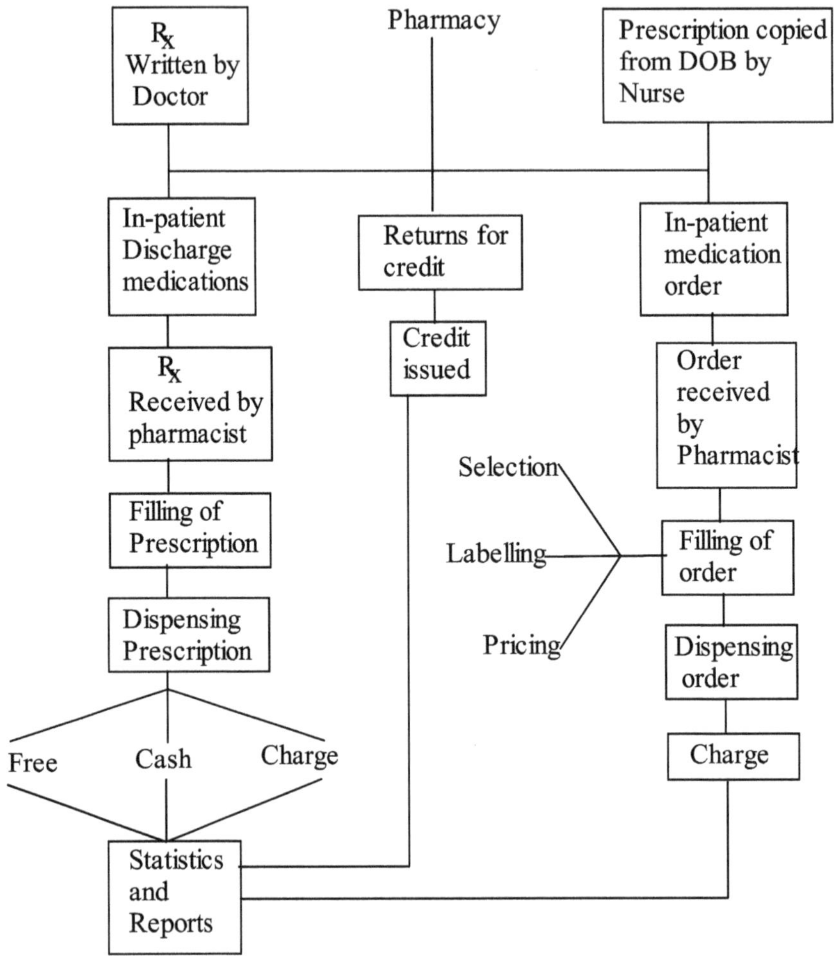

Chart 17.2 Inpatient activity

DISPENSING OF ANCILLARY

The practice in hospital pharmacy is the assumption of responsibility for the purchase, stocking and distribution of the different ancillary medical, surgical and laboratory supplies. The range of inventory for this type of article is extremely broad and may consist of costly surgical instruments, catheters, sutures, needles, syringes, sphygmo to nometers, and laboratory-ware. The whole process depends upon the individual pharmacist and the hospital administration. The administration of the hospital added special type of responsibility to the pharmacist is a clear indication of the administration's respect for his multiple talents. In addition, a few years of experience in handling these supplies will better qualify him to assume responsibility for the central sterile supply room or for the purchasing division if the occasion should ever arise. Definitely, in the small hospital such a responsibility is highly desirable for it may mean the difference between hiring a pharmacist or not hiring one on the basis of insufficient pharmaceutical works. There should be no doubt about the fact that the pharmacist is definitely capable of undertaking such a task for he, in all probability, will have had greater experience than the lay person who might be assigned the task. In addition, he will have a greater understanding relative to the use to which these items are to be put to and therefore may be able to act in an advisory capacity relative to the selection of one item over another. Hospital management hands over the responsibility to the pharmacist because of his experience in the handling and accounting of pharmaceuticals and also assured of proper control.

PURCHAGING

Ancillary supplies are usually purchased from sources other than a pharmaceutical house or drug wholesaler. For better quality and price, the pharmacist must acquaint himself with the various agencies, distributors and general wholesaler. The pharmacist is cautioned to take the time to ascertain the *integrity* and *reliability* of the vendor, as well as his ability and desire to be cooperative and render special services when called upon in an emergency situation because of high competition in this field. The general observation that many distributors have the agency for the same product and same quality but rate is very different. It is clear to purchase the many items through the quality and prize bid process with the open to all. In the process of purchasing the specifications and other service demands associated with the shipping, billing should be specified clearly. The all items are purchased through the most reliable vendors who can meet all the basic requirements. The purchasing of the supplies should not be mixed with the purchasing of pharmaceuticals and separate records and inventories should be maintained. Depending upon the scope of the ancillary supply inventory, some items may be extremely slow in turn-over. A separate physical inventory is maintained and recorded. It is possible to warp the true process of the drug part of the pharmacy by reducing the number of times of turn-over of the true pharmacy inventory. Pharmacists who take on the responsibility for the procurement, inventorying and distribution of ancillary supplies should give serious consideration to having the hospital join a successful group purchasing program. The institution can derive many benefits which include lower prices due to large purchasing. In some instances centralized storage and on-call delivery is very helpful in the following places-

- Easy to monitor on-going price fluctuations.
- Minimum space required in hospital.
- Elimination of sales personnel thereby conserving the pharmacist's time.
- Specifications and bids based purchasing.
- Availability of uniform products in use throughout the service area.
- Direct linked with group purchasing organization or a local wholesaler.

The pharmacist should give consideration to the following areas when dealing with a supplier:

1. FDA requirements, packaging and labeling must conform whenever necessary.
2. The company should not have a history of returning product recalls.
3. Supplier/manufacturers must provide data relating to analytical control, sterility testing, descriptions of test procedures for raw materials on request. They also provide all information of finished product which would confirm the safety and quality of the product.
4. Sutures and sterile fluids and catheters should be confined to a single lot number during the purchasing.
5. The expiration date should be sufficiently advanced to permit appropriate time for use and turn-over.
6. Unopened packages after the expiration date should be accepted and credited by Vendors.
7. Supplier should ship all merchandise freight prepaid and also provide inside delivery with a packing slip which indicates back ordered items.
8. Vendor must warrant to all products supplied by him and hold harmless the purchaser against any and all legal actions arising from claims by third parties relating to the supplies.

DISTRIBUTION

All the ancillary supplies can predict their rate of use and consequently order them from the pharmacy on a weekly or bi-weekly basis in the laboratories, pavilions and special service areas. The day on which these orders are positioned is arbitrary, but it is recommended that a specific day be selected in addition to a time deadline. There are two methods whereby the pavilions, laboratories and special service areas may be informed as to exactly what is carried in inventory. They are through a pre-printed requisition form which lists all the supplies or by issuing a catalogue printing on the form. The pre-printed form is ideal if the total number of items stocked is not too more and this type of system is the most practical. On the other hand, the best way to inform those who must requisition the supplies for their area is by means of a published format should be cross-indexed properly with its use and should show the unit size of the package to be dispensed. This types of process will save a great deal of time for the dispensing personnel as well as for the pricing clerk. In hospitals where a catalogue has been printed, a special requisition form must also be put into use. These types of form must be easy and be quite simple and yet capable of being used for any type of supply. All requisition forms should be prepared in duplicate by the department head. One copy may retain a copy of the original order as a receiving slip to make sure that all supplies ordered have been received. If any items will be out of inventory, it is advisable to put on the notice 'Out of stock Notice' to inform the requisitioning department. This form is initiated in duplicate by the pharmacist filling the requisition. The original is retained in the pharmacy and the duplicate is sent to the requisitioning department. When the supplies are again in inventory, it is a simple matter to give the information to the laboratory or ward without their issuing a new request.

Some times the pharmacist assumes the managerial responsibility for the dispensing of ancillary supplies, then he must utilize modern concept and technology to maintain control over the investment in inventory. During the handling of ancillary supplies pharmacist is required to apply the economic order quantity model. A number of financial order quantity models have been devised to help one in the control of inventory locked dollars. The mathematical models determine the optimum inventory level by calculating the optimum order quantity and re-order points.

ABC HOSPITAL

Requisition form for ward and Laboratory Supplies Only

For use in (Name of ward) : ____________________

Date : __________

Time : _________________________

Wanted		Description of Items	Availability	Cost
Amount	Size			

Required by : ________________________________

Approved by : ________________________________

Received by : _________________________________

Signature with date

Fig. 17.1 A requisition to the pharmacy for ward and laboratory supplies

WELFARE HOSPITAL

PHARMACY

Department : ____________________ Date : ____________

Name on original requisition : ________________________

We are temporarily out of the following :

Quantity	Items

When these items are available, your order will be completed

Note : Please 'DO NOT RE-ORDER'

Fig. 17.2 Out of Stock Notice

DISPENSING OF CONTROLLED SUBSTANCES

All system of medicine are based on natural drugs but a large number of synthetic drugs have found their way in the allopathic or the modern system of medicine. Some drugs like coca, hemp and opium are potent drugs but they are habit forming and have degenerative effect on the health of the user. Opium was brought under legislative control as far back as in 1857. The primary aim of the Opium Act was the protection of the public welfare by preserving health and eliminating undesirable social and moral effects commonly associated with indiscriminate use of this drug. Chinese are known to have almost unbroken record of addiction to opium since time immemorial. Hemp is very popular in Asia and Africa and in India particularly this drink is mentioned as the favourite drink of Lord Shiva, according to Hindu mythology.

Government of India passed the Dangerous Drug Act 1930 with a view to control certain operations in dangerous drugs and to centralize vest the same in Central Government. Another purpose of the Act was to increase penalties for certain offences relating to dangerous drugs and to render uniform all penalties relating to certain operations concerning the dangerous drugs. To keep pace with the changing times and overwhelming abuse of these dangerous drugs required a fresh legislation. This culminated into the enactment of the Narcotic Drug and Psychotropic substances Act and rules in 1985.

The Controlled Substances Act, has as its purpose to "amend the Public Health Service Act and other laws to provide increased research to :

- Prevention of drug abuse
- Drug dependence
- Provide for treatment and rehabilitation of drug abusers and drug dependent persons
- strengthen existing law enforcement authority in the field of drug abuse.

The Act is divided into four subjects:

1. Rehabilitation Programs Relating to Drug Abuse
2. Control and Enforcement
3. Important and Exportation; Amendments and Repeal of Revenue Laws
4. Report on Advisory Councils

Some important definitions

Addict : means a person addict to any narcotic or psychotropic susbstance.

Cannbis (Hemp) : means

a. **Charas** that is the separated resin, in whatever form, whether crude or purified, from the cannabis plant and also includes concentrated preparation and resin known as hashish oil or liquid hashish.
b. **Ganja** : means the flowering or fruiting tops of the cannabis plant (excluding the seeds and leaves when not accompanied by the tops) by whatever name they may be known or designated and
c. any mixture with or without any neutral material of any forms of cannabis or any drink prepared threform.

Coca derivative : means –

(a) crude cocaine, that is, any extract of coca leaf which can be used, directly or indirectly, for the manufacturing of cocaine.

(b) ecgonine and all the derivatives of ecgonine from which it can be recovered.

(c) cocaine, that is, methyl ester of benzyl-ecgonine and its salts; and

(d) all preparations containing more than 0.1 % of cocaine

Coca plant : means the plant of any species of the genus Erythroxylon.

Medicinal cannabis means any extract or tincture of cannabis (hemp);

Narcotic drug : means

coca leaf, cannabis (hemp), opium, poppy straw and includes all manufactured drugs;

Opium : means

(a) the coagulated juice of the opium poppy; and

(b) any mixture, with or without any neutral material of the coagulated juice of the opium poppy but does not include any preparation containing not more than 0.2% of morphine;

The word opium does not include any preparation. containing not more than 02% morphine. Coagulated juice of poppy is crude opium. Opium water is a mixture of water with capsules of poppy or with the juice of capsules of such poppy or its mixture with neutral materials.

Opium derivative :

(a) medicinal opium, that is, opium which has undergone the process necessary to adapt it for medicinal use in accordance with the' requirements of the Indian Pharmacopoeia' or any other pharmacopoeia notified in this behalf by the Central Government, whether in powder form or granulated or mixed with neutral materials;

(b) prepared opium, that is, any product of opium obtained by any series of operations designed to transform opium into an extract suitable for smoking and the dross or other residue remaining after opium is smoked;

(c) phenanthrene alkaloids, namely–morphine, codeine, thebaine, and their salts;

(d) diacetylmorphine, that is, the alkaloid also known as diamorphine or heroin and its salts; and

(e) all preparations containing more than 0.2% of morphine or containing any diacetylmorphine;

Morphine, being an alkaloid of opium, is a preparation of opium and, as such, it is opium:

The word 'prepared' designates a completed or manufactured article. It does not include an article in the process of preparation. If it can be used at the stage in which it is found, it is a prepared article. The word 'admixture' refers only to the completed articles and can be applied only after the mixing has been completed and not earlier. 'Opium water, collected from the washing of the opium pipes is not a mixture of such water. It is a dross or the residue of the smoked opium.

Opium poppy : means

(a) the plant of the species Papaver somniforum L; and

(b) the plant of any other species of Papaver from which opium or any other phenanthrene alkaloid can be extracted and which the Central Government may, by notification in the Official Gazette, declare to be opium poppy for the purpose of this Act.

AUTHORITIES AND OFFICERS

1. **Measures by Central Government**: To prevent and combat abuse of narcotic and psyhotropic substances and the illicit traffic therein, the Central Government may take measures with respect to the following matters:

   a. coordination of actions by various officers, State Governments and other authorities under this Act or under any other law for the time being in force in connection with the enforcement of the provisions of this Act;

   b. obligations under the International Conventions;

   c. assistance to the concerned authorities in foreign countries and international organizations to facilitate coordination and universal action for prevention and suppression of illicit traffic in narcotic drugs and psychotropic substances;

   d. identification, treatment, education, after care, rehabilitation and social re-integration of addicts; and

   e. such other matters as the Central Government deems necessary or expedient for the purpose of this Act and preventing and combating the abuse of narcotic drugs and psychotropic substances and illicit traffic therein.

   The Central Government is also empowered to constitute an authority or hierarchy of authorities for the purpose of exercising such powers and functions and for taking measures with respect to the matters mentioned above or specified in an order. Such authority or authorities may exercise the powers and functions and take measures, subject to the supervision and control of the Central Government and the provisions of such order, as if empowered by this Act to exercise those powers and take such measures.

2. **Officers or Government** : In addition to the above authorities, the Central Government shall appoint a Narcotics Commissioner and such other officers as it thinks fit for the purpose of this Act. The Narcotics Commissioner shall exercise all powers and perform all functions relating to the superintendence of the cultivation of the opium poppy and production of opium and shall exercise and perform such other Dowers and functions as may be entrusted to him by the Central Government. The officers shall be subject to the general control and direction of the Central Government, or if so directed by the Government, also of the Board or any other authority or officer. The Narcotics Commissioner may authorize any officer subordinate to him, to exercise all or any of his powers under the Rules. The Narcotics Commissioners and such other officers as may be appointed by the Central Government, may perform all or any of the function, or exercise any of the powers assigned under the rules to the officers subordinate to them.

3. **The Narcotic Drugs and Psychotropic Substances Consultative Committee:** This Committee may be constituted by the Central Government by notification in the Official Gazette, to advise the Central Government on such matters relating to the

administration of this act as are referred to it by the Government from time to time. The committee shall consist of a Chairman and such other members, not exceeding twenty, as may be appointed by the Central Government. It shall meet when required by the Central Government to do so and shall have power to regulate its own procedure. The Committee is also empowered, for the efficient discharge of any of its functions, to constitute one or more sub-committees, and may appoint to any such sub-committee, whether generally or for the consideration of any particular matter, any person (including a non-official) who is not a member of the Committee. The tenure of the office of, the manner of filling casual vacancies in the office of, and the allowances, if any, payable to the Chairman and other members of the Committee, and the conditions and restrictions subject to which the Committee may appoint a non-member as a member of its sub-committee, shall be such as may be prescribed by rules made by the Central Government

4. **National Fund for Control of Drug Abuse**: The Central Government may, by notification in the Official Gazette, constitute the National Fund for Control of Drug Abuse. The fund shall be applied by the Central Government to meet the expenditure incurred in connection with the measures taken for combating illicit traffic in, or controlling abuse of, narcotic drugs or psychotropic substances for specified purposes. The Central Government may constitute a Governing Body to advice the Government in regard to the application of the fund. The Central Government shall, as soon as may be, after the end of each financial year, cause to be published in the Official Gazette a report giving an account of the activities financed during the financial year, together with a statement of accounts.

5. **Officers of State Government :** The State Government may appoint officers with such designations as it thinks fit for the purpose of this Act. These officers shall be subjected to the general control and direction of the State Government, or if so directed by that Government, also of any other authority or officer.

PROHIBITION, CONTROL AND REGULATION

Prohibition of Certain Operations No person shall:

a. cultivate any coca plant or gather any portion of the coca plant or
b. cultivate the opium or any cannabis plant or
c. produce, manufacture, possess, sell, purchase, transport, warehouse, use, consume, import and export inter-State or tranship any narcotic drug or psychotropic substance; except for medical or scientific purpose and in the manner and to the extent prescribed or in accordance with the terms and conditions of a licence, permit, or authorization, if provided.

Provided that the prohibition against the cultivation of cannabis plant or the production of ganja or the production, possession, use, consumption, purchase, sale, transport, warehousing, inter-State import and export of ganja for any purpose other than medical and scientific, shall take effect only from the date specified by the Central Government.

Power of Central Government to Permit, Control and Regulate

Subject to the above provisions, the Central Government may, by rules,

(a) Permit and regulate-

- the cultivation and gathering of any portion (only on behalf of the Central Government) of coca plant, or the production, possession, sale, purchase, transport, inter-State import and export, use or consumption of coca leaves;
- the cultivation (only on behalf of the Central Government,) of the opium poppy;
- the production and manufacture of opium and production of poppy straw;
- the sale of opium and opium derivatives from the Central Government factories for export from India or sale to State Government or to manufacturing chemists;
- the manufacture of manufactured drugs (other than prepared opium) not including manufacture of medicinal opium or any preparation containing any manufactured drug from materials which the maker is legally entitled to possess:
- the manufacture, possession, transport, inter-State import and export. sale, purchase, consumption or use of psychotropic substances;

(b) prescribe any other requisite to render effective the control of the Central Government over any of the matters specified above.

Power of State Government to Permit, Control and Regulate

Subject to the provisions of the Act, the State Government may, by rules:

(a) permit and regulate-

- the possession, transport, inter-State import and export. warehousing, sale, purchase, consumption and use of poppy straw;
- the possession, transport, inter-State import and export. sale, purchase, consumption and use of opium,
- the cultivation of any cannabis plant, production, manufacture, possession, transport, inter-State import and export, sale, purchase, consumption or use of cannabis (excluding *charas):*
- the manufacture of medicinal opium or any preparation containing any manufactured drug from materials which the maker is legally entitled to possess;
- the possession, transport. purchase, sale, inter-State import and export. use or consumption of manufactured drugs other than prepared opium and of coca leaf and any preparation containing any manufactured drug;

- the manufacture and possession of prepared opium from opium lawfully possessed by an addict registered with the State Government on medical advice for his personal consumption.

Provided that unless expressly provided in the relevant rules, nothing shall apply to the inter-State import or export, transport. possession, purchase, sale, use or consumption of manufactured drugs which are the property and in the possession of the Government and that such drugs shall not be sold or otherwise delivered to any person who is not legally entitled to their possession.

(b) prescribe any other matter requisite to render effective the control of the state Government over any of the matters specified above.

Narcotic drugs and psychotropic substances are not liable to distress or attachment. No narcotic drug, psychotropic substance, coca plant, the opium poppy or cannabis shall be liable to be distained or attached by any person for the recovery of any money under any order or decree of any court or authority or otherwise.

SCHEDULES FOR CONTROLLED SUBSTANCES

Public Law is created the five schedules of controlled substances, known as Schedules 1, II, III, IV and V. The listings within each schedule must be updated and republished one year after the date of enactment and annually thereafter. The findings required for each of the schedules are as follows:

SCHEDULE I

- The drug or other substance has a high potential for abuse.
- The drug or other substance has no currently accepted medical use in treatment in the United States.
- There is a lack of accepted safety for use of the drug or other substance under medical supervision.

SCHEDULE II

- The drug or other substance has a high potential for abuse.
- The drug or other substance has recurrently accepted medical use in treatment in the United States or a currently accepted medical use with severe restrictions.
- Abuse of the drug or other substances may lead to severe psychological or physical dependence.

SCHEDULE III

- The drug or other substance has a potential for abuse less than the drugs or other substances in schedules I and II.

- (E) The drug or other substance has a currently accepted medical use in treatment in the United States.
- Abuse of the drug or other substance may lead to moderate or low physical dependence or high psychological dependence.

SCHEDULE IV

- The drug or other substance has a low potential for abuse relative to the drugs or other substances in schedule III.
- The drug or other substance has a currently accepted medical use in treatment in the United States.
- Abuse of the drug or other substance may lead to limited physical dependence or psychological dependence relative to the drugs or other substances in schedule III.

SCHEDULE V

- The drug or other substance has a low potential for abuse relative to the drugs or other substances in schedule IV.
- The drug or other substance has a currently accepted medical use in the United States.
- Abuse of the drug or other substance may lead to limited physical dependence or psychological dependence relative to the drugs or other substances in schedule IV.

APPLICATION FORMS

Individuals seeking registration under the Act are required to file special forms. A person applying for registration:

1. To manufacture or distribute controlled substances shall apply on specified Form only.
2. To dispense narcotic or non-narcotic, or to deduct research with non narcotic, or to conduct instructional activities with narcotic or non-narcotic controlled substances as per the list.
3. To conduct research with narcotic controlled substances listed in schedules II.
4. To conduct research with a controlled substance listed in schedule I, shall apply on prescribed Form in two copies of a research protocol describing the research project attached to the Form ..
5. To conduct instructional activities with a controlled substance listed in schedule I, shall apply as a researcher with detailed as nature of work, duration, uses of these substance, quantity etc.
6. To conduct chemical analysis with controlled substances listed in any schedule.
7. To import or export controlled substances listed in any schedule, shall apply on prescribed Form.

Applications for registration must include all of the complete information called for in the form, unless the item is not applicable, in which case this fact must be indicated. In addition, each application, attachment, or other document filed as part of an application, shall be signed by the applicant and other partners.

INVENTORY REQUIREMENTS

Every registrant, other than an individual practitioner, must on the day he is first registered and every two years there after, make a complete and accurate record of all stocks of controlled substances under his control. The record must indicate the date on which the inventory was taken and whether taken at the close or opening of business. The responsible person made complete inventory and be maintained at the location appearing on the registration for a period of two years.

LABELING AND PACKAGING REQUIREMENTS

Labeling and packaging requirements under this law are required that containers of controlled substances must meet the labeling requirements of the Drug and Cosmetic Act or the regulations to be promulgated by the Authority time to time. Each controlled substance manufactured after December 1, 1971 must have on its label a symbol designating to which schedule it belongs.

OFFENSES AND PENALTIES

1. Removing, changing or obliterating a symbol or label required by this title.
2. Dispensing controlled drugs without first becoming registered.
3. Refusing or failing to make, maintain or furnish any record, report, notification, declaration, order or order forms, statement, invoice or information required under this title.
4. Refusing an entry into any premises or inspection authorized by this title.

Finally, the section provides for various penalties for the various violations and range from fines, imprisonment or both depending upon the seriousness of the violation of the rules and basis requirement of the title.

CHAPTER 18

DRUG INFORMATION CENTRE

INTRODUCTION

Drug information is defined as the knowledge of facts acquired through reading, study or practical experience concerning any chemical substance intended for use in diagnosis, prevention and treatment of disease.

According to World Health Organizatin (WHO) a drug information center is an independent center that is accessible to any health professional to ask all questions about drug therapy. Drug information centers are defined by the following three criteria : (i) At least one dedicated and trained pharmacist must be available to answer queries; (ii) Sufficient information resources should be available to satisfy a broad range of querries., and (iii) specific room be set aside as location for drug information center.

The hospital setting provides a unique opportunity for the pharmacist to develop a comprehensive drug information service to the medical staff, residents, interns, medical students, nursing staff, nursing students, dentists and dental residents.

One of the hospital pharmacist's responsibilities includes 'furnishing information concerning medications to physicians, interns and nurses'. Not only is the hospital pharmacist called upon to provide pharmacological information, but he is also called upon to provide information on the physical and chemical aspects as well as biopharmaceutical information. He is in a position to bridge the gap between the biological and the pharmaceutical aspects of dosage forms. Pharmacists who are prepared to supply such information are highly esteemed by physicians, surgeons, medical students, nurses and others who may need such information.

Establishment of drug information centres creates the opportunity for pharmacists so inclined to become drug information specialist, in contrast to those who want to specialize in administration, manufacturing, drug distribution, radiopharmaceuticals, or other specialized areas of hospital pharmacy practice. The developing trend towards clinical pharmacy strengthens the need for and value of a drug information centre in the hospital pharmacy. An essential part of a clinical pharmacist's role is to deliver his knowledge about drugs at the patient's bedside and to the other members of the healthcare team. In ordr for him to do this, he needs the vast resources of drug literature. This palces a new significance on the development and expansion of the concept of drug information center.

The first drug information center was opened in 1962, at the University of Kentucky Medical Center and was intended to be utilized as a source of selected, comprehensive drug information for staff physicians and dentists to allow them to evaluate and compare drugs besides catering to the information needs of nursing staff. The staffs of the drug information center were likely to take an active role in the education of health professionals within the institution. The first formal survey was carried in 1973 and identified 54 drug information centers in the USA. In 1995, According to a report published, there were about120 full-fledged pharmacist-operated drug information centers in the United States, which accept a broad scope of requests from health care professionals.

The provision of accurate and timely drug information to health care professionals is an important mechanism to promote safe and effective drug therapy. Such type of service is poor in India. Hence, the purpose of the center is to provide accurate, current, and unbiased information for the promotion of rational drug therapy. The center also provides relevant information to physicians and faculty of the medical academy on evidence-based medicine at their request.

Table 18.1: The working model of drug information service

Books	**Journals**	**Formularies**	**Computer databases**	**World-wide web**
		Drug Information Services		
Access Callers				**Dissemination of Information**
• Physicians • Pharmacists • Nurses • Students • Researchers • Pharmacy and Therapeutic committee • Legal aides • Drug Industries • Marketing firms			• Reprint • Answer to telephone call • Computer retrieval system • Internet search • Publication and education • Drug policy decision • Cost benefit analysis • Sharing or debating • Information to patients	

Staff requirements for DIC depend on:

(a) Scope of services
(b) Hours of operation
(c) Monetary resources

Health care professionals' questions are easily answered with the help of five R's :

(i) Right drug
(ii) Right dose
(iii) Right dosage form
(iv) Right route, and
(v) Right patient.

The purpose of the Drug Information Center (DIC) is to serve health care professionals throughout India by answering critical questions on drug use and its possible side effects. The DIC routinely responds to inquiries such as –

1. Adverse reactions to drugs.
2. Information regarding appropriate therapy for specific patients.
3. Efficacy of drugs.
4. Drug interactions.
5. Intravenous additive incompatibilities.
6. Biopharmaceutic and pharmacokinetic parameters of drugs.
7. Dosing in renal failure.
8. Appropriate therapy for a disease state.
9. Identification of foreign drugs.
10. Information on investigational agents, and
11. Information on new drugs.

The purpose of the **drug information service** is to provide accurate, current and unbiased drug information in the promotion of rational drug therapy.

The hospital-based DIC will be doing the following activities:

1. Answering the in-house call
2. Assist in formulary decision
3. participate in drug use evaluation
4. Coordinate adverse drug reaction reporting
5. Publish a newsletter, provide in service education
6. Assist in P&T committee
7. Oversee investigational drug activity

Drug Information Centers in India

Recognizing the need to provide organized drug information to health care professionals as well as consumers, the WHO Country Office in collaboration with the Karnataka State Pharmacy Council (KSPC) supported the establishment of 5 drug information centres. The centres seek to provide authentic, unbiased drug information to healthcare professionals; provide tailor-made counseling and drug information to patients / consumers as well as monitor and document adverse drug reactions within the hospital.

The process of establishment of these centres included - identification of states, feasibility assessment studies and ascertaining the interest of selected states and training of individuals from each Centre amongst others. The selected centers have started functioning from January 2007 and are registered with International Register of Drug Information Services (IRDIS). The center is equipped with computer terminals, printed materials (current, periodicals, bound journal volumes, reference texts) and has access to Medline, the Internet and various other online drug and medical references. The center maintains subscriptions to nationally recognized journals and texts of Pharmacy and Medicine. Direct access to computerized on-line data searching, CD ROM databases and the World Wide Web are also available. Drug information requests may be initiated in person, by phone, fax, e-mail or by mail. The center is accessible by telephone 24 hours a day.

Service activities

- The staff answers questions on drug related matters, particularly to those related to safety of drug.
- The doctors, Pharmacists and patients could visit the center in person to get information.
- The literature searches are provided free of charge to all hospital faculty, clinicians, and pharmacy staff for patient specific issues and for research as well as teaching activities.
- Those services, which are not related to the activities of the university, are charged with a fee. The reimbursements for services are requested from organizations such as law firms, pharmaceutical companies and marketing firms.
- The center is accessible to undergraduate or graduate students working on special projects or patient care activities but does not provide services for students working on class assignments or preparing for tests.
- Since one of its aims is to promote physician-pharmacist-patient relationships it does not advertise to the lay public.
- General information is provided to patients requiring immediate information but they are strongly urged to consult with their treating physician.
- The center also provides written information in the form of articles, news-letters and journal columns to encourage and inform health professionals on rational drug therapy.

- An adverse drug reaction (ADR) monitoring and reporting program is in place which provides guidance for the monitoring, detection, reporting and evaluations of ADRs in the hospital. It also promotes ADR awareness and information dissemination to the medical, nursing and pharmacy staff. The data generated is used by the Pharmacy and Therapeutics Committee to ensure drug safety.
- The center also participates in the ADR reporting program of Food & Drugs Administration (FDA) and has 'The Product Problem Reporting' system to ensure drug safety by providing guidance in the event of a defect in the quality of drugs (for example: color change in tablet or particulate matter in infusion fluid).
- Evaluation of performance

Table 18.2 Drug Information Centres

S. No.	Drug information centre	Contact detail
01	Haryana (Sirsa)	Mr. Sameer Dhingra, Sr. Lecturer / Ms. Renu Kadian, Lecturer Lord Shiva College of Pharmacy, Near Civil Hospital, Sirsa-125055, Haryana, Tel: 01666-240057. E-mail: dicharyana@gmail.com, dicsirsa@yahoo.co.in
02	Chhattisgarh (Raipur)	Mr. Amber Vyas, Lecturer / Mr. Kamalesh Dashora, Lecturer Institute of Pharmacy, Chhattisgarh State Pharmacy Council, Quarter No. –77, Sector No. – 3, Geetanjali Nagar, Raipur, Chhattisgarh State, Tel: 0771 – 2444591. E-mail: dicraipur@gmail.com , dicraipur@yahoo.com
03	Rajasthan (Jaipur)	Mr. Manoj Dixit, Lecturer / Ms. Garima Joshi, Lecturer L.B.S.College of Pharmacy, Udaymarg, Tilaknagar, Jaipur. Tel: 0141-2620517, 3258229. E-mail: dicjaipur@gmail.com,dicjaipur@yahoo.com
04	Assam (Dibrugarh)	Mr. Ariful Hussain, Lecturer / Mr. Debajyoti Gogoi, Lecturer Institute of Pharmacy, Assam Medical College, Dibrugarh – 786 002, Assam. Tel: 0373 – 2300903. E-mail: dicassam@gmail.com , dic_amc@yahoo.com
05	Goa (Panaji).	Mr. Raj Vaidya, Community Pharmacist / Ms. Pooja Borker, Community Pharmacist Hindu Pharmacy, Cunha Rivara Road, P.B. No. 149, Panaji, Goa Tel: 0832-2223176; 2432903. E-mail: dicgoa@gmail.com, dicpanaji@yahoo.com

Enquiries made from Drug Information Centre by doctors during August 2000-January 2002 are presented in the following Table

Table 18.3 Enquirers form Doctors [August 2000-January 2002]

Category of Doctors	Number of queries	Percent of queries
Pediatricians	119	18.1
General Physicians	109	16.7
Gynecologists	70	10.6
Dermatologists	116	17.6
Pharmacologists	54	8.2
Dentists	22	3.3
Cardiologists	27	4.1
Anesthetists	17	2.5
Microbiologists	17	2.6
Psychiatrics	18	2.7
ENT specialists	19	2.8
Orthopaedecians	21	3.2
Pulmonologists	11	1.7
Oncologists	16	2.4
Pathologists	8	1.2
Endocrinologists	14	2.1

Independent DIC's in India

1. CDMU Documentation Center, Calcutta
2. Drug Information Center, Maharashtra State Pharmacy Council, Mumbai
3. Andhra Pradesh State Pharmacy Council, Andhra Pradesh
4. Karnataka State Pharmacy Council (KSPC), Bangalore, Karnataka
5. JSS College of Pharmacy, Ooty,
6. Pharma Information Center, Tamilnadu, Chennai

Hospital attached DIC's with Clinical Pharmacy Services

- Christian Medical College Hospital Vellore, Tamilnadu
- Drug Information Center, (KSPC), Victoria Hospital, Bangalore, Karnataka

- Drug Information Center, (KSPC), Bowring & Lady Curzon Hospital, Bengaluru, Karnataka
- Department of Pharmacy Practice, Chidambaram, Tamilnadu
- Department of Pharmacy Practice, National institute of Pharmaceutical Education and Research (NIPER), Chandigarh
- Jawaharlal Nehru Medical College Hospital (JNMC), Bengaluru, Karnataka
- JSS College of Pharmacy, Mysore, Karnataka
- N.R.S. Medical College & Hospital, Calcutta
- Kempagowda Institute of Medical Sciences (KIMS), Bangalore, Karnataka
- Kasturba Medical College (KMC), Manipal, Karnataka
- Poison Information Center, All India Institute of Medical Sciences (AIIMS), Delhi
- Poisons Information Centre, National Institute of Occupational Health, Ahmedabad
- Dept of Toxicology, (Incl. Poison Information & Laboratory Services) Amrita Institute of Medical Sciences & Research, Cochin
- Toxicology & IMCU Unit, Government General Hospital, Chennai
- Sri Ramachandra Hospital, Porur, Chennai
- Sri Ramakrishna Mission Hospital, Coimbatore, TamilNadu
- Trivandrum Medical College, Trivandrum, Kerala

WHO COLLABORATING CENTRES IN INDIA

(a) Communicable Diseases & Disease Surveillance

Sr. No.	Institute Name	Area of Work	Address	PI Name & Designation
1.	National Institute of Mental Health and Neurosciences (NIMHANS), Bengaluru	Reference and Research in Rabies	Department of Neurovirology P.B. No. 2900, Hosur Road Bengaluru – 560029, India	Dr S N Madhusudana Associate Professor
2.	Regional Medical Research Centre (ICMR), Port Blair, Andaman Nicobar Islands Email:- pblicmr@sancharnet.in; icmr@cal3.vsnl.net.in	Diagnosis, Reference, Research and Training in Leptospirosis	Indian Council of Medical Research Post Bag No. 13, Dollyganj Port Blair 744 101 Andaman Nicobar Islands, India	Dr P. Vijayachari Director

Contd…

3.	National institute of Communicable Diseases (NICD), New Delhi Email:- dirnicd@bol.net.in	Rabies Epidemiology	Directorate General of Health Services 22 Shamnath Marg, P.O. Box No. 1492, Delhi.110054, India	Dr Veena Mittal Joint Director & head Zoonoses Division
4.	National institute of Communicable Diseases (NICD), New Delhi	Epidemiology and Training	22 Sham Nath Marg Delhi – 110054 India	Dr S Venkatesh Joint Director & Head, Epidemiology Division
5.	National Institute of Epidemiology, Indian Council of Medical Research (ICMR), Chennai Email:- nieicmr@vsnl.com	Leprosy Research and Epidemiology	Indian Council of Medical Research Mayor V.R. Ramanathan Road, Chetpet, Chennai 600031 India	Dr. Vrinda Khole (Office I/C)
6.	Tuberculosis Research Centre, Chennai Email:- nrparanj@md2.vsnl.net.in	Tuberculosis Research and Training	Indian Council of Medical Research Mayor V.R. Ramanathan Road, Old Spur Tank Road, Chetput, Chennai.600031, India	Dr. P.R.Narayan Director
7.	National Tuberculosis Institute, Bangalore Email:- ntiindia@blr.vsnl.net.in	Tuberculosis Research and Training	(DGHS), Govt of India, Avalon, 8, Bellary Road Bengalure 560 003, Karnataka	Dr Prahlad Kumar Director
8.	National Institute of Virology, Pune Email: icmrniv@icmrniv.ren.nic.in	Arboviral and Haemorrhagic Fever Reference and Research & WHO H5 Reference Laboratory	20-A, Dr Ambedkar Road Post Box No. 14 Pune 411 001, India	Dr A.C. Mishra Director

Contd...

9.	Vector Control Research Centre (CVRC), Pondicherry Email:- vcrc@vsnl.com	Research and Training in Lympathic Filariasis and Integrated Methods for Vector Control	Indian Council of Medical Research Indira Nagar, Puducherry 605006 India	Dr. P.K Das Director
10.	National AIDS Research Institute (NARI), Pune	HIV Diagnosis and Monitoring of Antiretroviral Therapy	Indian Council of Medical Research G-73, M.I.D.C., Bhosari Pune - 411026	Dr Ramesh S. Paranjape Director

(b) Health Systems Development

Sr. No.	Institute Name	Area of Work	Address	PI Name & Designation
1.	School of Health System Studies, Tata Institute of Social Sciences Email:- director@tiss.edu ; hssdept@vsnl.com	Health Policy Research and Training	Post Box No. 8313 Sion Trombay Road Deonar, Mumbai-400088 Maharashtra	Professor S. Parasuraman Director
2.	Indian Institute of Health Management Research, Jaipur Email:- iihmr@iihmr.org	District Health System Based on Primary Health Care	1 Prabhu Dayal Marg, Opp. Sanganer Airport Jaipur 302011, Rajasthan, India	Dr S.D. Gupta, M.D. PhD Director
3.	Central Bureau of Intelligence, Directorate General of Health Services, Ministry of Health & Family Welfare dircbhi@nb.nic.in	Family of International Classifications	Room No. 404, A-Wing, Nirman Bhawan New Delhi	Mr. Ashok Kumar Director
4.	Community Health Department, Christian Medical College (CMC), Vellore Email: chad@cmcvellore.ac.in	Community Based Health Professions Education	Bagayam Vellore 632 002	Dr Jayaprakash Muliyil Professor & Head, Community Health Department

(c) Family & Community Health

S.No.	Institute Name	Area of Work	Address	PI Name & Designation
1.	College of Nursing, Christian Medical College and Hospital (CMC), Vellore deancon@cmcvellore.ac.in	Nursing and Midwifery Development	College of Nursing Christian Medical College and Hospital Vellore-632004 Tamil Nadu	Mrs Bharaty Jacob, Director
2.	National Institute of Nursing Education, College of Nursing, PGIMER, Chandigarh Email: principalpgi@yahoo.com;	Nursing and Midwifery Development	Postgraduate Institute of Medical Education and Research Sector 12 Chandigarh 1600012	Dr (Mrs) Indrajit Walia Principal
3.	Community Health Department, Christian Medical College (CMC), Vellore Email: chad@cmcvellore.ac.in	Community Based Health Professions Education	Bagayam Vellore 632 002	Dr Jayaprakash Muliyil Professor & Head, Community Health Department
4.	Genetic Unit, Department of Pediatrics, AIIMS, New Delhi Email: mkabra_aiims@yahoo.co.in	Training in Clinical & Laboratory Genetics in Developing Countries	Ansari Nagar New Delhi.110029	Dr Madhulika Kabra Addl. Prof. of Pediatrics & Officer-in-Charge
5.	National Institute of Cholera and Enteric Diseases (NICED), Kolkata Email: icmricd@ren.nic.in	Research and Traning on Diarrhoeal Diseases	P-33 C.I.T. Road, Scheme XM, Beliaghata, P.O. Box 177 Kolkata - 700 010	Dr G.B Nair Director
6.	Division of Neonatology, Department of Paediatrics, AIIMS, New Delhi Email: vinodkpaul@hotmail.com	Training and Research in Newborn Care	Ansari Nagar New Delhi	Dr Vinod Paul Incharge, Division of Neonatalogy

Contd…

7.	National Institute of Nutrition, Hyderabad Email: nin@ap.ap.nic.in	Nutrition Science in Primary Health Care	Indian Council of Medical Research, Jamai Osmania PO, Hyderabad-500007 Andhra Pradesh	Dr. B. Sesikeran Director
8.	M.S. University of Baroda, Gujarat Email: vc@msubernet.in	Anaemia Control and Diet, Related Non-Communicable Disease	Deptt of Food & Nutrition Vadodara 390002,	Professor Uliyar..V. Mani Director
9.	Department of Obstetrics and Gynaecology, AIIMS, New Delhi Email: dirirr@vsnl.com	Human Reproduction	All India Institute of Medical Sciences Ansari Nagar New Delhi - 110029	Dr Suneeta Mittal Professor and Head
10.	National Institute for Research in Reproductive Health (ICMR), Mumbai Email: dirirr@vsnl.com	Research and Training in Reproductive health	Jehangir Merwanji Street Parel, Mumbai 400012	Dr Vrinda Khole Director
11.	Department of Obstetrics and Gynaecology, PGIMER, Chandigarh Email: medinst@pgi.chd.nic.in	Human Reproduction	PG Institute of Medical Education and Research Chandigarh 160012	Dr Lakhbir Dhaliwal Programme Director

(d) Non-Communicable Diseases & Mental Health

S.No.	Institute Name	Area of Work	Address	PI Name & Designation
1.	L.V. Prasad Eye Institute, Hyderabad Email: ravithomas@lvpei.org	Prevention of Blindness	L.V. Prasad Marg, Banjara Hills Hyderabad 5000034	Prof Ravi Thomas Director
2.	Department of Epidemiology (NIMHANS), Banglore Email: mgd@nimhans.kar.nic.in	Injury Prevention and Safety Promotion	Department of Epidemiology NIMHANS Bengaluru. 560029	Dr G. Gururaj Professor & Head, Deptt of Epidemilogy

Contd…

3.	Diabetes Research Centre & M.V. Hospital for Diabetes, Chennai Email: ramachandran@vsnl.com	Research, Education and Training and Diabetes	4 Westmada Church Street Royapuram, Chennai Pin. 600013, T N	Dr. Vijay Vishwanathan Director
4.	Cardiothoracic Centre, All India Institute of Medical Sciences (AIIMS), New Delhi Email: ksreddy@ichealth.org	Epidemiology and Prevention of Cardiovascu lar Diseases	Cardiothoracic Centre AIIMS, Ansari Nagar New Delhi-110029	Dr. K. S. Reddy Director
5.	Radiation Standards Section Health Safety and Environment Group, Bhabha Atomic Research Centre	Secondary Standard Radiation Dosimetry	Bhabha Atomic Research Centre, Trombay, Mumbai - Pin: 400085	Dr V. Venkat Raj Head, Radiation Standards and Instrumentation Division
6.	Radiation Medicine Centre, Bhabha Atomic Research Centre, Mumbai Email: rmc@bom2.vsnl.net.in	Radiation Medicine	C/O. Tata Memorial Hospital Annexe Building Jerbai Wadia Road, Parel, Mumbai.400012	Dr N. Nair Head of the Centre
7.	Aravind Eye Hospitals and Postgraduate Institute of Ophthalmology, Madurai, Tamil Nadu Email: dr.nam@aravind.org	Prevention of Blindness	1 Anna Nagar, Madurai. 625 020 Tamil Nadu	Dr P. Namperumalsa my Director
8.	Dr. Rajendra Prasad Centre for Ophthalmic Sciences, AIIMS, New Delhi Email: pschiefrpc@yahoo.com	Prevention of Blindness	All India Institute of Medical Sciences Ansari Nagar New Delhi. 110029	Prof (Dr) Supriyo Ghose Director
9.	Indian Institute of Technology, New Delhi Email:dmohan@cbme.iitd.ernet.in	Research and Training in Safety Technology	Transportation Research and Injury Prevention Programme Hauz Khas	Professor Dinesh Mohan, Ph.D. Head of the WHO CC

Contd...

10.	Schizophrenia Research Foundation (India) (SCARF), Email: scarf@vsnl.com	Mental Health Research and Training	R/7A, North Main Road, West Anna Nagar Extension Chennai (Madras)-600101	Dr R. Thara Director
11.	Indian Institute of Mass Communication (IIMC), New Delhi	Health Promotion	Aruna Asaf Ali Marg, JNU New Campus New Delhi 110067	Mrs. Stuti Kacker Director
12.	Tata Institute of Fundamental Research, Mumbai Email: pcgupta@tifr.res.in	Training and Research in Tobacco Control	Homi Baba Road, Colaba Mumbai 400005	Prof. Mustansir Barma Director
13.	TATA Memorial Centre, Mumbai Email: dinshaw.tmc@vsnl.com	Cancer Prevention, Screening and Early Detection	Tata Memorial Hospital and Cancer Research Institute Dr Ernest Borges Marg, Parel Mumbai 400012	Dr K A Dinshaw Director
14.	All India Heart Foundation and National Heart Institute, New Delhi Email: padmavati@del12.vsnl.net.in	Preventive Cardiology	49, Community Centre East of Kailash New Delhi 110065	Dr S. Padmavati Director
15.	Dr. Mohan's Diabetes Specialities Centre, Chennai drmohans@vsnl.net	Noncommunicable Diseases Prevention and Control	6B,Gopalapuram Main Centre, Conran Smith Road, Gopalapuram, Chennai, 600086	Dr. V. Mohan Chairman
16	Department of Pulmonary Medicine, Postgraduate Institute of Medical Education and Research E-mail: skjindal@indiachest.org	Research and Capacity Building in Chronic Respiratory Diseases	Sector- 12 160012, Chandigarh	Prof S.K. Jindal Head of Department

(e) Sustainable Development & Healthy Environment

S.No.	Institute Name	Area of Work	Address	PI Name & Designation
1.	National Institute of Occupational Health, Ahmedabad Email: nichicmr@icenet.net	Occupational Health	Meghani Nagar Ahmedabad-380016	Dr H.N. Saiyed Director
2.	All India Institute of Hygiene and Public Health, Kolkata Email: alihph.cal@gems.vsnl.net.in	Disaster Preparedness	110 Chittaranjan Avenue, KOLKATA 700073 West Bengal, India	Dr Ranadeb Biswas Professor & Head

A well planned pharmaceutical library can play a major role in the continuation of medical education, the rapid dissemination of basic pharmacological research and as a source of research reference material. Library of a hospital pharmacy must be equipped with all reference material including books, journals, computer software, internet etc.

Hospital library and drug information centre are very useful to all the personnel in and outside the hospital, in general; and hospital personnel including patients, in particular.

UNIT - VII

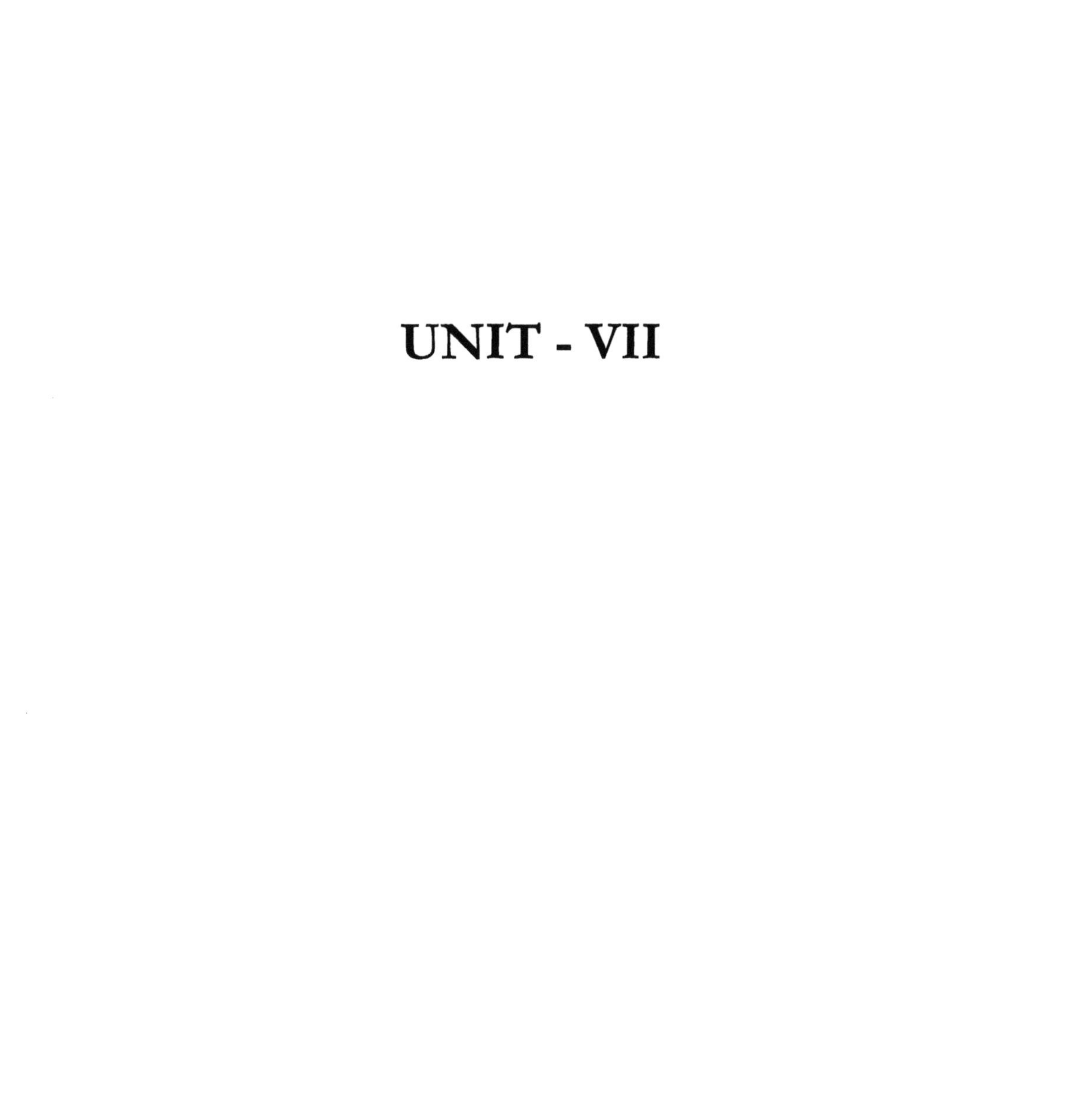

CHAPTER 19

HOSPITAL MANAGEMENT

BUDGET PREPARATION AND IMPLEMENTATION

Budget is defined as a financial or a quantitative statement prepared and approved prior to a period of time of the policy to be pursued during that period for purposes of attaining a given objective. It is considered to be a comprehensive plan of operations expressed in monetary and quantitative terms. It is more than a forecast of income and expenditure that reflects policy being implemented. The formulation of an ideal budget is essential to an optimal development of an organization.

Ideal Budget

While formulating a budget, there are certain essentials to be given due weightage.

(i) Identification and clear understanding of the hospital financial and services goal become important before the formulation of a budget.
(ii) Definite and accountable organization with clearly defined responsibilities for each department of the hospitals or healthcare organizations.
(iii) A system of accounting designed and maintained that would serve as a base for adequate reporting to provide a measure of performance and for holding the organization (department) responsible.
(iv) Represents a system of future accounts, stated in terms of organization responsibility. Thus there would be an active participation of hospital personnel in the preparation or formulation of the budget.
(v) Revealing the weaknesses and shortcomings.
(vi) Providing a strong base for coordinated working.
(vii) Lines of authority and responsibilities for execution of the tasks laid down are established.
(viii) Decentralisation of authority and responsibilities so as to place it as nearly as possible at the point of action.
(ix) Planning for the future is facilitated.

(x) The Plant and Equipment Budget (Capital Budget) consists of investment in assets to be acquired during the period of budget.

(xi) The estimates of operating revenues and expenses for next budget year and for that formulating the operating budget.

(xii) The formulation of cash budget for estimating the monetary requirements and the sources of funds for the budget period.

Formulation of a Budget

The formulation of an effective budget is essential for the sound development of hospitals and the healthcare organizations. An effective budget can't be prepared on imagination and hence different types of essential information are to be collected from different departments.

At the very outset, it is significant that written instructions regarding procedures to be followed are to be issued, which should be accompanied by illustrative forms and calculations and to be disseminated to all the personnel involved in the budget preparation. The different departments of hospitals then would formulate a budget for their own departments. Since we find salaries and wages accounting for at least 40 to 50 per cent of the total expenditure, it is pertinent that the budget is realistic or pragmatic. This focuses our attention on the compilation of a master list of the personnel in each department. Additional staff requirements, if necessary, are to be mentioned. Other expenses, such as drugs, food, supplies and expenses are to be projected on the basis of past year's expenses. Normally an increase of 10 per cent in a particular head is considered reasonable but keeping in view the inflationary pressure and other changes, it can fluctuate. While estimating the expenses on operation of plant and maintenance including depreciation, interest, some essentials are to be considered, such as any additional equipment like X-ray, laundry, sterilizer etc. are anticipated and acquisition of additional vehicles is to be contemplated besides the anticipation of a major renovation. The effect of free care is also an important consideration that requires due attention. Generally, the cost of free care is covered in the charges levied. An increase in the cost of free care is to be taken care.

Master Budget

The budgets formulated by the heads of different departments of hospitals are finally incorporated into a master budget.

We are well aware of the fact that formulation of an effective, realistic budget is a challenging task because it is based on a different types of information to be received from different sources and different departments of hospitals.

The preparation of the annual budget is one of the most important tasks in the economic operation of the department in the hospital. This important task requires serious consideration by administrators and pharmacists. It is not always acceptable submitted by the chief pharmacist. The preparation and implementation is described by the many administrators.

Budget is an instrument through which hospital administration, management at departmental levels, and the governing board can review the hospital services in relation to a prepared plan in a comprehensive and integrated form defined in financial terms. Budget of each and every department of hospital must be accurately prepared such that the over-all budget of the hospital could be developed. A properly developed and useful budget should have defined and ideal goals such as

- development of standards of presentation
- assessment of actual results with the standards so that deviations could be, identifying and determined
- Subsequent analysis of deviations useful to determine whether they are controllable or uncontrollable.

The budget has two main functions.

1. It estimates, as realistically as possible, the cost of completing the objectives identified in the proposal. The responsible person will use the budget details to determine whether the proposal is economically feasible and realistic.
2. The budget provides a means to monitor the hospital financial activities. In this way, it's possible to determine how closely the actual progress toward achieving the objectives is being made relative to the proposed budget.

Financial budget planning worksheet has proved to be an effective means to maintain a clear and concrete vision about the future of business and its performance in the financial year. Budget planning should be highly effective in controlling cash flow and helps in investing in useful and needful area in right direction.

The budget planning services include –

- Financial budget planning
- Budget planning worksheets
- Online budget planning and
- Long-term financial planning for cash flow

An ideal investment is required to preparing a realistic financial budget planning worksheet to help understand the financial implications, management of annual requirement, reduced long purchasing process, reduce storage problem, and also help in managing all types of problems.

Advantages of budget planning

1. Develop better financial planning
2. Gives a clear focus on decision-making to management of the hospital
3. Helps to focus on hospital priorities
4. Helps to prepare for contingencies or unforeseen expenses
5. Helps in taking secure financial strategies and decisions
6. Exposes domains of over expenditure
7. Creates additional resources to invest in core business activities
8. Effectively manage the finances of hospital
9. Make sure that budget is accurate and consistent
10. Enhance efficiency of staff and others

Responsibilities

General responsibilities of the Office of Budget and Analysis include the following functions :

1. Manage all types of small and big requirement of the hospital
2. Prepare the budget on behalf of hospital administration and with the help of Chief pharmacist
3. Maintain budget documentation for each financial year
4. Generate monthly analyses of expenditure including all
5. Informe the respective departments in case of line-item over-expenditures
6. Monitor the budget to ensure compliance
7. Supervise the preparation of the Research and maintenance

The pharmacist must be aware of the political aspects of the process, in order to participate more effectively in the budgetary process. Following factors are to be considered while preparing the budget :.

1. Institutional-philosophical pressures,
2. Personal considerations
3. Development of confidence among other officials, and
4. Demographic pressures

All these factors affect the power base of a department and, consequently, the strength of its bargaining position in the budgetary process. Personal thought, in the form of individual reputations, is important in any political process. An individual who has acquired a standing for having submitted previous budgets that have been thoroughly revised and supported by considerable system. The institutional-philosophical considerations in the budgetary process consist of the goals and objectives of the hospital and its various departments. In many state planning agencies require hospitals to submit the budget for upto 5 years plan with considering the budget of the financial year. Budget preparation is mainly two types on the basis tenure.

a. Short term budget (1 to 2 years)
b. Long term budget (5 to 10 years)

A budget is a short-range system for future handling and operations of various activities. It is essential to know the meaning and appropriate application of a budget and must be clearly understood by responsible persons who are working in managerial positions because their participation is required in its preparation and their cooperation. It is essential to management person to first identify the purpose of the unit, establish policies for its operation, and project the hospital's growth. The plan should be economic and attainable. It should not forecast results that are not possible under current and anticipated conditions.

Section of the budget

Every budget consists of three separate parts :

A. Revenue Accounts
B. Expense Accounts, and
C. Capital and Equipment budget

A. The Revenue Account

In the preparation of budget, total income of hospital is calculated. Either the department of pharmacy or the accounting department maintains a daily, weekly, monthly or annual total of the cost of the pharmaceuticals issued to the different patient services as well as to the special service departments. The true income of the department is the sum of the cost of pharmaceuticals issued to patient and the processing of patient prescriptions and requisitions of the department. In addition, there are other statistics that are of value in assisting management to accurately predict the volume of activity of the department of pharmacy. They are:

1. Total number of prescriptions dispensed per pharmacist.
2. Total hours of services.
3. Prescription volume per hour of service.
4. Per day medication cost of per patient.
5. Average supply cost per requisition.
6. Cost of medication per clinic visit.
7. Average cost of drug per prescription.
8. Average salary cost per prescription.

It is found that the income in the hospital pharmacy is limited to the sale of drugs to in-patients, out-patients and departments of the hospital. The total income of hospital depends upon the types of patient and their paying capacity. Generally following types of patients category is in the hospital such as -

1. Those who made full payment to the hospital.
2. Those who make partial payment
3. Those who make no payment at all
4. Staff of the hospital such as physicians and general employee

The total income obtained is summation of the above. It is required to separate income obtained from various parts for accurate appraisal and evaluation.

B. Expenditure Accounts

The total expenditure in hospital can be considered in following general categories :

1. Professional Care of Patients' expenses
2. Out-patient expenses
3. Administrative and general expenses
4. Emergency and Miscellaneous expenses

The department of pharmacy prepare the expenditure accounts detail on the following expenses.

1. **Expenses account Salary and wages**

   This is a recurring expenditure of department. The salaries criteria is not same. The chief pharmacist or other responsible person prepare a breakdown of the personnel in the department of pharmacy into the following categories:

   - Expenditure on permanent full-time positions
   - Expenditure on permanent part-time positions
   - Expenditure on temporary positions.
   - Expenditure on proposed new positions.
   - Expenditure on overtime requested.

   The total salary expenditure of financial year is the sum of all types of salaries paid to the staff including administrative, professional and non-professional staff. For detail It may be simple to prepare the date in a tabular form considering –

   - all full-time administrative staff
   - full time professional and non-professional pharmacy staff
   - part-time employees in each category

- New positions, if any
- Overtime expenditure

Total of all types of salary and wages represents the actual expenditure of the financial year under this category.

2. **Expenses of supplies and material**

   The responsible administrator or Chief Pharmacist should prepare a financial statement considering the requirement of amount in rupees for supplies and material with the help of latest available financial statement. It is also necessary to show the actual cost of materials and supplies. This actual mathematical process estimates what the actual expense will be for the present financial year. If the budgeted figure and the estimated actual figure are same, then the previously prepared budget was well done. On the other hand, if these two figures are different, it shows that the calculation is wrong or there was an error in the consideration of expenditure detail. True budget calculation needs investigation and evaluation of all the parameters. If the department is to be interested in an expansion program of service, *i.e.,* dispensing to new clinics, opening of a new wing, etc., then the administrator should determine the cost of the materials and supplies to be required for the new program and so provide for it in the new budget. The department of pharmacy is required to maintain the detailed records in order to achieve at the figures requested by the budget.

3. **Purchase Expenses**

   The budget of purchase expenses should include the cost of prescriptions purchased from an outside pharmacy.

4. **Drugs and Pharmaceuticals**

   Many drugs and pharmaceuticals are dispensed by prescription in the hospital pharmacy department. Some drugs and pharmaceuticals used in the outpatient and emergency departments should be charged there and not to this account.

5. **Miscellaneous Supplies**

   Expenses on many materials include labels, bottles, glassware, uniform of pharmacist, stationary, narcotic and alcoholic permit fees, printed forms and reference books, etc. Some parts of budget are required to repair and maintain equipment used by this department and repairs made by outside concerns to such equipment. If required separate sub-budget should be maintained for repairing of equipments.

C. EQUIPMENT AND CONSTRUCTION BUDGET

In hospitals where a separate budget is prepared for depreciation of physical plant and equipment, it is necessary that the actual cash for replacement or remodeling is made readily available. Budget for immediate arrangement for new model of equipment is also required. If proper budget in hospitals is not a policy, then construction and purchase of equipment creates a major financial problem. Equipment and construction of new section or renovation with time is essential for the modern arrangement and techniques. Hence, a well planned budget contains initial cost as well as maintenance and repairing expenditure.

IMPLEMENTATION OF BUDGET

The budget is the important tool of any hospital. The preparation as well as implementation of budget both need. The budget is prepared by groups of departments and compiled by one department. The implementation of budget is again very difficult task because in this process the money is directly attached with the final cost of product. Implementation is a difficult process and involves following parameters :

(i) Requirement of different department
(ii) Urgent need of different department
(iii) Actual fund position
(iv) Utility of particular item
(v) Cost of products
(vi) Quantity of products
(vii) List of manufacturers with quality of products
(viii) Purchasing skill

The budget is implemented in the hospital on the basis –

(i) Utilization of budget on individual activity
(ii) Utilization of budget on group activity
(iii) Centralize utilization of budget
(iv) Department wise utilization of budget
(v) Need based utilization of budget
(vi) Emergency based utilization of budget
(vii) Technology based utilization of budget

Many managerial committees and hospital administrator take decision for proper utilization of fund on the basis of need, requirement, emergency, technology and also consider the economic mode in all conditions.

2. HOSPITAL FORMULARY

The effective use of drugs is dependent upon the care of patients in hospitals and other health-care facilities. A sound program of drug usage is developed within the institution to ensure that patients receive the best possible care. In the benefit of patient care, the institution should have organized a program of objective evaluation, selection, and use of medicinal agents in the facility. This program is useful for appropriate and economical drug therapy. The formulary concept is a method for providing such a program and has been utilized as such for many years.

A **formulary** is a continually revised collection of pharmaceuticals and important ancillary information that reflects the current clinical judgment of the medical staff.

The **formulary system** is an important tool for assuring the quality of drug use and controlling its cost that are considered most useful in patient care. The formulary system provides for the procuring, prescribing, dispensing and administering of drugs under either their non-proprietary or proprietary names in instances where drugs have both names.

The Pharmacy and Therapeutics Committee is mainly responsible for formulary system and making liaison between the medical and pharmacy staffs. The pharmacist is one of the important members of this committee. The committee is answerable to the medical staff as a whole, and its recommendations are subject to sanction by the organized medical staff, as well as to the normal administrative approval process. This committee is also responsible for making all professional policies relating to drugs in institutions, including their evaluation of appraisal, selection, procurement, storage, distribution and safe use of medication.

GUIDING PRINCIPLES

The following principles will serve as a guide to physicians. Pharmacists, nurses, and administrators in hospitals and other facilities utilizing the formulary system:

1. A multidisciplinary Pharmacy and Therapeutics Committee is appointed for organization of various hospital days to day activities.
2. The formulary system shall be sponsored by the medical staff based upon the recommendations of the Pharmacy and Therapeutics Committee. The medical staff should adjust the principles of the system to the needs of the particular institution.
3. The Pharmacy and Therapeutics Committee shall adopt written policies and procedures governing the formulary system in the Institute.
4. These policies and procedures shall give guidance in the evaluation or appraisal. Selection, procurement. Storage, distribution, safe use, and other matters relating to drugs, and shall be in print in the institution's formulary of all members of the staff.
5. Non-proprietary name drugs should be included in the formulary.
6. The proprietary names may be in common use in the institution. Prescribers should be strongly encouraged to prescribe drugs by their non-proprietary names.
7. Limiting the number of drug entities and drug products routinely available from the pharmacy can produce substantial patient care and (particularly) financial benefits.

8. The benefits are greatly increased through the use of generic equivalents and therapeutic equivalents drug entity that are consider, have very similar pharmacologic and therapeutic activities.
9. The Pharmacy and Therapeutics Committee should establish the policies and procedures governing the dispensing of generics and therapeutic equivalent. These policies and procedures should include the following important parameters such as -
   - The pharmacist is responsible for selecting, from available generic equivalents, those to be dispensed pursuant to a physician's order for a particular drug product.
   - It is also essential that the prescriber has the option, at the time of prescribing, to specify the brand or supplier of drug to be dispensed for specific order.
   - The drug product entities are determined by the Pharmacy and Therapeutics Committee that shall considered therapeutic equivalents.
   - The conditions and procedure for dispensing a therapeutic change in place of the prescribed shall be clearly delineated.
10. The existing formulary system is informed to its entire medical and nursing staff. They should know the procedure governing its operation, and any changes in those procedures. Copies of the formulary must be easily available and accessible at all times.
11. The pharmacist shall be responsible for specifications as to the quantity, and source of supply of all drugs, chemicals, biological, pharmaceutical preparations used in the diagnosis and treatment of patients. Such products should meet the standards of the Indian Pharmacopoeia, as far as possible.

FORMULARY CONTENT AND ORGANIZATION

The main objectives of the formulary system are to give the hospital staff –

1. Information regarding the list of approved drugs for use by the Pharmacy and Therapeutics Committee.
2. Proper therapeutic information regarding each approved product.
3. Information policies and procedures governing the use of drugs in the hospital, and
4. Particular information about drugs such as –
   - Calculation of doses and nomograms
   - abbreviations approved by hospital
   - sodium content of various formulary items

On the basis of objectives the formulary is divided into three main parts :

1. Part I – Information on hospital policies and procedures concerning drugs.
2. Part II - Drug products listing, and
3. Part III- Special information

INFORMATION ON HOSPITAL POLICIES AND PROCEDURES CONCERNING DRUGS

The material considered in this section will depends upon the administration of the hospital. Following items may be included in this section -

1. Operation, membership and responsibilities of Pharmacy and Therapeutics Committee (PTC).
2. Detailed Formulary policies and procedures
3. Detailed list of restricted drugs use and procedures for addition of drugs to the formulary.
4. Hospital regulations for governing the prescribing, dispensing and administration of drugs. It includes –
   - drug orders and prescriptions,
   - controlled substances considerations,
   - generic and therapeutic equivalency policies and procedures,
   - automatic stop orders,
   - verbal drug orders,
   - patients' use of their own medications,
   - self-administration of drugs by patients,
   - use of drug samples,
   - policies relative to mentioned emergency drug orders,
   - use of emergency,
   - use of floor-stock items,
   - requests by staff for medications for their own use,
   - rules to be followed by medical service representatives,
   - standard drug administration time,
   - the reporting of adverse drug reactions, and
   - medication errors

   Other topics should be included as related to the prescription.

5. Pharmacy operating procedures : It includes such as –
    - service hours
    - out-patient prescription policies
    - pharmacy charging systems
    - prescription labeling and packaging practices
    - in-patient drug distribution procedures
    - handling of drug information requests and
    - specialized services of the pharmacy
6. Information on using the formulary : It includes following information-
    - how to arrange entries of formulary,
    - the information given in each entry,
    - procedure for a given drug product, and
    - Source of information regarding details on formulary drugs.

Drug Products Listing : This section is the main part of the formulary and consists of one or more descriptive entries for individual formulary item and indexes to make easy use of the formulary.

Entries of Formulary Item : The entries can be descried in several ways:

1. Common name (Brand Name)
2. Generic name in alphabetical order
3. Route of administration
4. Dosage form, packaging and strength
5. alphabetically within therapeutic class of drugs
6. Combination of two system such as generic and brand name
7. Special sections - Ophthalmic drugs, Dermatological, Diagnostic agents

The minimum information that must be included in each entry.

Generic name of the basic drug entity or product combination products may be listed by generic, common or trade name;

a. Common synonym(s) and trade name(s);
b. directions for use;
c. dosage form(s), strength(s), packaging(s) and size(s),stocked by the pharmacy;,
d. formulation (active ingredients) of a combination product; and
e. standard category (e.g. American Hospital Formulary Service) number, if any.

Additional information which may be part of the drug entries may include :

a. range of adult or pediatric dosage or both,
b. special cautions such as: “refrigerated”, or "do not administer i.v.", “do not store in refrigerator”,
c. controlled substances symbol,
d. Price of the product. This generally will be most useful where the therapeutic classification system is used or, alternatively, lists of similar drugs (e.g. oral steroids) may be presented showing comrative cost data.aof similar drugs, and

Indexes to the Drug Products Listing : For making the formulary useful to the users, two indexes can be included at the beginning or end of this section .

1. Generic Name-Brand/Synonym Cross Index : Some substances are very similar in the name hence reference to the proper page number should be included in each entry and may alsobe arranged in alphabetical order as shown below:
   - Camphorated Opium Tincture, : synonym for paregoric : page no.
   - Paragoric : page no.
   - Proparacaine : page no.
   - Ophthaine : brand of proparacaine
   - Opththetic : brand of proparacaine
2. Therapeutic/Pharmacologic Index : In this index all formulary items are included under each therapeutic category. It is useful in ascertaining what therapeutic alternatives exist for a particular situation or emergency such as patient allergy to a particular drug.

SPECIAL INFORMATION

The material to be included in this section varies from hospital to hospital. Special information section of hospital formularies should include some important information details useful to the hospital staff and not readily available from other sources. Examples of the type of items included in this section of special information are listed below.

1. Metric conversion scales and tables.
2. List of hospital-approved abbreviations.
3. Nutritional products.
4. Tables of equivalent dosages of similar drugs (e.g., corticosteroids).
5. Table of sodium content of antacids.
6. Rules for calculating pediatric dosages.
7. Sugar-free drug products.

8. Items available from central supply.- list.
9. contents of emergency carts.
10. dialyzable poisons.
11. Pharmacokinetic dosing and monitoring information.
12. Hospital form (blank or completed) such as prescription blanks, request for non-formulary drug forms and adverse drug reaction report forms.
13. Tables of drug interactions, drug interferences with diagnostic tests, and parenteral drug incompatibilities.
14. Poison control information.

FORMULARY - FORMAT AND APPEARANCE

The format (structure) and physical appearance of the formulary influences its importance and utility. are main part of the hospital pharmacy. The part depends upon the process and ability of the pharmacist to make suitable and effective formulary system. The most of the formulary related decisions are taken by the Pharmacy and Therapeutic committee. The formulary should be handy, visually pleasing, easily readable, and professional in appearance. Elaborate and expensive artwork and cosmetic appearance are unnecessary. Proper punctuation, correct spelling, grammar and neatness for better understanding enhcance the acceptance and usage of the formulary. Format or arrangement of formularies may differ but a typical formulary must have the following composition :

1. Title page
2. Names and titles of the members of the Pharmacy and Therapeutics Committee
3. Table of contents
4. Information on hospital policies and procedures concerning drugs
   - How to use the formulary
   - Formulary system - objectives and operation
   - The Pharmacy and Therapeutics Committee of a particular hospital
   - Regulations and procedures of hospital for prescribing and dispensing drugs
   - Hospital pharmacy services and procedures
5. Products accepted for use at a particular hospital
   - Items added and deleted since the previous edition
   - Generic-brand name cross reference list
   - Pharmacologic/therapeutic index with relative cost codes
   - Descriptions of formulary drug products by pharmacologic therapeutic class

6. Appendix
    - Rules for calculating pediatric doses
    - Nomogram for estimating body surface area
    - Central service equipment and supply list
    - Schedule of standard drug administration times

The appearance and ease of use of the formulary can be further improved employing following techniques :

1. Different color paper used for each section of the formulary
2. Using an edge index
3. Making the formulary pocket size, and
4. Printing the generic name of each drug in boldface type or highlighting the same using some other method.

FORMULARY - DISTRIBUTION

All necessary steps should be taken and the copy of the formulary should be available with all responsible people involved in health care administration of patients in hospital. Each division of the pharmacy such as in-patient dispensing, out-patient dispensing, drug information service and others should receive a copy of the formulary. Heads of departments in their administrative capacity should directly receive the copy of the hospoital formulary. Copies of the formulary should be placed in all relevant places such asin each patient care unit, including clinics and other outpatient care areas such as the emergency room. It must be insured that the medical and nursing staff are familiar with the existence of formulary system in the hospital and how should it be used.

An effective mechanism must be evolved so that the formulary can be kept update. Thus, provision should be made for addition or deletion of formulary items, its periodic revision and the relevant mechanism should be widely circulated to all concerned. This enchances the utility of the hospital formulary in the real and practical sense.

FORMULARY SYSTEM - THE LEGAL BASIS

A written and signed medication or a written and signed prescription in the Doctor's Order Book (DOB) is the only legal permit to administer or dispense a prescription drug.. The pharmacist may dispense the desired preparation using a generic or chemical name or therapeutic equivalent for a prescritption or medication order, and there will be no legal legal problems irrespective of whether or not the hospital has adopted a formulary system.

If a formulary system is operating in the hospital then all prescribers are morally and ethically bound to prescribe the medication according to the formulary system. The problem usually arises when the hospital has in effect a formulary system yet the prescribers continue to use a proprietary name for the drug desired. In many instances, the prescriber is conscious of the information that the hospital is operating under the formulary system but, through routine, writes for brand-named drugs. Under these circumstances, if the prescriber had previously agreed to the policy that all prescriptions and medication orders will be dispensed without reference to brand identity, then the pharmacist may so dispense. On the other hand, if there had been no earlier permission to the policy by the physician, the pharmacist is professionally and ethically duty bound to honor the prescriber's wishes as to brand.

In order to avoid such situations, hospitals should devise methods of obtaining the prescribers' consent to the hospital formulary system.

The most common method is to print the statements like 'Dispensed according to hospital formulary system', or 'Generic Equivalent Permitted' on the prescription forms itself. In various hospitals, the permission statement is often followed by a check box with a "Yes" or "No," so that the physician can exercise an option each time he prescribes.

The second method of obtaining prior medical consent to the operation of a hospital formulary system is to incorporate the basic policy and procedures governing its use in the medical staff by-laws or in the rules and regulations

The third method of obtaining prior medical consent to the operation of a hospital formulary system is to express the policy and procedures governing the formulary system in a separate document and taking signatures of all physicians.

It is quite clear that whenever a physician accepts an appointment to a hospital staff he agrees to the medical staff as a whole so far as his practice in that hospital is concerned. As long as he admits to and treats patients in the hospital, he can not disregard or willfully circumvent the accepted by-laws of the staff or the hospital.

PRESCRIPTION WRITING

Prescription writing is the mechansism establishing the contact of the pharmacist with the patient by the mediation of the prescriber. Prescription writing in a hospital pharmacy differes slightly from that in community pharmacy or private clinics. It is essential that all prescriptions have the following information written correctly, clearly, and neatly :

1. Name and address of the patient
2. The date of prescription writing
3. The medication prescribed, its strength and total amount to be dispensed (as per format prescribed format in the Formulary)
4. The signa, containing the instructions to the patient, should be in clear, concise and simple terminology, avoiding confusing statements like 'Take/Use as directed'.
5. The physician should avoid mixing Latin and English abbreviations.

6. Refill information. Prescription shall not be refilled unless this information is clearly indicated by the prescriber.
7. Signature, name, registration number of the prescriber.

Additional important data such as (a) normal laboratory values, (b) Tables for the calculation of percentages, milliequivalents and dosages, (c) Tables of heights and weights, (d) Formulae of various diagnostic stains and reagents in common use in the hospital, and (e) other factual information; may also be included.

However whatever information is to be written on prescription should be considered, evaluated and decided by the Pharmacy and Therapeutics Committee of the hospital.

3. PURCHASE AND INVENTORY CONTROL

The word **purchse** mens "to obtain by paying money or its equivalent; to buy for price".

The word **inventory** is defined as "an itemized list of good with their estimated worth; specificlly an annul account of stock taken in any business".

The word **control** is defined as "to exercise, directing, guiding, or retraining of power over".

The purchase and inventory control of pharmaceuticals is a special and important phase of the operation of a successful hospital pharmacy. The main purpose of purchase is to ensure constant flow of raw materials of right quality, quantity and at low price. The purchasing procedure is not a simple job. Judicious purchasing in a hospital pharmacy requires short listing of accurate sources of reputed suppliers whose dealing should be reliable, honest, sharp and timely. Another parameter of purchasing is the avoidance of duplication and wastage with respect to various items purchased.

Who should purchase : Pharmacist or purchasing officer?

The purchase of drugs and pharmaceuticals is a specialty, which can be carried out to the best advantage by a pharmacist trained in managing a hospital pharmacy. This is the only department in the hospital in which it is not advisable to have purchasing done by a general purchasing agent. Since the pharmacist has the responsibility for the compounding, dispensing and manufacture of the drugs used in the hospital, he should also have the authority to specify the drugs to be purchased. If the hospital decides to purchase drugs through a purchasing officer even then the specifications must be obtained from the pharmacist. Best option, legally as well ethically, would be to purchase the drugs and pharmaceuticals through a pharmacist.

Common methods of purchasing in hospitals are described below :

a. Department wise purchasing
b. Centralized purchasing
c. Need based purchasing

d. Monthly purchasing
e. Annual purchasing
f. Emergency purchasing

It is very difficult to justify why one type of purchasing is good and more useful as compared to others. The main objective of purchasing is to obtain the required product at right time and right price. Some important parameters considered during purchasing known as 5 R are described below :

1. **Right Quality :** It is important part of purchasing and means the quality which is required according to the particular items. All items have some standards specified in the standard values such as specification, grade, brands, trade name, durability, physicochemical characteristics, application, arrangement etc. The quality must be checked with the authentication of the particular products.
2. **Right Quantity :** Timely, adequate and constant supply of material on the basis of need is required to be maintained throughout the year. If purchasing is in excess then the problems about storage and maintenance may arise hence the right quantity is an important parameter of purchasing. On the basis of previous experience the need of a particular material to be purchased in right quantity may be established avoiding shortage, excess or wastage..
3. **Right Price** : It is well known that the cost of same material varies from supplier to supplier. For right price, quality and quantity call quotation on the basis of price and quality bids. The tender should be checked carefully before considering all terms and conditions including supply condition, taxation, transportation and maintenance /warranty of the product etc.
4. **Right Source :** Some supplier gives their rate very low for consideration of the quotation and order but at the time of purchase supplier reputation and working process should be checked. It is one of the most important activities to place order of final products. Hence selection of right supplier is one of the important parts of purchasing.
5. **Right Time :** It means considering all situations including political, social, climatic and emergency conditions like floods, strikes, accidents etc. because these factors may also deviate lead time of order. Lead time means, the total time period required from the placing of order to supply of materials. Number of time demands of particular items is increased in the market hence right time consideration of purchasing is one of the most important parts.

It would be advantageous that the hospital pharmacist assumes the following duties relating to the purchase of drugs and pharmaceuticals.

1. Maintaining a lsit of names, addresses, telephone numbers, fax number, email id of manufacturers, wholesalers and their local representatives.

2. Preparing detailed specifications for drugs, chemicals and biologicals.
3. Preparing request for purchase forms.
4. Preparing Receipt Memo if the drugs are received directly by the pharmacy.
5. Preparing Return Goods Memo, if applicable.

PURCHASE PROCEDURE

Proper purchase of items in hospital pharmacy may be facilitated with the help of the following steps–

A. Requirements of Items : The pharmacist or authorized person should complete the requirements of materials to be purchased for particular period. The requirements of items are well planned for the purpose of their regular and continuous use. The purchase requisition is generally completed by departmental heads and other responsible person in the prescribed format such as –

(i) List of material

(ii) Quantity of material

(iii) Time of requirement

B. Source of Supply : The Pharmacy and Therapeutic Committee sets satisfactory standards for the purchase of quality drugs. The material is generally obtained from the following process in the store.

- Medical Store
- Direct from whole sellers
- Direct from manufacturers
- From Directorate General of Supplies and Disposals (DGS & D)
- Large supply by inviting tenders
- Specific items or emergency purchases from local suppliers

C. Purchase Order : The Pharmacy and Therapeutic Committee or Chief Pharmacist, after confirming the supplier prepares a **purchase order** containing detailed description, specification, quantity, packaging unit, price and quantity needed of the items. All purchasing order should be in written form with all terms and conditions specified in the order. The number of copies of order depends on the regulation of a particular hospital. The general process of purchasing order requires multi copy snap-out form so as to supply copies as follows :.

(i) One copy to the vendor (supplier)

(ii) Second copy to account section

(iii) Third copy to the purchasing number file

(iv) Fourth copy to the initiating department

(v) Fifth and sixth as receiving reports, sent to the receiving department, and

(vi) Seventh copy to guard file or master file (history copy) to be retained by the purchasing agent.

For timely supply of order it is essential to follow-up the purchase order regularly.

D. Receipt of Acknowledgment: Number of times the supplier may complain about not receiving the order sent by couriers or by any other means. The order to supplier must be confirmed by sending a copy of purchase order in duplicate. The supplier should send back the copy with signature and confirm the acceptance of order. It is also important that in case of any confusion or misunderstanding regarding order or supply condition, every thing must be cleared while accepting the purchase order.

E. Receipt of Drugs : The material should be checked to confirm the (a) quantity of material, (b) quality of material, (c) price of material, (d) original package of product, and (e) verification of specification

The same person is also responsible for checking the availability of material in stocks, date of expiry, description, quantity, batch number, as given in the Order Form. Some time random sampling can be conducted to make sure that product is in original position. There should be no change in colour, odour and other physical as well as chemical properties. If any change is observed during the storage the matter should be informed in writing to medical superintendent and concerned Drugs Inspector of the area. These stocks should never be used until the Drugs Inspector's permission is granted and even the information should be given to the supplier and manufacturer. After the examination of drugs by the officer, they should give "No objection" to accept the supply in writing on the hospital copies of delivery challans or invoices by putting signature and date. The invoice received from the supplier is sent to accounts section for verification and for payment. All types of payment should be by cheque or by Draft, not cash.

F. Distribution of Drugs : The drugs are received from manufacturer in the original packing. It is not possible to deliver the material in original packing in the wards of the hospital. Drugs should be distributed in clean containers so that the integrity and original properties can be preserved. On the label following detail should be mentioned – Name of drug, quantity, date of expiry etc. It is always desirable that appropriate precautions should be taken to dispose off original empty containers and to avoid their misuse. It is also required to prepare written statement for disposal of container in the presence of responsible person also puts date and signature on the written statement. Chief pharmacist should visit wards to check the storage condition, cleaning and arrangement of the system.

Purchase or Repair Request Form

PQRS Hospital, Nanded

Date : ________________

Purchase / Repair of Equipment

Department Name : _________________________________
Purchase order no. : _________________________________

Date of Supply : _________________________________

Suggested Vendors : 1. ___________________________________
2. ___________________________________
3. ___________________________________

No.	Description-Specification-Packaging	Price per unit	Units Needed	Total Price	Quantity	
					On hand date	Used per month

Required by : _____________________ Approved by : __________________

Fig 19.1 Purchase or Repair Request Form

INVENTORY CONTROL

Management of Inventory

The actual meaning of the word inventory focuses our attention on cataloguing the materials related to stores. It is a list or schedule of articles. Inventory is considered to be an ideal resource that possesses economic values. It is nothing but a stock of goods that we maintain to facilitate the continuous production of goods or services. Like other organizations, the hospitals also need to manage inventory because a large number of materials are used by hospitals for which we find an independent materials and stores department. It is the prime responsibility of a material manager that he/she in consultation with the hospital manager manages inventory in such a way that possibilities of misuse of materials are checked. In a majority of the government hospitals, we find mismanagement of inventory which has been very much instrumental in the waste, misuse, theft and pilferages resulting into the huge financial looses. The mismanagement of inventory increases the cost of healthcare services. In an age of information technology, it is easier to manage the inventory in a right fashion. A material manager with the support of computers would be successful in cataloguing the materials and proper documentation would be made regarding the issue of inventory to the persons and departments. The management of inventory thus paves the avenues for optimizing the costs of Medicare services besides making available materials to the patients which increase the quality of healthcare services. It is in this context that we need to go through the problem of management of inventory.

An inventory can be described as the sum of the value of raw materials, finished product, parts of maintenance, consumables, semi-processed materials and finished goods stock of a hospital. Inventories are primarily maintained for smooth running of system. Inventory management is essential to maintain a large size inventory for efficient and smooth working. It also minimizes a firm's investment in inventory with a view to gain maximum profit. For proper management of all activities it is evident that neither excessive nor inadequate inventories are kept.

Objectives of Inventory Control

The main purpose of having an inventory control is :

1. To supply the drug in time.
2. To give maximum customer service.
3. To reduce or minimize inventory investment.
4. To maintain plant operation at low cost.
5. To avoid stock out and shortages.
6. To use capital profitably.
7. To avoid wastage.

Techniques of Inventory Controls

Different techniques commonly used to control the inventory are planning, acquisition, control of material and storage. The following techniques are commonly used -

1. ABC analysis
2. Economic Order Quantity (EOQ)
3. VED analysis
4. Perpetual inventory system
5. Review of slow and non-moving items
6. Setting of various levels
7. Use of material budgeting
8. Establishing an effective purchase procedure.
9. Computerization of inventory control
10. Buffer stock

<table>
<tr><td rowspan="7">Hospital</td><td>ABC (Always Better Control)</td><td rowspan="7">Inventory Control</td></tr>
<tr><td>HML (High, Medium, Low)</td></tr>
<tr><td>VED (Vital, Essential, Desirable)</td></tr>
<tr><td>FSN (Fast Moving Slow Moving Non Moving)</td></tr>
<tr><td>SDE (Scarce Difficult Easy)</td></tr>
<tr><td>GOLF (Government Ordinary Local Foreign)</td></tr>
<tr><td>SOS (Seasonal Off-Seasonal)</td></tr>
</table>

Fig 19.2 Inventory Control Methods

1. ABC ANALYSIS

ABC analysis is very common tool in drug stores where large inventory items are stocked.

A- means **A**lways

B- means **B**etter

C- means **C**ontrol

In this technique, the materials are divided into three groups A, B and C according to the cost of the materials and money value of consumption.

A Class : This group includes some of the costly items, which may not be more than 10-15% of the total items but account for about 70-80% of the total budget of inventories. These types of items require proper storage conditions. Only necessary quantities of these inventories are purchased and stocked, over stocking is always avoided.

B Class : This class is intermediate between A and C in terms of the cost of the items. The items in Class B constitute 20-25% of the total quantity of the inventories while account for 20% of the total expenditure of inventories.

C Class : The items in Class C are relatively cheaper in cost and represents 60-70% of the total quantity of the inventories. About 5-10% of the total expenditure of inventories is spent on these items.

Advantages of ABC Analysis

Following are the main advantages of ABC analysis -

- The investment in inventory can be maintained and funds can be used in the best possible manner.
- Easy to control on costly items
- Suitable for maintaining safety of total stock value
- Easy to maintain stock and turnover rate
- Fully tested method for high stock

2. **Economic Order Quantity (EOQ)**

This technique is very useful to ascertain how much of the inventory is to be ordered. The correct quantity to buy is the quantity at which the ordering cost and the inventory carrying cost will be minimum.

The ordering cost consists of the cost of stationary, salary of employee, storage, follow-up, receiving, inspection etc. This method is useful for avoiding some expenditure which are generally not required.

Mainly three methods are used for determination of EOQ -

1. Tabular determination of EOQ
2. Graphic presentation of EOQ
3. Determination of EOQ by an algebraic formula.

Here, EOQ determination is discussed by using the following formula –

$$EOQ = \sqrt{\frac{2A \text{ x } B}{CS}}$$

Where, A = annual consumption, B = buying cost per order, C = cost per unit of material, and S = storage and other inventory carrying costs.

After calculation of EOQ value the frequency or number of items to be purchased can be determined by dividing the annual requirement by the order.

3. VED Analysis

This system is based on the utility of the material in the drug store. It is very useful in controlling and maintaining the stock of various types of formulations of a particular group of drugs. In this method all items in the different brands of drug formulation are classified into anyone of the following categories: ***V***ital, ***E***ssential, and ***D***esirable. For example, Aspirin tablets are available as Disprin, Anacin and Micropyrine. If there is great demand of Anacin tablets then it is considered as vital item, Disprin may be considered under essential items because of its lesser demand and Micropyrine may be considered as desirable item because there are hardly a few prescriptions for this brand. According to this example, there should be maximum stock of Anacin tablets, followed by Disprin and then very less number of Micropyrin tablets in the drug store inventory.

4. Perpetual inventory system

Maintaining a perpetual inventory is an ideal method provided the record keeping is up to date. In small pharmacies, at the end of the day, the pharmacist can summarise all drugs, charge slips and make appropriate postings in the perpetual inventory file. One of the methods is called the 'peg board' that requires a peg board and requisition forms with holes evenly spaced and punched along the top. The large hospitals may require mechanized operations through equipment marketed by IBM (International Business Machines) or Remington Corporation.

In this method store balance is checked after every receipt and issue to facilitate regular checking and to prevent closing down for stock-taking. The perpetual inventory system comprises of three parts –

1. Bin card
2. Stores ledger
3. Continuous stock-taking

Bin card : This document is maintained by the store-keeper to keep record of all items of materials and goods in his store. This serves as is a ready reference. It shows quantities of each material received, issued and in stock. A bin card is applied for each material. Each receipt, issue or return is recorded on bin card in a sequential order and the latest balance is given in each receipt and issue.

XYL Hospital Pharmacy., Bhopal

BIN CARD

Description of material :

Bin No. :

Code No. :

Normal quantity to order :

Stores ledger folio No. :

Maximum stock level :

Re-order stock level :

Date	Receipt		Issue		Balance
	G.R. No.	Quantity	S.R. No.	Quantity	Quantity

Fig 19.3 Format of Bin card

Store Ledger : It is a very useful inventory control system. The store ledger contains loose leaf cards for easy removal and insertion. It is used to maintain all costly items.

XYL Hospital Pharmacy., Vijaywada
STORE LEDGER ACCOUNT

Description of material :	Maximum stock :
Code No. :	Minimum stock :
Bin No. :	Re-order stock level :
Location :	Ordering quantity :
Unit :	

Date	Receipt				Issue				Balance			Stock Verified		
	G.R. No,	Qty.	Rate	Amt.	G.R. No,	Qty.	Rate	Amt.	Qty.	Rate	Amt.	Date	Int.	Rem.

G.R.No. means Goods Receipt Number; S. R. No. means Stock Receipt Number

Fig. 19.4 Format of Stores Ledger Account

Continuous stock-taking : In this system limited number of items are verified on a day. The items are selected of the on the basis of utility. All items are checked at least a certain number of times in a year while checking of a particular item is evenly distributed during the period. The selected numbers of items are counted every day and matched with the bin card and also by the store ledger.

5. Review of slow and non-moving items

Inventory is an important constituent of total cost and as such a proper system of inventory control. It is divided in three parts –

1. Periodic report : Periodic report consists of monthly or quarterly report of stocks of non-moving items. It shows purchase, consumption and balance in hand of such items.

2. Obsolete items : Obsolete items list may consist of slow and non-moving items. It is useful to control the purchasing these items.
3. Moving ratios : This shows the turnover of slow moving items, inactive and dead stocks. The moving ratio may be calculated periodically.

6. Setting of various levels

This method is useful to maintain inventory control to decide upon various levels of materials. These are **maximum**, **minimum** and **reorder** levels. The level of the particular items may be changed on the basis of demand. The level of the maximum stock is fixed by considering the following points.

1. Nature of material
2. Restrictions of Government
3. Rate of consumption of material
4. Market trend
5. Storage space available
6. Amount of capital needed
7. Amount of capital available
8. Fashion habits
9. Risk involved due to accident
10. Lead time from the date of placing the order

Maximum level = Re-order level + Re-order quantity + Minimum consumption

Minimum consumption = Minimum consumption (per week) x Minimum re-order period

7. Use of material budgeting

In this method purchase budget of both the whole-stock and the individual items is prepared. Following factors are to be considered during the preparation of material budget.

- Sales status - increase or decrease in previous month as compared with the previous year.
- Management of over buying or under buying during the previous month or year.

These information is made it is subtracted from the balance of the purchase budget maintained in a separate purchase record. On the basis of data the purchase of inventory will come to know whether buying is too much or is less by referring to purchase budget.

8. **Establishing an effective purchase procedure.**

   In this method, the purchase procedure starts with the recognition or realization of the need of an item. The requirement is given in the prescribed form in writing. On the basis of items, the sources are identified and suitable suppliers are selected. The order is placed with the selected supplier and monitored thoroughly. After verification of invoice, payment is made accordingly.

   Every business organization prepares its own purchasing manual, which prescribes the purchase policies and procedures. The purchasing policies differ from company to company. It is true that good purchase policies and inventory control are interlinked with each other. If applied properly in purchasing these policies are effective in controlling the inventories.

Controls on Purchases

Putting monetary restrictions on the purchase of drugs and pharmaceuticals in hospital pharmacy by the administrators is unjustified and unscientific method of management.

In order to control such purchases a modern and reliable method of **Computation of inventory turnover** can be safely adopted in hospital pharmacy. It can be computed by dividing the cost of goods sold during a financial year (fiscal period) by the average of opening and closing inventories. Thus one can calculate the number of times the inventory has been 'turned' over during the financial year. A low turnover indicates (a) duplication of stock, (b) large purchase of slow-moving items, and (c) dead inventory. Similarly a high turnover of inventory would small volume purchasing and failure to take advantage of the maximum quantity discounts.

In general, a turnover of six to eight times a year is considered satisfactory for most of the hospitals, depending on available cash reserves.

Purchase volume and inventory can be controlled by the hospital pharmacist following the time of the Economic Order Quantity (EOQ) and Reorder Quantity Level (RQL). RQL is the inventory level that must be reached before additional stock can be ordered but zero stock must be avoided because it may cause serious problems. An easy way of avoiding this is by building into the system "safety factors" for various vendor lead times, as explained in the following Table.

Safety Factors for Various Vendor Lead Times

Vendor Lead Time(VLT), Weeks	*Safety Factor*
0 to 2	1.0
2 to 5	1.5
5 to 8	2.0
8 to 11	2.5
11 to 15	3.0

The RQ can be determined by dividing the **average usage rate** per month in units of issue by thirteen weeks, and then multiplying this figure by the average **vendor lead time** plus the safety factor.

$$RQL = \frac{\text{Average usage rate per month}}{13} \times \text{Average supply lead time} + \text{safety factor}$$

Under certain conditions the hospitals may have to evolve their own EOQ, RQL, SLT and Safety Factors for example when there are uncertainties of availability of raw materials, power crisis, labour crisis etc.

9. Modern Computerization of Inventory Control

In these days, the all types of purchasing and inventory control are made by computer application. Many software agencies are involve working on the inventory control system. They have also established many type of software for this purpose. National Informatics Centre (NIC) has developed software for maintaining inventory control throughout the year including day to day facilities. Computerized system is highly useful as compared to other system of inventory control due to following advantages.

- Very fast system
- Multiplies the data in shortest period of time
- Minimum investment required
- Minimums space required
- Easy to handle using pen-drive, CD etc.
- Minimum wastage
- Very fast supply of items
- Very fast payments
- Minimum main power required

10. BUFFER STOCK

This is useful in the emergency to meet the unexpected demands. It means to maintain at least the minimum quantity of a particular item in the stores at all times. Buffer stock requires following factors for consideration.

- Lead time
- Nature of item
- Speed of consumption
- Availability of substitutes
- Re-order level
- Stock out cost

4. ORGANIZATION OF DRUG STORE

LAYOUT DESIGN

Mainly three factors are responsible for success of drug store/wholesale store.

1. Location
2. Professional management
3. Strong financial support

Other factors such as – design, placement of article, display, supporting staff, advertisement etc, are also important.

Common Design of Drug Stores

It is very difficult to classify the design of drug store because it depends on the size of drug store and organization according to product as well as cutomers. Some common designs are given here.

a. I shape counter : Very common, needs less space, most suitable for small drug store
b. L Shape counter : Very common, needs more space as compare to I shape for semi drug store
c. T shape counter : Not very common but most suitable if delivery place is different
d. U shape counter : Very common but need big space, most suitable in big drug store
e. F shape counter : In big cities and also in shopping moll, have separate cash counter with modern technology, very useful and also minimize the theft.
f. E Shape counter : not very common but most common in shopping moll where purchasing, delivery and payment counter all are not at common place.

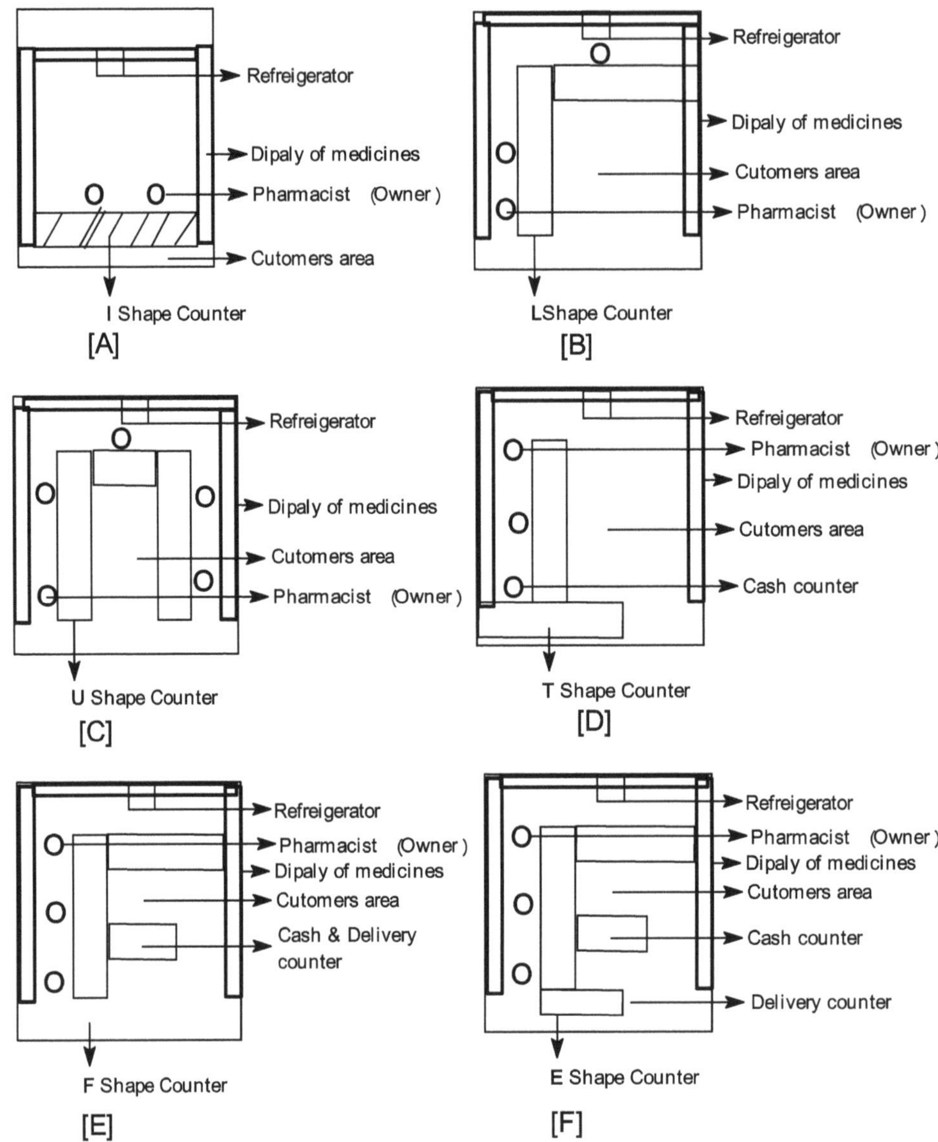

Figure 19.5 A to F Common designs of Drug Stores

Main purpose of a good layout design

The main aim of a good layout design is to achieve the following objectives :

a. To provide maximum facilities to customers so that purchasing is increased from each customer entering inside the store.

b. To draw more attention of customers toward the drug store.
c. Full on display including new products for kids growth and ladies requirements.
d. All schemes and professional leaflet for introducing new common product (not required prescription)
e. Some other specific objectives includes
   - Fixed cost of articles
   - Availability of professional image
   - Provide customers satisfaction and convenience
   - Provide sufficient parking place near to store
   - Properly attending the customer upto the satisfaction
   - Proper utilization of space
   - Provide hygienic place and drinking water facility

Characteristic of good layout design of Drug Store

A good drug stores layout design should have the following characteristic :

1. There should provide sufficient and properly ventilated space inside the store and comfortable to customers.
2. There should have air conditioner/cooler in side the drug store.
3. There should be adequate lighting, ventilation and partitioning of areas, as required.
4. There should be soft light (not irritating) in side of the store.
5. The wall and roof should be painted properly using light colour because of pleasant nature of light colours.
6. Sufficient number of wooden or steel racks should be arranged for storage of storage of drugs.
7. Maintain dust free environment using glass paneling and proper transparent gate with door closure.
8. Use proper stainless steel stool or stair to pick the material stored at upper part of shelves at height inside the store.
9. Sufficient waiting space should be provided for the customers if required arranged comfortable chairs.
10. Delivery counter /Cash Counter should be well maintained with decorative material and also depicting instructions, if any.
11. Used suitable carry bags paper/poly materials with instruct ion slip helpful to patient.
12. Maintained the computerized billing system.

LEGAL REQUIREMENTS FOR ESTABLISHMENT OF DRUG STORES

Under the Sale of Goods Act the term 'sale' is defined as 'a contract for sale of goods is a contract whereby the seller transfers or agrees to transfer the property in goods to the buyer for a price'. The drugs reach the consumers from the manufacturers by retail through shopkeepers. Manufacturers generally sell their goods to the stockiest who in turn sell the same to the shopkeepers. This transaction between the stockiest and the shopkeepers is the wholesale. Under the Drugs (Prices Control) Order, 1987 'wholesaler' means a dealer or his agent, or a stockiest appointed by a manufacturer or an importer for the sale of his drugs to a retailer; and a retailer means a dealer carrying on the retail business of sale of drugs to customers.

Sale of drugs being a specialized job, different from the sale of common goods, the Drugs and Cosmetics Act, 1940 and the Rules thereunder provide for a licence for the purpose. If drugs are sold or stocked for sale at more than one place, separate licence should be taken in respect of each such place. However, this is not applicable to itinerant (travelling from place to place) vendors. For the purposes of issuing licences, the State Government is empowered to appoint Licensing Authority (LA) for specified areas. A LA may, with the written approval of the State Government, delegate the powers to sign licences and other specified powers to any person under his control.

Sale of Drugs

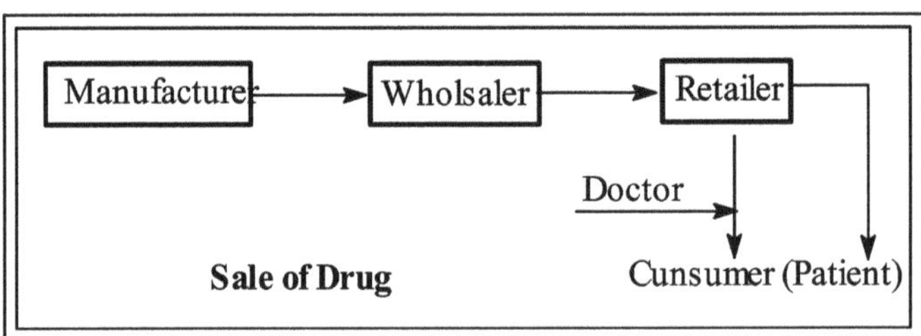

Sale of Drug

Dispensing and compounding of drugs

For the purposes of the Drugs & Cosmetics Act and Rules, *"Pharmacy"* means and includes every store or shop or other place –

(i) where drugs are dispensed *i.e.* measured, weighed or made up and supplied; or

(ii) where drugs are prepared; or

(iii) where prescriptions are compounded; or

(iv) which by sign, symbol or indication gives the impression that the operations mentioned or

(v) which has upon it or displayed within it or affixed to or used in connection with it a sign bearing the word or words 'Pharmacy', 'Pharmacist', 'Dispensing Chemist', or 'Pharmaceutical Chemist', *or*

(vi) which is advertised in these terms.

In granting license for a *pharmacy* the licensing authority may have regard to (i) average number of licenses granted during the period of 3 years immediately preceding; *and* (ii) the occupation, trade or business ordinarily carried out by such applicant during the preceding 3 years.

Supply of any drug other than those specified in Schedule X on a prescription of a RMP should be recorded at the time of supply in a prescription register maintained fur the purpose and the serial number of the entry in register should be entered on the prescription. Following particulars should be entered in the register:-

(1) Serial number of the entry

(2) The date of supply

(3) Name and address of the prescriber

(4) Name and address of the patient/owner of the animal if the drug is supplied for the veterinary use

(5) Name and quantity of the drug

(6) In case of Schedule H and X drugs the name of manufacturer, its batch number and expiry date, if any

(7) Signature of the registered pharmacist under whose supervision the medicine was made or supplied.

If the drugs are not compounded in the premises and supplied in the original container, then particulars specified in (1) to (6) above may be entered in a cash or credit memo book.

In the case of refill prescriptions it shall be sufficient if the new entry in the register included a serial number, the date of supply, the quantity supplied and a reference to the entry when the drug was dispensed on the previous occasion.

It is not necessary to record the particulars in the register or cash or credit memo in respect of-

1. Drugs supplied against prescriptions under the Employee's State Insurance Scheme if all the particulars are given on the prescription, and
2. Any drug other than those specified in Schedule C and H if it is supplied in the original container.

STORAGE OF DRUGS

In general, drugs should be stored in manner prescribed under the Drugs & Cosmetics Act and Rules as well as the instruction given by the manufacturer on the label.

a. Storage of Schedule X drugs

Substances specified in Schedule X should be stored under lock and key in cupboard or drawer reserved solely for the storage of these substances or in a part of the store separate from the remainder of the store and to which only responsible persons have access.

b. Storage of veterinary drugs

Veterinary drugs should be stored:-

(i) In a cupboard or drawer reserved for storage of veterinary drugs; *or*

(ii) in a portion of the premises separated from the remainder of the premises to which customers are not permitted to have access.

c. Maintenance of record of Wholesale and Retail drug stores

Proper record should be maintained of sale and purchase of wholesale and retail drug store.

d. Record of purchase of Drugs

The records should be maintained under the following headings:

(i) Date of purchase with bill number

(ii) Name and quantity of the drug its batch number

(iii) Name of the manufacturer of the drug

(iv) Licence number of seller with validity

RECORDS OF SALE OF DRUGS

Sale of drug specified in Schedule X

Schedule X means list of drugs whose import, manufacturing and sale, labeling and packaging are governed by special provisions. For sale and purchase a bound, serially numbered register should be maintained and separate pages for each drugs be provided. In the register following particulars are maintained:

1. Date of purchase
2. Name of the drug
3. Quantity of the drug supplied
4. Name and address of the supplier
5. Licence number of the supplier
6. Manufacturer's name and batch number

7. Name and address of the purchaser
8. Quantity received
9. Detail of prescription in which the drug used
10. Bill number and date of receipt of purchase
11. Signature with date of the person under whose supervision the drugs have been sold

Sale of drug other than those specified in Schedule X

The following particulars are required to be entered in a prescribed register maintained for the purchase or credit memo.

1. Serial number of entry
2. Date of supply
3. Name and address of the prescriber
4. Name and address of the patient (if the drug is supplied for veterinary purpose, name and address of the owner should be maintained).
5. Name of drug with quantity should be mentioned in the register
6. Name of manufacturer and its batch number, expiry date are required if Schedule H and C drugs.
7. Signature of the registered pharmacist under whose supervision the drugs supplied.

5. PATIENT COUNSELING

The pharmaceutical sciences are developing rapidly all over the world. The responsibility of the pharmacist towards proper utilization of this scientific knowledge in the proper use of modern medicine, is also gradually improving. The pharmacist has to perform dual role –

a. Counseling and educating the patient
b. Monitoring of drug levels and also providing relevant information to the physicians.

Patient counseling is defined as providing medication information to the patients or their representatives orally or in written form for proper use of medicament. Following precaution are essential to take while counseling the patient.:

(i) Use language that the patient understands
(ii) Use appropriate counseling aids such as diagram, photos, pictures, videos, computer that may be easily understood by the patient.
(iii) Present facts and concepts in simple words and in logical order
(iv) Use open ended questions.

Patient counseling consists of mainly three stages :

1. Introduction
2. Satisfaction of patient and family person curiosity
3. Technical part and revision

1. Introduction

a. Introduce your self and discuss purpose of counseling
b. History taking of the patient – present and past history of patient and family persons, if required
c. Review the patient's record and family history.
d. Obtain drug related information
e. Assess the patient's understanding of the reasons for therapy
f. Assess any actual and / or potential concerns or problems of importance to the patient.

2. Technical part

(i) The medicine's generic and brand name and how it helps the patient.
(ii) How to be taken- with or without milk, before or after meal, and breakfast etc.
(iii) How long it takes to begin working and duration of therapy
(iv) How long it will be necessary to take the medicine
(v) What to do if you missed a dose
(vi) Restrictions on activities while taking the medicine
(vii) When to seek help if there are problems
(viii) How long to wait before reporting no change in symptoms
(ix) The cost of the medicine
(x) How to have your prescription refilled, if necessary

3. Technical part and revision

(i) How to remove the drug from the package
(ii) How to administer certain medication such as ENT preparations, rectal/vaginal products
(iii) Importance of medication for patient's well being.
(iv) Side effect medications
(v) Drug interactions (drug-drug, drug-food) and adverse reactions
(vi) Storage condition of dosage forms
(vii) Precautions to be taken during the treatment

(viii) Supply medication reminder chart

(ix) Necessity to complete the course.

Management of drugs

Proper management of drugs is essential because the mismanagement, in addition to the financial losses, would also be dangerous if not rightly administered. The WHO documents focus on the problem of drug management in hospitals. Making productive use of drugs and regulating the waste of drugs are the important objectives of drug management and therefore a hospital pharmacist should take necessary steps to the management of drugs. There are a number of factors found instrumental in increasing the waste of drugs and some of them are the following:

Causes of Hospital waste

A non-optimal use of drugs results into waste. We find cases where a number of drugs are administered on one patient when he/she requires an optimal dose. This results into waste and in addition to the side-effects, we also find non-availability of drugs for the needed patients.

Some of the doctors develop a craze for using expensive drugs when we find low-cost drugs equally effective. This draws our attention on brand loyalty resulting into a waste, and an increase in the Medicare costs.

'Just to try it' or 'Trial and Error" method has been found common. A large number of drugs, though not necessary for the patients, are prescribed by the doctors. This in addition to an increase in the cost of treatment also the generates side-effects. It is really amazing that some of the doctors just to get commission from the dispensaries adopt such a practice which results into the waste of drugs, vis-à-vis over medication.

Disproportionate dose also results into a waste. We also find cases where the doctors administer a larger dose of drugs when even smaller dose would have been equally effective.

Prescribing drugs to those patients who don't use and throw them, or to the patients not serious to the management of treatment and avoid to use the drugs regularly, also resulting into the waste of drugs.

Over-supply also results into a waste. We also find cases that just to get commission, the over supply of drugs is practiced and we have no option but to throw them after the expiry date.

Inadequate provisions for preserving the expensive and sensitive drugs also result into a waste. This is due to the fact that proper refrigeration or preservation facilities are not made available. Vaccines in a majority of the cases are no longer effective and are to be discarded.

Mismanagement of drugs also occurs due to improper steps such as exposing drugs to sunlight of heat.

A non-optimal supply by the stores also results into a waste.

The aforesaid reasons generate huge financial losses and in addition also increase the costs on treatment. It is against this background that hospital administrators and pharmacists should appreciate and endeavour a scientific management of drugs so that cases of waste are checked and financial losses to the hospitals are regulated. It is the prime responsibility of a material/stores/hospital manager to take due care of drugs so that the increasing cases of waste are checked.

Sensing Patients about Drugs

To be more specific in the Indian society where we find the rate of literacy low, it is the prime responsibility of a hospital manager to educate and sense the patients in a right fashion so that the increasing cases of over-medication are checked. It is really amazing that in the Indian society, a majority of us believe that taking more drugs and expensive drugs would solve their problems but in lieu of getting relief from the medicines, they face the problem of side-effects and invite a number of serious health problems. This makes it essential that we educate and sense the masses and patients with creative slogans and messages so that they come to know about the side-effects of wrong or over-medication. It is against this background that we talk about innovating the promotional measures or revolutionizing the process of healthcare communications. The following steps are to be effective in sensing the patients.

Narrating the Facts: The prescription should be written carefully. At the very outset, it is the responsibility of doctors attending on the patients to explain to the patients or their attendants certain facts about drug usage. Let them know about the side-effects of excess dose and over-medication. It is essential because in a number of cases we find patients and attendants believing in the principle of taking excess dose of medicines.

Explaining Facts in Catalogue: In the library of hospitals, we find catalogue detailing the list of medicines. It is considerably important that a hospital manager with the consultation of doctors explain the dose and duration to be followed by the patients and attendants believing in the principle of taking excess dose of medicines.

Displaying Signposts: For sensing the patients and attendants, it is also pertinent that some of the selected medicines, often prescribed by the doctors, be mentioned in the signposts detailing the dose and duration, besides the side-effects. At different important places of the hospitals where patients and attendants assemble in a large number, the display of signposts would be instrumental in informing and sensing them. Since the hospital managers are supposed to know about creativity in messages and slogans, the task of sensitizing the patients and attendants in a right fashion would be found easier.

Informative Packaging: In addition, the pharmaceutical industry also bears the responsibility of informing and sensing the patients and attendants with the help of detailed information regarding the dose, duration and the side effects. If the patients and attendants come to know about the details, there would be less scope for taking the excess dose.

Social Advertising to be Promoted: Besides, The media, pharmaceutical industry, health department, social organization, leading hospitals bear the responsibility of promoting social advertising. This would let the patients and attendants know about the side-effects and over-medication due to the excess dose of medicines. To be more specific in the Indian society, we find it essential because the masses are illiterate and they don't know about the harmful effects of taking excess dose and over-medication.

Explaining the Use Drugs; It is pertinent that we explain to the patients the right way of using the medicines. Each drug has a particular effect in a particular condition and therefore a drug taken by an individual will not help another. They should be made clear that the optimal dose of medicines plays an important role. If it is too little, the effects are very slow and if it is too high the reactions and side-effects can't be avoided. The dose for children is found different. They should be made it clear that regularity or continuity in treatment plays an effective role because it helps in maintaining the required dose of medicines in the body. We find treatment as a course and the patients need to complete the full course. If the course remains incomplete, the possibilities of relapse resulting into an even more dangerous condition can't be ruled out. The place for drugs should be out of the reach of the small children who may use it and the effects may be very dangerous.

Explaining The Use Of Life Saving Drugs

While sensing the patients it is also significant that we explain to them the importance of the live saving drugs.

In a few cases we find the condition of the patients so acute that immediate use of drugs is found essential since a delay in the uses of drugs may results in irreparable losses.

The material and stores manager should be advised to keep the stock of the life saving drugs.

It is essential that they are made available a list of vital or a life saving drug and place them in a shelf.

The shelf is required to be checked frequently

The aforesaid facts make it clear that patients and attendants are required to be sensed in a right way so that effect of medicines helps them in quick recovery besides the side-effects are also checked. To be more specific in the Indian condition we find it essential because the masses are illiterate and they don't know about the right and proper use of medicine help they believe that medicine are to be taken and a minor change in the dose and duration carries no meaning for them where as the realities are found something different. We find the medicine essential but at the same time we can't negate side effects to be more dangerous because the side effects are resulting into even the irreparable losses. We find frequent cases of over- medication especially at places where the patients are not conscious. Of course, this also requires proper education to the doctors who prescribe the medicines. The practice of trial and error has been found resulting into hazardous side effects. The doctor, in a few cases, doesn't know about the importance of dose and duration. While educating and training, they should be made clear that side effects and over- medication are more dangerous

In the management of hospital, we find marketing of hospital services significant and while explaining the promotional measures we have gone through the problem in detail. It is in the context that we talk about healthcare communications. Educating, informing and sensing the patients or even the masses are found important, especially in the Indian condition where the doctors take it very lightly. Proper instruction or guidelines to patients are found essential to counter the possibilities of the hazardous side effects. In a true sense, it is a major problem requiring due attention of almost all segments. The doctors, the media, the social organizations, the Red Cross societies need to understand the importance of use of drugs or medicines to get the positive effects and remove the side effects.

Types of Materials Stocked

In the drug store proper racks open and closed should be available in sufficient number for storage of drugs. The mobility area and circulation space should be sufficient. Safety arrangement such as – ABC Fire Extinguisher, BC Fire extinguisher and CO_2 fire extinguishers should be placed at strategic points along with fire buckets for immediate control of fire near to the store. Following materials are stocked.

(i) Tablets, Capsules, Syrups, Mixtures, Liquid dosage form, Semi solid dosage form etc.

(ii) Sterile products such as ophthalmic, parenteral etc.

(iii) Antibiotics, biological stored in refrigerator.

(iv) Narcotics and psychotropic substances stored under lock and key.

(v) Alcohol and alcohol containing preparations

(vi) Vaccines, sera and other thermolabile drugs stored under cold (2-10^{0}C)

(vii) Vitamins, antibiotics, liver preparations stored at cool temperature (15-20^{0}C)

(viii) Schedule X drugs stored separately under lock and key.

(ix) Large bulk items on bottom.

(x) Poisons stored in separate closed rack, labelled as 'POISON'.

Storage Conditions

a. Cold temperature : 2-8^{0}C

b. Cool temperature : 8-25^{0}C

c. Room temperature : temperature in working area around 25-30^{0}C

d. Warm : 30-40^{0}C

e. Excessive heat : Above 40^{0}C

Table 19.1 List of Some Drug Products to be Stored in Cold Conditions (2-8^0 C)

Sera	**Cobra Venom in Solution**	**Schick test Toxin**
Vaccines	Viper Venom in Solution	Cholistin Sulphamethate Injection
Whole Human Blood	Insulin Preparations	Suxamethonium Chloride Injection
Normal Human Plasma	Oxytocin Injection	Human Gamma Globulin Injection
Thrombin	Vasopressin Injection	Corticotropin Zinc Oxide Injection
Thromboplastin	Corticotropin Gelatin Injection	Posterior Pituitary Injection

Table 19.2 List of Some Products to be Stored at Cool Tmperature (8-25^{0}C)

<table>
<tr>
<td>Blood Preparations
Dried plasma
Human fibrin foam
Human fibrinogen
Human Serum Dried
Human Thrombin</td>
<td>Vitamins Preparations
Vitamin B Complex Elixir, Vitamin B Complex Injection, Vitamin K Injection
Vitamin K preparations
Other preparations containing Vitamin A, B_1, B_2, B_6 and Vit. C and D containing products</td>
<td rowspan="2">Other Preparations
Anaesthetic ether
Chlorambucin
Chlorhexidine
Choline Theophyline Preparations
Injection
Dextran, Dextran Sulfate, Dextrose and sodium, Dextrose
Dihydrotachysterol
Dimercaprol Heparin,
Hyaluronidase, Injection
Domiphen Bromide
Glyceryl Trinitrite Tablets
Halothane
Liver Injection crude
Pancreatin
Paraldehyde
Trichloroethylene</td>
</tr>
<tr>
<td>Antibiotic Containing Products
Cephaloridine, Neomycin, Neobiocin, Nystatin, Viomycin, Cycloserine preparations
Benzethine Penicillin, Eloxacillin, Methicillin, Ampicillin, Streptomycin Sulphate and Chloride Preparation, Chloramphenicol, Tetracycline, Oxytetracycline, Chlortetracycline and Dimethyl Chlortetracycline, Bacitracin and Zinc Bacitracin Preparations</td>
<td>Hormone Preparation
Corticotropin, Oxytocin Tablets
Chorionic Gonadotropin, Betamethasone Sodium Phosphate Injection
Prednisolone Sodium Phosphate Injection
Arsenicals Preparations
Neoarsphenamine Injection
Sulpharsphenamine Injection
Tryprsanide Injection</td>
</tr>
</table>

The life periods of drugs under Schedule P of Drugs and Cosmetics Act and Rules mention the periods in months if the drugs are stored under prescribed conditions.

6. ROLE OF PHARMACIST IN COMMUNITY HEALTH CARE AND EDUCATION

Health is a very well known word but it carries a lot of complications and troubles. According to the WHO, health is a state of complete physical, mental and social well-being and not merely absence of any illness. Health care system depends upon a health care team. A health care team is the group of community who contribute to a common health goal and common objectives determined by community needs. India with the greatest cultural diversity, health though an important issue has been neglected due to many hindrances. The condition is worsened due to inadequate drug use problems. It is in the hands of the pharmacist particularly the community pharmacist, to take up the challenge for providing better health care and better outcomes reasonably. Although community pharmacist is of key importance in providing better healthcare. In India, Pharmacist does not command due recognition in the healthcare system as compare to other well-developed countries. The community pharmacist can take part in health promotion campaigns, locally and nationally, on a wide range of drug related and health related topics. A community pharmacist involvement could play an important role in the following areas of health care.

Pharmacists are dynamic, patient-oriented professionals committed to fulfilling the health care needs of their patients. Pharmacy is a profession that is expanding in new directions to meet the health care needs. There is a movement amongst pharmacists beyond the traditional compounding and dispensing of medication, towards a more professional advisory and primary health care role. Pharmacists can apply their knowledge and skill to become directly involved in the healing and education of patients. Pharmacists form an integral part of the community and serve as an important source of knowledge. A modern-day pharmacist should be trained in providing the knowledge concerning:

- Optimal drug therapy for patients with a focus on drug interactions and potential side effects
- Counselling on various disease conditions
- Education and promotion of the general health of the public
- Information on immunization.

World over pharmacist is one of the important member of the health-team including clinical research. If Indian pharmacist is not fulfilling this role, then he should be appropriately trained and be oriented as a health - care provider to the vast rural population. He can be used intelligently as an alternative manpower towards the sacred goals as i) a communicator, ii) a quality drug supplier, iii) a health promotera collaborator, and v) a trainer and supervisor.

The WHO report on "The role of the pharmacist in the healthcare system" states that the competence of the pharmacist is already proven and evident:

- In the direction and administrative of pharmaceutical services
- In drug regulation and control
- In the formulation and quality control of pharmaceutical products
- In the inspection and assessment of drug manufacturing facilities

- In the assurance of product quality through the distribution chain
- In drug procurement agencies, and
- In National and institutional formulary committees.

The main role of community pharmacist

A. As Pharmacist and health promoter

a. Immunization
b. Minor dressing
c. Preventing tropical diseases
d. Providing drug-information
e. Monitoring adverse drug reactions
f. Monitoring and minimizing adverse drug interactions
g. Preventing misuse of drugs
h. Preventing medication errors

B. Health educator

1. Nutrition counseling
2. Individualization of drug therapy
3. Family Planning
4. Alcohols, drug abuse and smoking cessation
5. Sexually transmitted diseases-AIDS
6. Rational use of drugs
7. Women welfare-pregnancy and infant care

1. Nutrition Counseling

Community pharmacist can play significant role in assuring adequate nutrition by advising his patients about basic food needs, keeping to correct improper food habits in children, advising on special requirements, suggesting special diet instructions for diabetic patients and people with food allergy and participating in school lunch programs and schemes like mid-day meals etc. in rural areas. There are certain facts such as women who often eat fish or 3-fatty acids are less likely to suffer stroke, symptoms of hyper vitaminosis result in irregular menstrual cycle and excessive intake during pregnancy may cause birth defects. .

2. **Women Welfare-Pregnancy and Infant Care**

   Women health care is the first priority in India. Women are the corner stone for effective public health and investing in women translate into investing in family, community and the Nation. The pharmacist who understands the normal course of pregnancy and infancy is at a distinct advantage as he or she can guide the mother in simple matters of hygiene and management. The community pharmacist can encourage breast feeding and can play a major role by guiding the mother for the protection of the child by following proper immunization schedule. Efforts are definitely underway in this area.

3. **Rational Use of Drugs**

   A community pharmacist can also discuss with administration on the medication, provide information on the storage of the medication and wherever necessary he can counsel the patient. Drug information system should be set up and access to adverse drug reaction (ADR) system should be made. A community pharmacist should do therapeutic drug monitoring and he should have a sound knowledge of genotype reporting i.e. predictive pharmacology. How many amongst the common people know that drugs such as Vicks Action 500, Coldarin can increase blood pressure in patients having hypertension. Even pain shows difference between men and women; women respond better to the opiods such as morphine, pentazocine and pethidine men respond better to the non-steroidal anti-inflammatory drug, ibuprofen. In a nut shell there should be rational use of drug i.e. right drug in right patient in right dose at right time. A community pharmacist is one of the inevitable members of the health care team who can help to achieve the goal of rational use of drugs.

4. **Sexually Transmitted Diseases-AIDS**

   India has 3.5 million HIV positive cases, which is about 10% of the global HIV cases and barely second to South Africa. HIV drugs are expensive and beyond the reach of common man. Huge resource of community pharmacist can educate people in the prevention and information of HIV/AIDS. A sensitive issue is the increasing number of women patients suffering from AIDS. The number rose from 7% in 1985 to 18% in 1995. Explaining to what HIV is, its transmission, risk reduction, patient counseling are the components of the counseling that a community pharmacist can provide.

5. **Alcohols, Drug Abuse and Smoking Cessation**

   The pharmacist can play an important role to help individuals who become dependent upon alcohol. Drug abuse is similar to alcoholism yet different because it has been gaining more acceptance among young people. Annual mortality from tobacco use exceeds that from all other causes combined. Smoking is the greatest single preventable cause of morbidity and mortality in India. The pharmacist can advise on the products available to assist the patient in giving up smoking. Counseling sessions can be made by the community pharmacist to stop smoking.

6. **Family Planning**

   Currently, India's annual population growth rate is 1.74%. India is the second most populous country in the world, contributing about 20% of births worldwide In 1952, the Indian Government was one of the first in the world to formulate a National Family Planning Programme, which was later expanded to encompass maternal and child health, family welfare, and nutrition. All problems are associated with tremendously increasing population in India. The community pharmacist plays a very important role in this case to educate the people and advise various methods available in the market helpful in family planning.

7. **Individualization of Drug Therapy**

   Today the latest concept in medicine is towards individualization of drug therapy. Where judicious patient care is needed individualization of drug therapy becomes a need and a pharmacist can play a vital role in this. A physician who is preoccupied with patient diagnosis and treatment may not spare time for patient counseling regarding pharmaco-economics, drug information, alternative therapy, moral supporting etc. A pharmacist can set up a separate consultation room and provide counseling to the patient.

IMPORTANT TERMS

Drug includes, all medicines for internal or external use of human beings or animals and all substances intended to be used for, or in the diagnosis, treatment, mitigation or prevention of any disease or disorder in human beings or animals, including preparations applied on human body for the purpose of repelling insects like mosquitoes

Bulk drug means any pharmaceutical, chemical, biological or plant product including its salts, esters, stereo-isomers and derivatives, conforming to pharmacopoeial or other standards specified in the Second Schedule to the Drugs and Cosmetics Act, 1940, and which is used as such or as an ingredient in any information.

Scheduled bulk drug means a bulk drug specified in the First Schedule;

Non-Scheduled bulk drug means a bulk drug not specified in the First Schedule;

Formulation means a medicine processed out of, or containing one or more bulk drug or drugs with or without the use of any pharmaceutical aids, for internal or external use for or in the diagnosis, treatment, mitigation or prevention of disease in human beings or animals.

Scheduled formulation means a formulation containing any bulk drug specified in the First Schedule either individually or in combination with other drugs, including one or more than one drug or drugs not specified in the First Schedule except single ingredient formulation based on bulk drugs specified in the First Schedule and sold under the generic name;

Non-Scheduled formulation means a formulation not containing any bulk drug specified in the First Schedule.

Dealer means a person carrying on the business of purchase or sale of drugs, whether as a wholesaler or retailer and whether or not in conjunction with any other business, and includes his agent.

Distributor means a distributor or his agent or a stockist appointed by a manufacturer or an importer for stocking his drugs for sale to a dealer.

Retailer in relation to the sale of any goods means a dealer carrying on the retail business of sale of drugs to consumers.

Wholesaler means a dealer or his agent or a stockiest appointed by a manufacturer or an importer for the sale of his drugs to a retailer, hospital, dispensary, medical, educational or research institution purchasing bulk quantities of drugs.

Retail price means the retail price of a drug arrived at or fixed in accordance with the provisions of the Drugs Prices Control Order and includes a ceiling price.

Ceiling price means a price fixed by the Government for Scheduled formulations in accordance with the provisions.

Manufacture includes any process or part of a process for making, altering, finishing, packing, labelling, breaking or otherwise treating or adapting any drug with a view to its sale and distribution, but does not include the compounding or dispensing of any drug or the packing of any drug in the ordinary course of retail business, and 'to manufacture' shall be construed accordingly;

Maximum retail price means the retail price arrived at or fixed in accordance with the provisions of the Drugs Prices Control Order and includes a ceiling price, at which the drug may be sold to the ultimate consumer and where such price is mentioned on the pack, the words "Maximum or Max. Retail Price Inclusive of all taxes" shall be printed on the pack;

Local taxes means any tax or levy (except excise duty included in retail price) paid and/or payable to the Central Govt. or State Govt. or any local authority under any law, by the manufacturer or his agent or dealer:

Goods means goods as defined in the Sale of Goods Act, 1930 and includes (i) products manufactured, processed or mined in India, (ii) shares and stocks including issue of shares before allotment,

Price in relation to the sale of any goods or to the performance of any services, includes every valuable consideration whether direct or indirect, and includes any consideration which in effect relates to the sale of any goods or to the performance of any services although ostensibly relating to any other matter or thing.

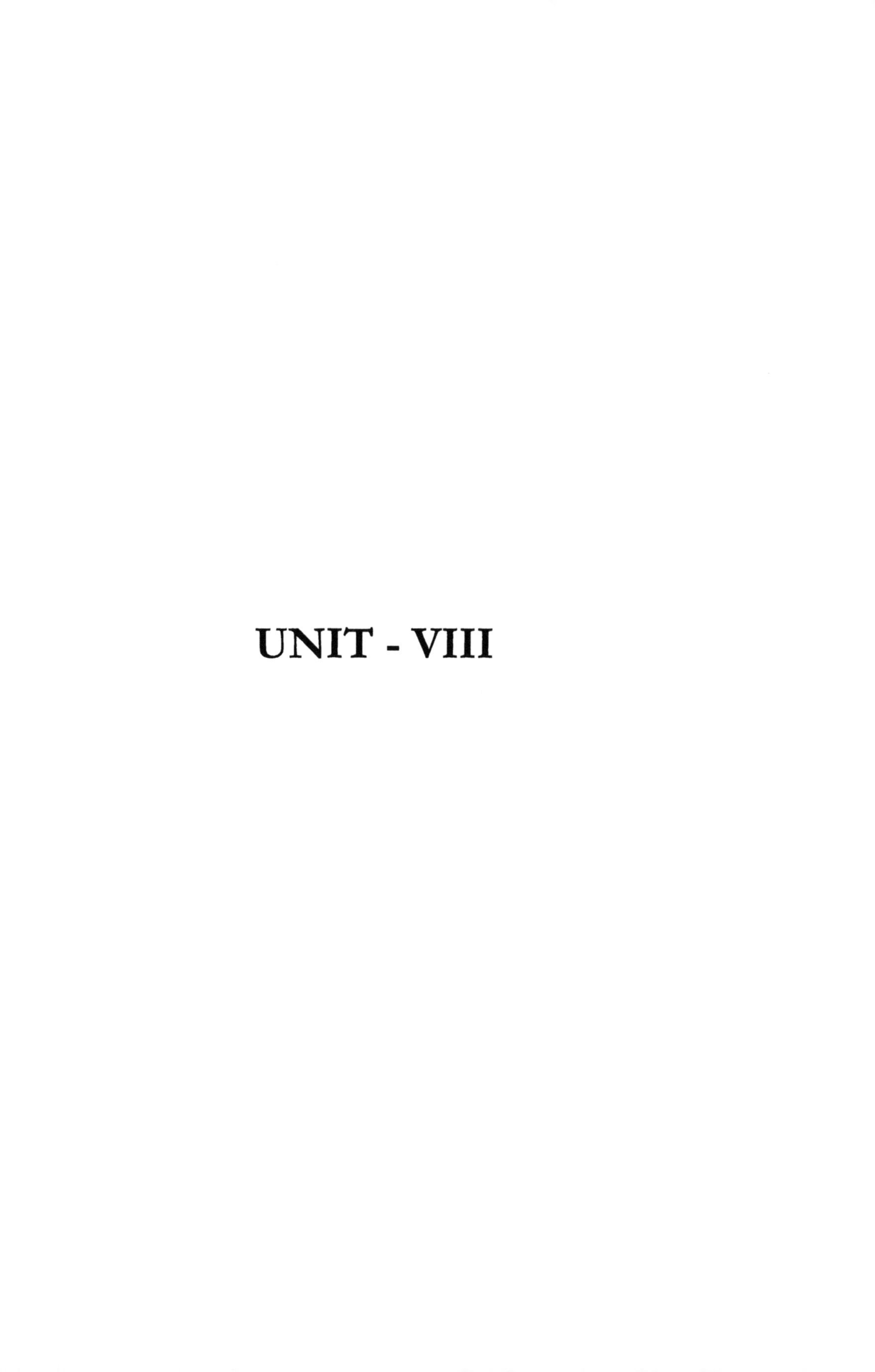

UNIT - VIII

CHAPTER 20

RECORDS

1. PRESCRIPTION FILLING

All prescriptions from health care provider are received by the pharmacist.. Submission of the paper slip of prescription and receiving the final dosage form such as tablet, capsule, mixture, creams etc is not an easy process. A slip of paper prescription must contain all the detailed information. Sometime it may be necessary to buy the medication from various sources. Essential factors to consider before perusing the filling of the prescription are given below.

a. Prescription must be handled by the registered and qualified pharmacist
b. Types of prescription
c. Type, severity and symptoms of diseases
d. Location of pharmacy
e. Working hours of pharmacy
f. Cost of the medications
g. Insurance coverage

Although it may appear to be simple enough yet prescription filling is a detailed process designed with all precaution and safety. The process or prescription filling can be separated into five phases:

1. Prescription drop-off
2. Patient profile review
3. Order entry
4. Final check, and
5. Pick-up the filled prescription.

1. **Dropping off the Prescription**

On receiving a prescription form the physician, a pharmacist must ensure that it is complete and correct in all aspects. Laws governing filling of prescription may vary from country to country and from State to State. The prescription order must be checked by the pharmacist before starting to fill it. Following information must be clearly available on the prescription –

1. Patient's full name
2. Age, sex and weight of patient
3. Symptoms and type of diseases
4. Medication and dosage
5. Directions for use
6. Physician's signature, and
7. Refill information

In case of any doubt or discrepancy in the prescription the pharmacist should contact the physician for clarification before filling the prescription.

2. **Patient Profile Review**

Once the prescription authorized by the physician is found to be complete in all aspects, the pharmacist may require asking some questions about the patient personal and medical background. Some of the more common questions asked by the pharmacist are given below.

- What is your name?
- What is your date-of-birth?
- What is your address?
- What is the duration of problem?
- Do you have prescription insurance?
- Do you have any drug allergies?
- Are you taking/have you been taking any other medications?

All or some of the question may be asked at each visit even if the patient is an established customer. Date-of-birth is often used to confirm patient's identity in the case of similar names. Address is required as identifier of the patient. Insurance policies are dependent on time hence it is essential to ask any change for an update. Any new allergies can develop at any time, and the pharmacist should maintain current records of all medications taken by the patient. All of this information is for the benefit and safety of the patient. The pharmacist uses it to determine if the new drug is compatible with other medications and also safe and appropriate to the condition of the disease. This process is known as **drug utilization review** and is one of the pharmacist's most important responsibilities.

A prescription is completed by the pharmacist and a label is generated, the medicine is counted on a counting tray or poured into a bottle, and the label is affixed, along with any small warning labels, such as drowsiness cautions, etc.

3. **Order Entry**

After collecting all the necessary information, the pharmacist is required to enter all the information into the record. In these days all the entries should be made by the pharmacist into a computerized system. Other systems rely on manual entry via keyboard. Selection and pricing of product are also done at this stage. To save time, doctors may use pharmaceutical abbreviations or symbols when writing prescriptions. The pharmacists and pharmacy technicians are well trained in the use of this medical shorthand without any mistake. The pharmacies may also employ an internet connection to send information to the insurance company. The insurance company decides what portion of the prescription is covered and what part of prescription is not covered. If prescription is not covered by insurance the total payment is made by the patient. The cost of a prescription typically includes the medication, supplies, and the pharmacist's expertise. The pharmacist or technician selects a product from available inventory. Depending on state regulations, the pharmacist may be allowed to substitute a generic equivalent unless the physician has specified otherwise.

4. **The Final Check**

The final product will be transferred by the pharmacist or technical person in an appropriate container and labeled according to legal requirements. The pharmacist then reviews the order during a process called the **final check**. During the final check the pharmacist must check the following information regarding the filled prescription–

- The drug name
- Strength
- Dosing directions, and
- Appearance of the medication

It is very important to ensure that the prescription has been filled for the correct patient. During this check, any discrepancies between the physician order and the final product should be noted and corrected immediately.

5. **Prescription Pick-Up**

The pharmacist presents the filled prescription to patient and offers counseling about the prescription. During pick-up pharmacist should ask any questions to reconfirm that the prescription is delivered to the right patient. Each step in the prescription filling process is very useful to ensure that the prescription is complete, appropriate, safe, and correct. It is designed to provide careful and safe delivery of medication to the patient and is well explained to the patient or his representative. Some important point for collection of prescription by the patient should be duly publicised.

- Be prepared to wait for at least an hour if a pharmacy is particularly busy.
- It may be best to drop off your prescription and pick it up later in the day.
- If your prescription is for a narcotic, be ready to provide positive identification in the form of a government-issued ID, such as a driver's license or military ID card.
- depending on how quickly the doctor supplies the information that the insurance company has requested, the prior authorization process can take several days,
- Federal law states that once you have accepted the prescription and taken it home, it may not be returned to the pharmacy to be re-dispensed.

PRESCRIPTION FILING

Original prescriptions can be maintained and preserved using a variety of prescription files. Suitably partitioned drawers can be used for filing of prescription orders. The partitions may be placed between every 100, 200 or 300 prescription orders, plainly marked with the numbers of orders filed in that section. This method has the advantage that a single sheet can be removed without preventing ready access to others. The drawers are esthetic in appearance and can be designed to enhance the décor of the pharmacy.

Metal or cardboard units, which can store about 1ooo prescription orders, are the most common. The orders are first punched, slipped onto two metal rods firmly attached to the file, and placed in a selected compartment for safe storage and rapid retrieval.

Modern pharmacies employ microfilming and computer software for filing and retrieving prescription orders. This method helps in minimizing the cost as well as space occupied.

Prescription orders for narcotic drugs and psychotropic substances, as well as Schedule X drugs should be separately filed as per the requirement of the relevant Act and Rules.

STORAGE OF PRESCRIPTION

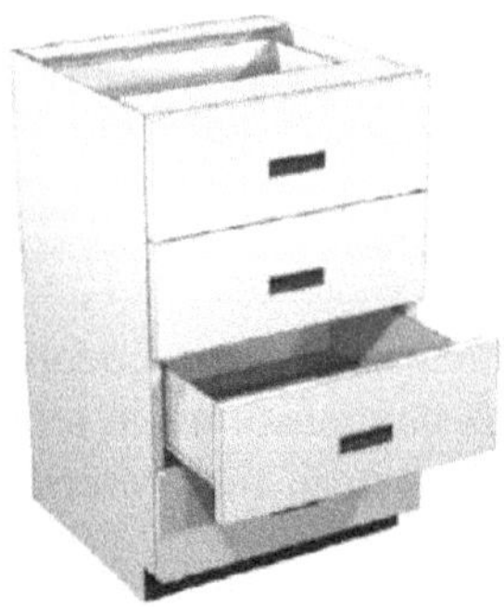

a. Prescription File Cabinet

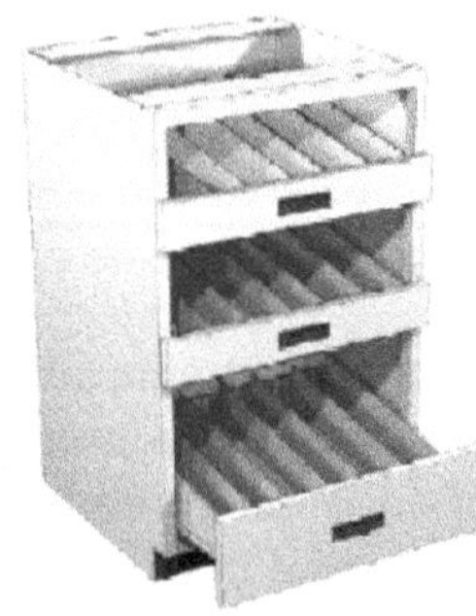

b. Bottle Dispenser

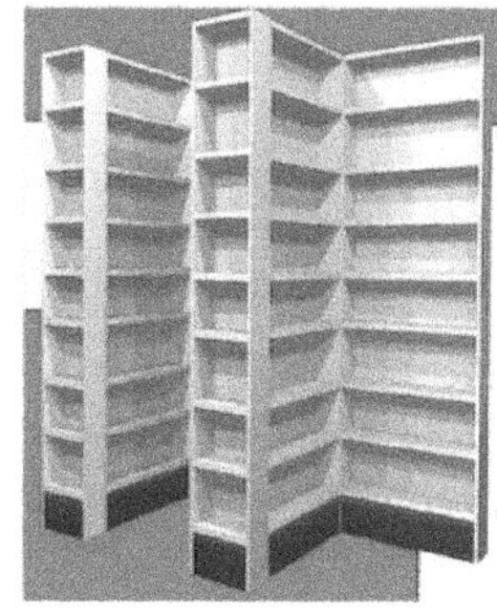

c. Classic Rx Shelving Features

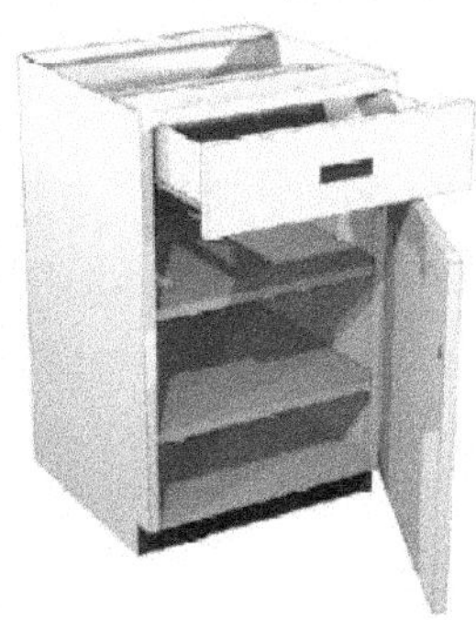

d. Closed Storage Cabinet

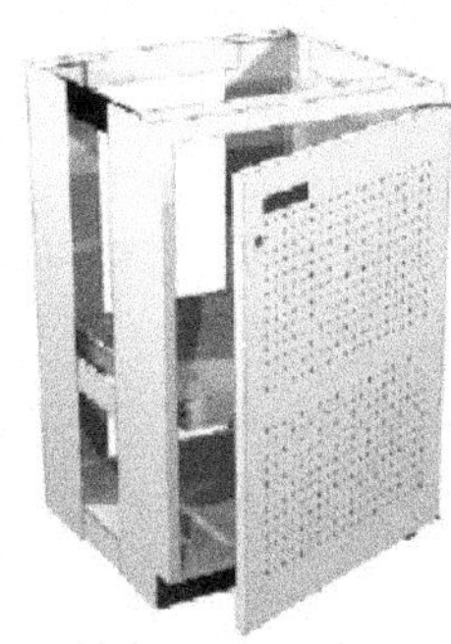

e. Pharmacy Computer Cabinet

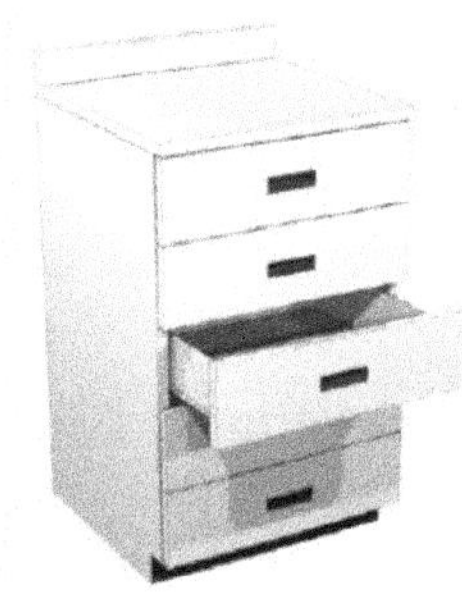

f. Five Drawer Undercounter Cabinet

2. DRUG PROFILE

Drug profile presents a summary of the characteristics of a drug or drug family. The drug profile is important to know about the drug and its properties and is generally provides information under following heads –

1. Introduction
2. Classification
3. Category
4. Dosage
5. Indication
6. Contraindication
7. Side effect
8. Special precautions
9. Drug Interaction

Examples of drug profiles of few drugs are given below.

1. **Drug Profile of Aspirin**

   It is acetylsalicylic acid which is potent anti-inflammatory and good analgesic.

   Category : Anti-inflammatory and analgesic

   Indications : Analgesic (headache, backache, myalgia, joint pain, toothache, neuralgias, dysmenorrhoea) antipyretic, acute rheumatic fever, rheumatoid arthritis, osteoarthritis, postmyocardial infarction and post stroke patients, coronary bypass, transient Ischaemic attacks.

   Dosage : Analgesic antipyretic: 0.3-0.6 g three times.

   Acute rheumatic conditions: 4-6 g or 75-100 mg/kg/day in divided doses.

   Post myocardial infarction and post stroke patients - 50-300 mg daily.

   Contra-ndications: Hypersensitivity, peptic ulcer, liver disease, bleeding tendencies and haemophilia; Children suffering from chicken pox or influenza; Pregnancy; avoided in diabetics and in juvenile rheumatoid arthritis and should be stopped before surgery.

   Special-precautions: Aspirin may precipitate bronchospasm and induce asthmatic attack in susceptible subjects. It may induce gastro intestinal haemorrhage, occasionally major. *Use with caution in subjects with gout.*

   Paediatrics : Not recommended under 12 years.

   Pregnancy : Contraindicated

   Lactation : Use with caution.

   Elderly : No special problem.

   Side-effects: Nausea, vomiting, epigastric distress, occult blood loss in stools, dizziness, tinnitus, vertigo, impairment of hearing and vision, excitement and mental confusion, hyperventilation and electrolyte imbalance.

   Drug Interactions : PABA may increase serum levels; Urinary alkalisers, antacids, corticosteroids may increase excretion; may potentiate the effects of anticoagulants, hypoglycaemics, methotrexate, tricyclic antidepressants; may antagonise uricosurics, spironolactone and tetracyclines.

2. **Drug Profile of Indomethacin**

   It is a potent anti-inflammatory and promptly acting antipyretic but it relieves only inflammatory or tissue injury related pain.

   Category : anti-inflammatory

   Dosage : Adult – 25-50 mg 2 to 4 times daily

Indications : Rheumatoid arthritis not controlled by aspirin, ankylosing spondyliitis, destructive arthropathias and psoriatic arthritis, acute gout.

Contraindication : Machinery operators, drivers, psychiatric patients, epileptics, kidney disease or hepatic dysfunction.

Paediatrics : Usually not prescribed for children under 14 except for patent ducts arteriosus in neonates

Pregnancy : Not prescribed

Lactation : Unsafe

Elderly : Reduced dose is necessary

Side effects: Gastric irritation, nausea, anorexia, gastric bleeding, diarrhea, frontal headache, dizziness, mental confusion, hallucination, depression, psychoisis, can induce asthma.

Drug Interaction : Salicylates, lithium, anticoagulants, corticosteroids, diuretics, ß-blockers, probenecid.

3. Drug Profile of Tenoxicam

It is NSAID of the oxicam class, having anti-inflammatory, analgesic and antipyretic activity. It is a potent inhibitor of prostaglandin biosynthesis by inhibiting the enzyme cyclooxygenase.

Category : anti-inflammatory, analgesic and antipyretic

Dosage : 20 mg daily. Not recommended for children

Indications: Osteoarthritis, rheumatoid arthritis, ankylosing spondylitis, gout, Non -articular rheumatic conditions.

Contraindications: Acute peptic ulceration, G.I. bleeding, severe gastritis.

Special Precautions: Monitor long term therapy (especially with G.I. disease). Renal, hepatic and cardiovascular functions.

Paediatrics : Not recommended.

Pregnancy : Contraindicated.

Lactation : Contraindicated.

Elderly : Reduced dose necessary

Drug Interactions: Antacids, anticoagulants, other NSAID's, lithium, hypoglycaemics.

Side-effects: Dyspepsia, nausea, abdominal pain, constipation, diarrhoea, flatulence, indigestion, oedema, headache, rashes, blood dyscrasias, visual disturbances, raised liver enzymes.

3. PATIENT MEDICATION PROFILE

The patient medication profile is one of the most important parts of medication. The aim of the Patient Medication Profile (PMP) is to reduce the risk of medication-related adverse events by assisting people to better understand and manage their medications, including prescription, over-the-counter and complementary medicines. The provision of a PMP service through community pharmacies is expected to improve patient confidence in self medication management, and support communication between the patient and other health professionals, especially on admittance to hospitals or nursing homes. The medication profile gives pharmacy personnel the opportunity to actively participate in monitoring patient care. The form used for the profile is designed locally and may vary from one hospital to another, but the information contained on the form should be similar.

Mechanism of Idiosyncratic drug toxicity

The possible mechanism of idiosyncratic drug toxicity is as –

1. Abnormal receptor sensitivity
2. Abnormal biological system that is only apparent in the presence of drug.
3. Abnormality in drug metabolism
4. Immunological
5. Multifactorial

The patient medication profile is divided into six sections.

a. Diagnosis and Pre-existing Conditions
b. Scheduled Medications
c. Nonscheduled/nonrecurring medications
d. Ward stock/floor stock medications

a. **Patient Information :** Following information is compulsory to know in detail for safety and proper consideration of medication.
    - Name of patient
    - Age
    - Sex
    - Weight of patient
    - Social security number
    - Ward, and
    - Bed number

b. **Allergy Information :** It is important to know of any allergies the patient has/had to allow the pharmacy to make sure the patient is not being given medication to which he is allergic. The physician should have checked this before ordering the medication but this allows for one more safety check.

c. **Diagnosis and Preexisting Conditions:** It allows the pharmacy to check for medications, which may be harmful to patient because of an ailment currently being treated, a different ailment, or other drugs the patient is taking for the diagnosed condition. It is essential to make sure by the pharmacy if any pre-existing conditions are also receiving treatment. An example, a patient is required surgery who also has high blood pressure for which he is taking medication. The detailed information can be notified and informed to physician. The pharmacy must be aware of this condition.

d. **Scheduled Medications :** This portion of the profile is a major safety check for the patient. All medications are required to be check for drug interactions. The medications identified on this part of the form are those ordered by the physician. Scheduled medications are those that are prescribed to be given at definite intervals.

e. **Nonscheduled/Nonrecurring Medications** : This type of medication is one that is ordered for a one-time administration or as needed. This types of medications do not have a specific time-span between doses. On the prescription label, it stat that indicate non-recurring medications.

f. **Floor stock/Ward stock Medication :** Some medications are already on the wards as per the local Standard Operating Procedure They are managed by the bulk drug order section of the pharmacy.

RECORDS

Unless you are aware of your mistakes, you can't remove them. Unless you know the intensity of effectiveness of your diagnostic and treatment plans, you can't adopt them. You are supposed to manage the present; you are supposed to manage the future. You are required to file; you are required to document. You need to make use of your records and you also need to make them useful to the researchers and medical scientists. You need to sort out the records of no use and to destroy them. Testifying its instrumentality as a clinical, scientific, legal and managerial document relating to patient care and other important matters, the management of hospital records has been found gravitating the attention of managers, medical scientists and researchers which in a majority of the hospitals has not been given due weightage. It is against this background that a hospital manager needs to assign due priority to the management of hospital records.

In the context of hospitals, we find record a clear, concise and accurate history of the life and illness which is written from the health and medical point of view. The statement of patients, observations of nurses and comments of doctors are mentioned in the medical records. The medical sections of record consists of history sheet, physical examination sheet, provisional diagnosis, investigation reports, physicians' order sheet, treatment record, anaesthesia and operation records, obstetric records, consultancy report, progress report, discharge summary and in case of death, the cause of death and autopsy report.

There are different categories of records, such as vital records which are required to be protected and preserved for the long time; important records which are not of current use but are to be retained for future reference, useful records which are found of current use but are to be retained for future reference, useful records which are found of current use and transit record found useful only for a short period. A hospital manager is required to identify the nature and uses of records and to be more specific the information technology has added a new dimension in the management of records because the process of documentation is now found easier.

<table>
<tr><td rowspan="8">Records</td><td>Vital Records</td><td></td><td></td><td rowspan="8">Types</td></tr>
<tr><td></td><td colspan="2">Protected for long time</td></tr>
<tr><td>Important records</td><td></td><td></td></tr>
<tr><td></td><td colspan="2">To be useful in Future</td></tr>
<tr><td>Useful records</td><td></td><td></td></tr>
<tr><td></td><td colspan="2">Correspondence</td></tr>
<tr><td>Transit records</td><td></td><td></td></tr>
<tr><td></td><td colspan="2">Useful for short period</td></tr>
</table>

PATIENT RECORD OF MEDICATION PROFILES

A. Introduction

The patient record of medication profiles allows for immediate and easy recovery of information necessary to the dispensing pharmacist for identifying medication previously dispensed and for counseling purposes before the current prescription order is dispensed.

B. Patient Medication Identification

1. The following patient information should be available for medication identification and counseling.
   a. Name of the patient
   b. Address with telephone number
   c. Date of birth or age of the patient
   d. Patient gender (sex- male or female)
   e. All information of the patient five years immediately preceding the most recent sentry. The list should show the following :
      (i) Name of the medication
      (ii) Prescription no.
      (iii) Name and strength of the medication

(iv) Quantity
(v) Date of dispensed
(vi) Name of the prescriber
(vii) Indication for use

f. A record of the pharmacist's comments relevant to the patient medication therapy including any information relevant to the patients or to any medication currently being dispensed, such as –

(i) Identification of caregiver
(ii) Counseling documentation
(iii) Refill instruction
(iv) Missed dosages history
(v) Record of counseling offered
(vi) Pharmacist - prescriber interaction

C. Prospective Drug Review Information

The pharmacist shall record information pertaining to the patient's medical history obtained from the patient or the patient's caregiver for use in future drug review including the following.

a. Allergies
b. Adverse drug reaction, if any
c. Idiosyncrasies
d. Chronic conditions
e. Diseases
f. Currently used prescription medications
g. Currently used over-the-counter medications
h. Currently used medical devices

D. Documentation Requirements

1. The patient record of medications profile shall be maintained for a period of not less than five years from the date of the last entry in the profile record
2. This record may be maintained in a hard copies or a computerized form
3. Reasons of not counseling must be recorded. This includes refusal due to prescriber request or in response to the patient/caregiver.

E. Administrative and financial information

a. Tax records
b. Insurance records
c. Billing information

Table 20.1 Sample of Medication Profile

Patient Medication Profile					
Name : ______________________			Date completed :		
Date of Birth : ______________________			______________________		
Height : _______ Weight : _________			Sex : Male /Female		
Drug Allergies					
☐	None	☐	Compazine	☐	Percocet
☐	Amoxycillin	☐	Darvon	☐	Phenobarbital
☐	Ampicillin	☐	Demerol	☐	Opiates
☐	Aspirin	☐	Epinephrine	☐	Sulfa
☐	Bactrim	☐	Ibuprofen	☐	Talwin
☐	Biaxin	☐	Keflex	☐	Tetracycline
☐	Ceclor	☐	Penicillin	☐	Tylenol
☐	Cipro	☐	Percodan	☐	Valium
☐	Codeine	☐	OTHERS	☐	OTHERS
☐	OTHERS	☐		☐	
MEDICAL CONDITIONS					
☐	Anxiety	☐	Epilepsy	☐	Hypertension
☐	Arthritis	☐	Glaucoma	☐	Kidney/renal problems
☐	Asthma	☐	Gout	☐	Multiple scierosis
☐	Cancer	☐	Heart disease	☐	Organ transplant
☐	Cystic fibrosis	☐	Hepatitis /Liver disease	☐	Psychiatric disorder
☐	Depression	☐	High cholesterol	☐	Thyroid
☐	Diabetes	☐	HIV/AIDS	☐	Ulcer
☐	OTHERS	☐	OTHERS	☐	OTHERS
☐		☐		☐	
Current Medications					
1.		5.		9.	
2.		6.		10.	
3.		7.		11.	
4.		8.		12.	
					Signature

PATIENT PLANNING RECORD

This patient planning record will help appointment of patient and ensure discussions with the pharmacist. This information is also important to get early appointment.

Table 20.2 Patient planning Record Form

<table>
<tr><td colspan="3">Name: ____________________
Date of Birth :______________
Height : _______ Weight : _________</td><td colspan="3">Date completed : _______________

Sex : Male /Female</td></tr>
<tr><td>Name of medicine</td><td>Why do I take it</td><td>How much do I take (1 tablet, 1 lbs, etc)</td><td>When do I take it? (breakfast, lunch, dinner etc.)</td><td>Where do I store it? (bathroom cabinet, kitchen pantry etc.)</td><td>Question about this medicine</td></tr>
<tr><td></td><td></td><td></td><td></td><td></td><td></td></tr>
<tr><td></td><td></td><td></td><td></td><td></td><td></td></tr>
<tr><td></td><td></td><td></td><td></td><td></td><td></td></tr>
<tr><td></td><td></td><td></td><td></td><td></td><td></td></tr>
<tr><td></td><td></td><td></td><td></td><td></td><td></td></tr>
<tr><td></td><td></td><td></td><td></td><td></td><td></td></tr>
<tr><td colspan="6">Questions :</td></tr>
<tr><td colspan="6"></td></tr>
<tr><td colspan="6">I (name) __________________ consent to having my medication history reviewed. I consent to pharmacist and any of my health-care professionals discussing issues in relation to my medications and providing information to each other in relation to my medications.

Signed ______________________ Date ___________ Witness _______________</td></tr>
</table>

4. ADVERSE DRUG REACTIONS

Adverse Drug Reaction (ADR) is an expression that describes harm associated with the use of given medications at a normal dose. The meaning of this expression differs from the meaning of "side effect", as this last expression might also imply that the effects can be beneficial. The study of ADRs is the concern of the field known as **pharmacovigilance**.

An adverse drug reaction may be defined as "any pathological condition precipitated by a drug regardless of its nature or the circumstances of its occurrence, i.e. toxicity caused by over-dosage (therapeutic, accidental, homicidal); hypersensitivity; allergy; or injury from improper technique of administration, use of the wrong dose, error in compounding, labeling, or packaging, or from other error in the manufacture of the drug, or in its preparation for use in the hospital. Reactions caused by blood and plasma products need not be reported unless a chemical agent other than the basic substance is responsible."

The simplest definition of ADR would be "Any untoward or unintended effect of drug treatment".

ADRs are more common in patients taking large number of drugs. In general, more than 3 per cent of the admissions to medical wards occur because of the ADRs and this per cent is increasing at an alarming rate because of multi drug prescribing habits of the physicians.

Classification

I. ADRs may be classified by – A. Cause of disease, and B. Severity of disease

A. Cause of disease

1. Augmented pharmacologic effects - dose dependent and predictable
2. Bizarre effects (or idiosyncratic) - dose independent and unpredictable
3. Chronic effects
4. Delayed effects
5. End-of-treatment effects
6. Failure of therapy

B. Seriousness and Severity

The FDA defines a serious adverse event as one when the patient outcome is any of the following.

1. Death
2. Life-threatening
3. Hospitalization (initial or prolonged)
4. Disability –
    - significant
    - persistent or permanent change
    - impairment
    - damage or disruption in the patient's body function/structure
    - physical activities or quality of life.

5. Congenital anomaly
6. Requires Intervention to Prevent Permanent Impairment or Damage
7. Severity is a point on an arbitrary scale of intensity of the adverse event in question. The terms "severe" and "serious" when applied to adverse events are technically very different. They are easily confused but can not be used interchangeably, require care in usage.
8. A headache is severe, if it causes intense pain. There are scales like visual analog scale that help us assess the severity. On the other hand, a headache can hardly ever be serious, unless it also satisfies the criteria for seriousness listed above.

II. Adverse effects may develop promptly after prolonged usage of medication or some times stoppage of the drug. They are very common using multiple drug therapy. Adverse drug effects have been classified in many ways and may be divided into –

1. Predictable reactions (Type A) : These are based on the pharmacological properties of the drug such as – side effect, toxic effect and drug withdrawal symptoms.
2. Unpredictable reactions (Type B) : These are based on the peculiarities of the patient and not on known drug action such as – allergy and idiosyncrasy. This type of reaction can be prevented if the generic basis is well known.

Drug Risk

No any official system exists to describe the drug risk but drug risk rating system is a five colour rating scale such as -

1. Red (High Risk)
2. Orange (Elevated Risk)
3. Yellow (Guarded Risk)
4. Blue (General Risk)
5. Green (Low Risk)

Ideally an adverse drug reaction of a drug should have a profile consisting of the following elements.

- Manifestation
- Severity and seriousness
- Mechanism of action
- Frequency of occurrence
- Causality
- Predisposing factors
- Therapy, if any
- Reversibility of sequelae

Prevention of ADR

The adverse drug effect can be minimized by taking the following precautions –

a. Minimum use of drug and avoiding all types of inappropriate drugs
b. Use proper dose, route and frequency of administration.
c. Study allergic history of the patient before administration of dosage form
d. In combine drug therapy check the rationality among the drugs and their suitability.
e. Apply correct route of administration
f. Proper monitoring of the patient during the therapy.
g. Proper storage of drug.

Table 20.3 Drugs generally causing allergic reactions

Allopurinol	Local anesthetics	Quinolones
Antitubercular drugs	Methyl dopa	Salicylates
Carbamazepine	Penicillins	Sulfonamides
Cephalosporins	Phenothiazines	Tetracyclines
Hydralazine	Phenylbutazone	

Examples of adverse effects associated with specific medications –

1. Abortion, miscarriage or uterine hemorrhage associated with Misoprostol (Cytotec), a labor-inducing drug (this is a case where the adverse effect has been used legally and illegally for performing abortions)
2. Addiction to many sedatives and analgesics such as diazepam, morphine etc.
3. Birth defects associated with Thalidomide and Accutane.
4. Bleeding of the intestine associated with aspirin therapy
5. Cardiovascular disease associated with COX-2 inhibitors.
6. Deafness and kidney failure associated with Gentamicin (an antibiotic).
7. Death, following sedation in children using Propofol (Diprivan).
8. Depression or hepatic injury caused by Interferon.
9. Diabetes caused by atypical antipsychotic medications.
10. Diarrhea caused by the use of Orlistat (Xenical)
11. Erectile dysfunction associated with many drugs, such as antidepressants.
12. Fever associated with vaccination (BCG and Poliomyelitis)
13. Glaucoma associated with corticosteroid-containing eye drops
14. Hair loss and anemia may be caused by chemotherapy, leukemia, etc.
15. Headache caused by spinal anesthesia.

16. Hypertension associated in ephedrine users.
17. Insomnia caused by stimulants, Ritalin, etc.
18. Lactic acidosis associated with the use of Stavudine (for anti-HIV therapy) or Metformin (for diabetes)
19. Liver damage from Paracetamol
20. Melasma and thrombosis associated with use of estrogen-containing hormonal contraception such as the combined oral contraceptive pill.
21. Irreversible peripheral neuropathy associated with the use of Fluoroquinolone medications.
22. Seizures caused by withdrawal from Benzodiazepine
23. Drowsiness or increase in appetite due to antihistamine use.
24. Stroke or heart attack associated with Viagra when used with nitroglycerine.
25. Suicide, increased tendency associated to the use of Fluoxetine and other SSRI antidepressants
26. Tardive dyskinesia associated with long-term use of Metoclopramide and many antipsychotic medications

Pharmacists stand at the crossroads of drug therapy, where they have the responsibility of providing professional services to patients receiving drugs prescribed by physicians and also to patients' self medicating with non-prescription drugs. Computer software is already available to screen patients' medication regimens for potential drug-drug, drug-diet and drug-disease interactions.

5. IDIOSYNCRATIC CASES

Adverse drug reactions are a major problem of modern drug therapy. Many serious adverse reactions occur in patients with diseases which in themselves are not necessarily life-threatening, such as depression and epilepsy, but do require long-term drug treatment. It is therefore essential to understand more related to such reactions. Adverse drug reactions may be classified as follows:

Type A: These reactions are predictable in terms of the primary and secondary pharmacology of the drug and are usually dose-dependent. Examples - hypoglycaemia with oral hypoglycaemics and hypotension with anti-hypertensives. This type of reactions can be eliminated by change of dose.

Type B : Unpredictable from a knowledge of the basic pharmacology of the drug and do not show any simple dose-response relationship. This type of reaction is also known as idiosyncratic. These reactions occur in only a small percentage of the population but are often serious and account for many drug-induced deaths.

Type C: These reactions are associated with long-term drug therapy, examples of which include benzodiazepine dependence and analgesic nephropathy.

Type D: These types of reaction showed delayed effects such as carcinogenicity and teratogenicity.

Idiosyncratic drug reactions (IDR) are a specific type of drug toxicity characterized by their delayed onset, low incidence and reactive metabolite formation with little, if any, correlation between pharmacokinetics or pharmacodynamics and the toxicological outcome. Examples of drugs include trovafloxacin, zileuton, troglitazone, tolcapone and felbamate. IDR also known as type B reactions, are drug reactions which occur rarely and unpredictably amongst the population. These reactions are often serious and are a major cause of iatrogenic disease and yet the mechanisms involved are, in general, poorly understood. Such reactions are not detected by preclinical toxicology testing in animals and indeed cannot be reproduced in animal models. The mechanisms involved is therefore nearly always dependent on retrospective clinical analysis. The clinical characteristics of such reactions are often suggestive of drug allergy or drug hypersensitivity. Idiosyncratic reactions are of major concern both in medical practice and for present and future drug development. It is not possible to evaluate new drugs for their potential to cause idiosyncratic reactions, and such adverse reactions are only detected at a relatively late stage in drug development.

Table 20.4 Product withdrawls due to Idiosyncratic Drug Reactions

Alcofenac	Hypersensitivity reactions
Althesin, Glafenine, Zomepirac	Anaphylaxis
Benoxaprofen	Hepatotoxicity, Nephrotoxicity
Fenclofenac	Toxic epidermal necrolysis
Ibufenac, Tienilic acid, Temafloxacin	Hepatotoxicity
Nomifensine	Haemolytic anaemia
Practolol	Oculo-mucocutaneous syndrome
Zimeldine	Guillain-Barre Syndrome

It is therefore important to study and elucidate the chemical, biochemical and immunological mechanisms of idiosyncratic adverse drug reactions in order to explain the chemical and cellular basis of the toxicity. Perhaps the most important goal of such studies should be to define the individual factor(s) responsible for the idiosyncratic nature of the adverse reaction.

Such information could then be used prospectively to avoid drug toxicities in several ways. First, identification of patients who have a genetically determined susceptibility to certain classes (chemical or biochemical) of drugs, and development of a simple method for genotyping such individuals. This may reveal chemical or biochemical links between unrelated drugs not previously suspected. Secondly, cells derived from patients phenotyped for drug sensitivity could be used in the preclinical evaluation of a new drug, or a new analogue of a drug, that has been withdrawn because of an idiosyncratic reaction. Thirdly, a knowledge of the chemical mechanism of drug toxicity could lead to the design of an analogue which retains the efficacy of the parent drug but cannot produce the (idiosyncratic) toxicity.

Mechanism of Idiosyncratic drug toxicity

The possible mechanism of idiosyncratic drug toxicity is as –

1. Abnormal receptor sensitivity
2. Abnormal biological system that is only apparent in the presence of drug.
3. Abnormality in drug metabolism
4. Immunological
5. Multifactorial

CLINICAL MANIFESTATIONS

The clinical pattern of idiosyncratic reaction can be remarkably variable even with respect to the same drug. Many of these reactions, although rare, are life-threatening and have resulted in the withdrawal of potentially useful drug. The most common site for idiosyncratic drug reactions are the skin, the blood and the liver, while the kidney and the nervous system may also be affected. The primary drug-induced lesion may be accompanied by general manifestations such as lymphadenopathy, fever, arthralgia and eosinophilia suggestive of a hypersensitivity reaction.

(a) Hepatotoxicity

Many drugs are reported to cause hepatic injury. The pattern of liver injury is variable and includes hepatitis, steatosis, granuloma, cirrhosis and neoplasia. Idiosyncratic hepatotoxicity may be due to direct toxicity of a chemically reactive metabolite, so-called 'metabolic' idiosyncrasy or secondary to an immune reaction. The clinical presentation of drug-induced hepatotoxicity is also variable, ranging from asymptomatic elevation of liver enzymes to hepatic failure. Over hepatic dysfunction due to drugs is uncommon, with drugs accounting for about 2% of all cases of jaundice. For the most severe form of liver injury, i.e. hepatic failure, idiosyncratic drug reactions account for approximately 20% of cases being exceeded only by paracetamol over dosage and viral hepatitis.

Table 20.5 Drugs reported to cause idiosyncratic hepatotoxicity

Drugs	Toxic metabolite	Postulated Mechanism	Comments
Halothane	Acyl halide	Neoantigen	Predisposition may lie with immunehyper-responsiveness
Amineptine	Epoxide	Immune-mediated	Genetic predisposition
Pheytoin	Eposide	Immune-mediated	Possible deficiency of microsomal epoxide hydrolase
Sodium valproate	Diene	Enzyme inhibition	commonest in infants
Amodiaquine	Quinoneimine	Immune-mediated	May be associated with leucopaenia
Dapsone	Hydroxylamine	Immune-mediated	May be part of the sulphone syndrome
Erythromycin	Nitroso derivatives	Immune-mediated	Can occur with estolate, ethyl succinate and proprionate derivatives
Isoniazid	Monoacetyl hydrazine	Protein alkylation	Non associated with acetylator status
Sulphonamide	Hdroxylamine	Immune-mediated	Unknown genetic predisposing factor
Allopurinol	Unknown	Immune-mediated	
NSAID	Unkown	Immune or toxic dependent on compound	Commonenst with benoxaprofen and phenylbutazone, least common with fenamates

(b) Blood dyscrasis

Drug-induced haematological toxicity can affect either platelets, red cells, white cells or all the cellular elements of the bone marrow leading to thrombocytopaenia, haemolytic anaemia, agranulocytosis or aplastic anaemia respectively. The most serious of these reactions, because of its high mortality is aplastic anaemia. Drug-induced thrombocytopaenia and haemolytic anaemia may be immune-mediated. In addition, haemolysis may occur because of an underlying metabolic abnormality, for example, glucose-6-phosphate dehydrogenase deficiency. The presentation of a patient with aplastic anaemia may be dependent on which cell line is most severely affected, and thus, fever, sore throat (agranulocytosis), tiredness (anaemia) or bruising and gastrointestinal haemorrhage (thrombocytopaenia) may all be presenting

(c) Cutaneous reactions

In clinical practice the most of the drugs reported to cause cutaneous toxicity. In the majority of cases, the skin reactions are mild and only require withdrawal of drug for resolution. The pathogenesis of such reactions is unknown although with certain drugs, for example, phenytoin, dose-dependency has been demonstrated. With mild cutaneous reactions, patients may have no systemic symptoms suggestive of hypersensitivity.

RISK FACTORS

(a) Chemistry of the drug

An adverse reaction must be a function of the biology of the individual and the chemistry of the drug. The idiosyncratic reactions must be caused by the presence of certain functional groups within the drug molecule or a metabolite. The chemical mechanism may provide a means of designing a safer drug, provided the functional group is not essential for activity, and also the possibility to identify susceptible individuals by the development of non-invasive techniques. The hypersensitivity reactions associated with penicillins and cephalosporins is attributed to the presence of the strained beta-lactam ring which is directly reactive, in a chemical sense, to nucleophilic groups on proteins. This chemical reactivity is an integral part of the antimicrobial activity of the drugs but will also produce drug antigen in all individuals.

(b) Variation in receptor function

Malignant hyperthermia, a metabolic disorder of skeletal muscle which is inherited as an autosomal dominant trait can be triggered in susceptible individuals by anaesthetic agents such as halothane and succinylcholine. It has been postulated that malignant hyperthermia results from disruption in the control of intracellular free calcium the primary defect being in the calcium-induced calcium release channel of skeletal muscle.

(c) Variation in drug metabolism

The genetic polymorphisms in various types of drug biotransformations have been described including those in drug oxidation, hydrolysis, acetylation and glutathione conjugation. The pharmacological and toxicological implications for the phenotype with a reduced ability to clear the drug and/or metabolite have been reviewed.

(d) Age

It is well known that adverse drug reactions occur more frequently in the elderly than in other age groups. Following are the main possible reasons -

First : the elderly take more drugs and are therefore more likely to be subjected to polypharmacy; secondly : age-related decline in renal function and hepatic metabolism may lead to toxicity through excess drug accumulation as was noted with the anti-inflammatory drug benoxaprofen and thirdly : it is possible that there are age-related declines in drug detoxication processes and in cellular and DNA repair mechanisms. For example, valproic acid causes an idiosyncratic reaction primarily in children under the age of 2 years.

CHAPTER 21

DRUG INTERACTION

The problem of drug interaction is the one of most serious concern to physicians, pharmacists, nurses and other related professional persons. The complexity of drug treatment and consequently eve greater risk of the patient may be attributed to the introduction of an overwhelmingly large number of potent medicaments particularly in last three decades. The knowledge of drug interactions is most useful to a pharmacist in developing the best medication. In the past, drug interactions were considered as those interactions which occured both in vivo and in vito and could be of physical or chemical nature. Today drug interaction is defined as the phenomenon which occurs when he effect(s) of one drug are modified by prior o simultaneous administration of other drug(s). These interactions may arise either from alteration of the absorption, distribution, metabolism or excretion of one dug by another; or from combination of their actions or effects. The risk of clinical consequences from drug-drug interaction is higher with some drug categories than with others. Drug categories commonly involved in clinically important drug interactions include anticoagulants, cardiac glycosides, oral hypoglycemics, sympahomimetic amines, antihypertensives, anticonvulsants or cytotoxic dugs. Common manifestations are haemorrhage, hypotension, cadiac arrhythmias, severe hypertension, convulsive seizures or hypoglycemia.

Drug interactions are usually considered as undesirable, as detrimental exaggerations or diminutions of the action of the drug upon another on account of the frequency and the clinical importance of adverse drug interactions. Equally important is the fact that the drugs are also used concurrently to enhance or improve their clinical effect. Thus a desirable drug interaction is defined as either a beneficial drug effect that is enhanced or a detrimental drug effect that is mitigated by the concomitant use of another drug.

The term 'incompatibility' should be reserved for those reactions which occur in vitro.

It should be remembered that the greatest information available is about those interactions in which the effects of interaction are readily measurable. There may be many more interactions which remain in the practice of clinical medicine and often attributed to patient idiosyncracy or the underlying disease. A glaring example is that of phenylbutazone and coumarin anticoagulants which wee given concomitantly to many patients over a period of several years before the adverse interaction was detected.

Classification

Drug interactions may often involve more than one mechanism but a simple classification of drug interaction mechanisms is as follows:

(A) **Pharmacokinetic (ADME) interactions** - Where the absorption, distribution, metabolism and excretion of one drug is affected by another drug. Pharmacokinetic interactions are those in which GI absorption of a drug is affected, plasma protein binding is affected, drug metabolism is either stimulated or inhibited; and urinary excretion is either enhanced or inhibited.

(B) **Pharmacodynamic (Pharmacologic) interactions** - Where drugs may have additive or synergistic or antagonistic affects and may or may not involve action on the same receptor.

(C) **Miscellaneous** - Where the interaction cannot be assigned to any of the above classifications.

Drug interactions may be caused due to i. interaction(s) with other drugs, ii. Endogenous physiologic chemical agents, iii. With components of the diet; and iv. Chemicals used in diagnostic tests or the results of such tests.

The clinical significance of any drug interaction depends on i. the patient factor e.g. disease state, renal function, hepatic function, serum protein levels, urinary pH, dietary factors, environmental factors, pharmacogenetic factors, age etc; and ii. The drug administration factors e.g. order and route of administration, duration of therapy, dose of dug and dosage forms etc.

A discussion of common categories of drug interaction with suitable examples is presented below.

1. **Modification of intestinal absorption**

   The drugs being mainly weak acids or bases, ionise depending on the pH of the GI tract and hence their absorption is affected. It should be remembered that the non-ionised forms of drugs are more lipid-soluble and absorbed more rapidly than the ionised ones.

   (a) **Antacid-Aspirin :** Aspirin being weakly acidic, it is expected to be primarily absorbed from the stomach and hence antacids would decrease its absorption. However, since aspirin produces GI side effects it is quite often administered concurrently with antacids. According to some investigators aspirin is less readily absorbed from buffered products and its absorption may, in fact, decrease.

Aspirin dissolves faster in alkaline pH though it is in the ionised form. This probably explains the use of aspirin with antacids.

(b) **Antacid - Penicillin G:** Penicillin G being acid sensitive, its absorption from the stomach will be a function of the pH of the stomach.

(c) **Antacid-Phenobarbital :** Phenobarbital remains in a non-ionised form in acidic medium and hence its absorption is decreased when antacid is given. Antacid administration will raise the pH of the stomach.

(d) **Antacid-Pseudoephedrine :** Being a basic drug, the absorption of pseudoephedrine will be enhanced with the simultaneous administration of antacids as the drug remains in a non-ionised form.

(e) **Antacid - Enteric coated medicines :** If enteric coated medicines are given with antacids, they will disintegrate and cause irritation and vomiting e.g. bisacodyl.

2. **Effect on transport system :**

(a) **Food - Antibiotics** : The presence of food slows the process of stomach emptying and affects the dissolution rate. Hence food may influence the absorption of many drugs. Antibiotics like penicillins, tetracyclines, erythromycin and lincomycin are recommended to be given 1 hr before or 2 hr after meal to permit maximum absorption.

(b) **Griseofulvin - Phenobarbital :** Phenobarbital may increase the secretion of bile and increase peristalsis. This would decrease the transit time in upper portion of the GI tract where griseofulvin is absorbed most efficiently. This phenobarbital reduces the absorption of griseofulvin.

(c) **Cathartics** - These agents increase the motility of GI tract and influence the passage of other drugs through the tract. The drugs with slow absorption and requiring longer contact may thus be absorbed slowly when given with cathartics.

(d) **antimuscarinics** - As these agents decrease the peristalsis, their gastric emptying time is prolonged. The drug may remain in contact with the stomach for a longer time and its absorption may be increased from the stomach or the small intestine. Riboflavine is absorbed from the small intestine. When given with the anticholinergic propantheline, the initial absorption of riboflavine is delayed due to its accumulation in the stomach but subsequently as the drug reaches he small intestine its absorption becomes greater. This may be attributed to inhibitory peristalsis, delayed gastric emptying and longer duration of contact of the drug with the intestine.

(e) **Antimuscarinics- Levodopa :** The antimuscarinics which are used in Parkinson's disease may have some synergistic effect when administered alongwith levodopa. In such cases the levodopa is poorly absorbed. The greater portion of levodopa is metabolised prior to absorption and hence antimuscarinics should be given in the smallest dose when administered alongwith levododa.

3. **Complex formation**

Complexation should be considered in a broader perspective and may involve drug-drug, dug-additive or even drug-container interactions. Complexes may be soluble or insoluble and may affect the drug absorption.

(a) **Tetracycline - Metals :** It is well established that the absorption of tetracyclines is reduced in presence of certain metals like calcium, aluminium, magnesium, bismuth and iron. Antacids containing the slats of these metals would also reduce the absorption of tetracyclines. As milk contains calcium it may also reduce absorption of tetracyclines. However, the absorption of newer tetracyclines like doxycycline and minicycline is not affected by calcium but aluminium may affect. The inhibition of tetracycline salts due to complexation with iron in descending order is as follows ferrous sulphate, ferrous fumarate, ferrous succinate, ferrous gluconate, ferrous tartrate. Thus, inhiobition is minimum in a more stable iron complex as sodium edetate.

(b) **Lincomycin - cyclamates :** Food beverages containing sodium or calcium cyclamates reduce the absorption of lincomycin possibly due to formation of a complex. To facilitate the absorption of lincomycin it is recommended hat nothing should be given orally except water for a period of 1 to 2 hr before and after oral administration of the drug. The problem has been solved due to introduction of clidamycin which is better tolerated and has the same spectrum of activity.

(c) **Cholestyramine :** Cholestyramine may complex with various agents and drugs e.g. bile salts, thyroid hormone, vitamin K, warfarin etc. Thyroid hormone and cholestyramine should be given at an interval of 4 hours. An interval of 6 hr is necessary for the optimum absorption of warfarin. Prolonged therapy of cholestyramine decreases the absorption of vitamin K.

(d) **Sodium fluoride :** In presence of a large quantity of calcium the absorption of sodium fluoride may be reduced due to complexation. Hence an interval of 1 hr before and 2 hr after the meal is recommended.

(e) **Antidiarrhoeal mixtures :** These mixtures essentially absorb toxic substances causing diarrhoea but then there also exists a possibility of absorption of other medicines. This is evidenced from the finding that the rate and extent of absorption of promazine is decreased by concurrent administration of a mixture of attapulgite and citrus pectin. Lincomycin is reported to be absorbed by kaolin mixture.

4. **Displacement of drug from storage tissue components**

   (a) **Drug - Drug :** Drugs may be bound to protein and this binding may be competitive or non-competitive. The binding sites being fewer in number there will be a competition for binding and the drug having greater affinity will displace the other having lesser affinity. There will exist an equilibrium between the bound and non-bound drug. Such an interaction is significant when one dug is prone to get bound in a larger quantity and is given with another drug which is able to displace the first one room its site of binding.

   (b) **Phenylbutazone - Warfarin :** Because of its greater affinity for binding, phenylbutazone displaces warfarin from the binding site. Thus more free drug is available for the action resulting in haemorrhage. Combination of the two drugs should be avoided. However, the two drugs may be indicated simultaneously as in superficial venous thrombosis.

   (c) **Chloral hydrate - Warfarin :** It is reported that prolonged chloral hydrate therapy requires less warfarin during the induction phase of an anticoagulant therapy. But other conflicting reports indicate that chloral hydrate decreases the anticoagulant activity.

   (d) **Bilirubin - Sulphonamides :** Bilirubin gets bound with albumin but may be displaced by a number of drugs from the binding sites. Sulphisoxazole and salicylate are reported to have such affect.

   (e) **Indomethacin with oral anticoagulants -** The anticoagulant response is increased due to displacement from protein binding sites.

5. **Modification of drug action at receptor site**

   (a) **Physiological antagonism :** This implies that two endogenous substances antagonise the effect of each other by acting at different receptors. Examples are adrenaline and histamine, adrenaline and acetylcholine etc.

   (b) **competitive antagonism :** It involves the competition between against and antagonis for the same receptors and the extent to which the antogonist opposes the pharmacological action of the agonist is determined by relative number of receptors occupied by the two receptors.

   (c) **Non-competitive antagonism :** Non-competitive antagonism occurs when the agonist and antagonist act on completely different receptors to produce antagonism e.g. acetylcholine and papaverine.

   (d) **International at receptor site :** The increased effect of warfarin in the presence of d-thyroxine is attributed to increased affinity of the drug for the receptor site brought about by d-thyroxine. The anabolic stroids like dianabol, norethandrolone and oxymetholone are also reported to increase the affinity of warfarin for the receptor site.

6. **Interaction at adrenergic neuron**

   (a) **MAO inhibitors-Sympathomimetics :** Concurrent administration of MAO inhibitors and sympathomimetics is of potential danger. Hence the patients being treated with MAO inhibitors should be advised to avoid using products containing these sympathomimetic agents. Amphetamine and MAO inhibitors when given simultaneously cause severe headache, hypertension and cardiac arrhythmias.

   (b) **MAO inhibitors - Tyramine :** Although this is not considered to be of serious consequences, yet such an interaction cannot be overlooked. When monoamino oxidase is inhibited, large quantities of unmetabolised tyramine can accumulate resulting in release of noradrenaline from adrenergic neurons.

   (c) **MAO inhibitors - Tricyclic antiderpressants :** It is recommended that therapy with a MAO inhibitor or a tricyclic antidepressan (amitryptiline, nortryptiline, imipramine etc.) should not be initiated until at least two weeks after the therapy with the other dug has been discontinued.

   (d) **Guanethidine - Tricyclic antidepressants :** Tricyclic antidepreseants can inhibit the uptake of guanethidine. A reversal of hypotensive effect of guanethidine following administration of desipramine and protryptiline is also reported.

   (e) **Guanethidine - Sympathomimetic agents :** Amphe'amine, ephedrine and mehylphenidae antagonise he effect of guanethidine. Amphetamine acts in a way similar to tricyclic antidepressants and in addition it may cause the release of guanethidine from its storage sites in the neuron.

   (f) **Guanethidine Antipsychotic agents:** Chlorpromazine, haloperidol and thiothixene can markedly reverse the antihypertensive response of guanethidine by the same mechanism as tricyclic antidepressants.

7. **Biotransformation**

   (a) **Enzyme inhibition -** chloramphenicol is reported to inhibit the metabolism of bishydroxycoumarin, tolbutamide and diphenylhydantoin due to inhibition of microsomal enzymes. Disufiram has been used in alcohol addicts due to its inhibitory effect on the enzyme aldehyde dehydrogenase. MAO inhibitors enhance the effect of drugs like babiturates, alcohol, sedatives, hypnotics, tranquillisers and other CNS depressans due to the inhibiion of the liver enzyme system. Allopurinol inhibits the enzyme xanthine oxidase and may increase the effect of mercaptopurine azathiopurine etc. as the same enzyme is involved in their metabolism.

   (b) **Enzyme stimulation (induction) :** Barbiturate, chloral hydrate, glutethimide and griseofuvin may cause enzyme induction. Chlordiazepoxide, diazepam and other benzodiazepines donot interfere with the barbiturate action. Decrease in the effect of diphenylhydantoin, steroidal hormones and digitoxin is reoported on simultaneous administration due to enzyme induction. Chlorinated hydrocarbons reduce the effect of barbiturates whereas MAO inhibitors increase the effect of barbiturates due to enzyme induction.

It is suggested that pyridoxine accelerates the decarboxylation of levodopa in peripheral tissues and hence less amount of levodopa crosses blood brain barrier and less dopamine is formed in the brain. This ultimately causes a reduction in therapeutic effect.

In alcoholic subjects increased rate of excretion of phenobarbital, meprobamate and increased rate of metabolism of tolbutamide, diphenydantoin and warfarin is reported. This has been attributed to increased activity of liver enzymes.

8. Alteration of urinary excretion

An acidic pH is required for the activity of methenamine but in the same condition there is danger of precipitation of sulphonamides resulting into crystalluria.

In case of drugs such as salicylates there will be large proportion of non-ionised form in acidic urine with increased reabsorption and intensified activity. On the same analogy, for a basic drug e.g., amphetamine, quinidine, pseudoephedrine etc. there will be increased proportion of non-ionised form in basic urine with increased reabsorption and intensified activity.

The antiinfective agentsemployed for the urinary tract infections are effective in a particular urinary pH. Tetracyclines, nitrofurantoin, methenamine are most active at urinary pH of 5.5 or even less. On the contrary an alkaline pH is required for kanamycin, streptomycin and chloramphenicol.

Antibacterial spectra of many drugs can be modified by appropriate reaction of urine. Thus, erythromycin is active against gram positive bacteria but its spectrum can be expanded to include gram negative organisms by making the urine alkaline. Novobiocin can be made active against gram negative organisms if urine is name acidic.

The acidification of urine enhances the excretion of methadone but its metabolite is less affected by urinary changes. In a number of drugs reabsorption and excretion are influenced by the urinary pH.

9. Direct effect on kidney

Probenecid, phenylbutazone, sulphapyrazone, aspirin, indomethacin etc. are reported to increase the half-life of penicillin by blocking its tubular excretion. Probenecid apart from penicillin also increases the half-life of aminosalicylic acid, sulphonamides and dapsone. It also increases the half life of acetoheximide and causes hypoglycemia. This is attributed to the interference in the renal excretion of hydroxyhexamine, the active metabolite of acetohexamide.

It has been suggested that high doses of salicylates should be given cautiously when administered alongwith frusemide as there is a competition between these drugs for renal excretory sites and patients may experience salicylate toxicity at lower dose.

Sodium depletion enhances lithium toxicity. It is suggested that lithium carbonate should not be given to the patient on diuretic therapy.

10. Increase or decrease of synthetics

Antibiotics like chloramphenicol, neomycin, tetracyclines and sulphonamides enhance the anticoagulant effect due to the interference with the synthesis of vitamin K by micro-organisms in GI tract. Similarly, quinidine enhances anticoagulant effect by suppressing prothrombin formation.

INDEX

I

J

L

M

O

P

R

S

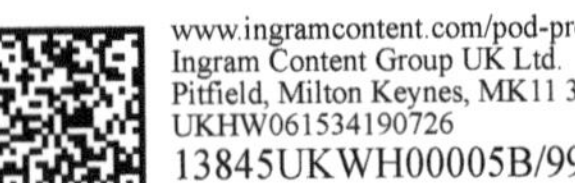

www.ingramcontent.com/pod-product-compliance
Ingram Content Group UK Ltd.
Pitfield, Milton Keynes, MK11 3LW, UK
UKHW061534190726
13845UKWH00005B/99